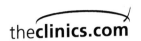

PSYCHIATRIC CLINICS
OF NORTH AMERICA

Obsessive-Compulsive Spectrum Disorders

GUEST EDITOR
Dan J. Stein, MD, PhD

June 2006 • Volume 29 • Number 2

SAUNDERS

An Imprint of Elsevier, Inc.
PHILADELPHIA   LONDON   TORONTO   MONTREAL   SYDNEY   TOKYO

W.B. SAUNDERS COMPANY
A Division of Elsevier Inc.

1600 John F. Kennedy Boulevard • Suite 1800 • Philadelphia, PA 19103-2899

http://www.theclinics.com

PSYCHIATRIC CLINICS OF NORTH AMERICA   Volume 29, Number 2
June 2006   ISSN 0193-953X
Editor: Sarah E. Barth   ISBN 1-4160-3515-X

Reprints. For copies of 100 or more, of articles in this publication, please contact the Commercial Reprints Department, Elsevier Inc., 360 Park Avenue South, New York, New York 10010-1710. Tel.: (212) 633-3813 Fax: (212) 462-1935 e-mail: reprints@elsevier.com

The ideas and opinions expressed in *Psychiatric Clinics of North America* do not necessarily reflect those of the Publisher. The Publisher does not assume any responsibility for any injury and/or damage to persons or property arising out of or related to any use of the material contained in this periodical. The reader is advised to check the appropriate medical literature and the product information currently provided by the manufacturer of each drug to be administered, to verify the dosage, the method and duration of administration, or contraindications. It is the responsibility of the treating physician or other health care professional, relying on independent experience and knowledge of the patient, to determine drug dosages and the best treatment for the patient. Mention of any product in this issue should not be construed as endorsement by the contributors, editors, or the Publisher of the product or manufacturers' claims.

Psychiatric Clinics of North America (ISSN 0193-953X) is published quarterly by W.B. Saunders, 360 Park Avenue South, New York, NY 10010-1710. Months of publication are March, June, September, and December. Business and Editorial Offices: 1600 John F. Kennedy Blvd., Suite 1800, Philadelphia, PA 19103-2899. Accounting and Circulation Offices: 6277 Sea Harbor Drive, Orlando, FL 32887-4800 Periodicals postage paid at New York, NY and additional mailing offices. Subscription prices are $180.00 per year (US individuals), $305.00 per year (US institutions), $90.00 per year (US students/residents), $215.00 per year (Canadian individuals), $370.00 per year (Canadian Institutions), $250.00 per year (foreign individuals), $370.00 per year (foreign institutions), and $125.00 per year (international & Canadian students/residents). Foreign air speed delivery is included in all *Clinics'* subscription prices. All prices are subject to change without notice. **POSTMASTER:** Send address changes to *Psychiatric Clinics of North America*, Elsevier Periodicals Customer Service, 6277 Sea Harbor Drive, Orlando, FL 32887-4800. Customer Service: 1-800-654-2452 (US). From outside of the US, call 1-407-345-4000.

Psychiatric Clinics of North America is covered in *Index Medicus, Current Contents/Social and Behavioral Sciences, Social Science Citation Index, Embase/Excerpta Medica,* and PsycINFO.

Printed in the United States of America.

GUEST EDITOR

DAN J. STEIN, MD, PhD, Professor and Head, Department of Psychiatry and Mental Health, University of Cape Town, Cape Town, South Africa

CONTRIBUTORS

JONATHAN S. ABRAMOWITZ, PhD, Associate Professor and Director, OCD/Anxiety Disorders Program, Department of Psychiatry and Psychology, Mayo Clinic, Rochester, Minnesota

EMILY R. ANDERSON, MS, University of Nebraska-Lincoln, Lincoln, Nebraska

AUTUMN E. BRADDOCK, PhD, Postdoctoral Fellow, Department of Psychiatry and Psychology, Mayo Clinic, Rochester, Minnesota

MARIA CONCEIÇÃO ROSÁRIO CAMPOS, MD, PhD, Research Fellow, Department of Psychiatry, University of São Paulo Medical School, São Paulo, Brazil

DODANID CARDONA, MD, Child and Adolescent Psychiatry Fellow, The Children's Hospital of Philadelphia, Philadelphia, Pennsylvania

DAVID J. CASTLE, MSc, MD, MRCPsych, Chair of Psychiatry, St. Vincent's Hospital and University of Melbourne, Melbourne, Australia

DAMIAAN DENYS, MD, PhD, Department of Anxiety Disorders, Rudolf Magnus Institute of Neuroscience, Department of Psychiatry, University Medical Center, Utrecht, The Netherlands

CHRISTOPHER FLESSNER, MS, University of Wisconsin-Milwaukee, Milwaukee, Wisconsin

MARTIN E. FRANKLIN, PhD, Associate Professor of Psychiatry, University of Pennsylvania School of Medicine, Philadelphia, Pennsylvania

DANIEL A. GELLER, MBBS, FRACP, Director, Pediatric Obsessive Compulsive Disorder Program, Division of Pediatric Psychopharmacology, Massachusetts General Hospital; Assistant Professor, Department of Psychiatry, Harvard Medical School, Boston, Massachusetts

WAYNE K. GOODMAN, MD, Professor and Chairman, Department of Psychiatry, University of Florida School of Medicine, Gainesville, Florida

JON E. GRANT, JD, MD, MPH, Associate Professor, Department of Psychiatry, University of Minnesota Medical School, Minneapolis, Minnesota

BRIAN H. HARVEY, BPharm, PhD, Division of Pharmacology, School of Pharmacy, North-West University, Potchefstroom, South Africa

SÎAN M.J. HEMMINGS, PhD, Postdoctoral Fellow, Department of Medical Biochemistry, Faculty of Health Sciences, University of Stellenbosch, Tygerberg, South Africa

JILL HENRICKSEN, MA, Bio-Behavioral Institute, Great Neck, New York

ANA GABRIELA HOUNIE, MD, PhD, Research fellow, Department of Psychiatry, University of São Paulo Medical School, São Paulo, Brazil

SCHAUN KORFF, MSc, Division of Pharmacology, School of Pharmacy, North-West University, Potchefstroom, South Africa

MICHAEL KYRIOS, PhD, Professor of Psychology, Department of Psychology, Faculty of Life & Social Sciences, Swinburne University of Technology, Hawthorn, Australia

CHRISTINE LOCHNER, PhD, MRC Unit on Anxiety Disorders, University of Stellenbosch, Stellenbosch, South Africa

DAVID MATAIX-COLS, PhD, Departments of Psychological Medicine and Psychology, King's College London, Institute of Psychiatry, London, United Kingdom

EURÍPEDES C. MIGUEL, MD, PhD, Associate Professor of Psychiatry, Department of Psychiatry, University of São Paulo Medical School, São Paulo, Brazil

TANYA K. MURPHY, MD, Associate Professor of Psychiatry and Chief, Department of Psychiatry, University of Florida School of Medicine, Gainesville, Florida

FUGEN NEZIROGLU, PhD, ABBP, ABPP, Bio-Behavioral Institute, Great Neck, New York

MARC N. POTENZA, MD, PhD, Associate Professor, Department of Psychiatry, Yale University School of Medicine, New Haven, Connecticut

SUSAN ROSSELL, PhD, Associate Professor, Mental Health Research Institute of Victoria, Parkville, Victoria, Australia

MUHAMMAD W. SAJID, MD, Assistant Professor of Psychiatry, Department of Psychiatry, University of Florida School of Medicine, Gainesville, Florida

ROSELI GEDANKE SHAVITT, MD, PhD, Research Fellow, Department of Psychiatry, University of São Paulo Medical School, São Paulo, Brazil

DAN J. STEIN, MD, PhD, Professor and Head, Department of Psychiatry and Mental Health, University of Cape Town, Cape Town, South Africa

ODILE A. VAN DEN HEUVEL, MD, PhD, Department of Psychiatry, VU University Medical Center, GGZ Buitenamstel, Amsterdam, The Netherlands

MICHAEL R. WALTHER, BA, University of Pennsylvania School of Medicine, Philadelphia, Pennsylvania

CHAD T. WETTERNECK, MS, University of Wisconsin-Milwaukee, Milwaukee, Wisconsin

DOUGLAS W. WOODS, PhD, Associate Professor of Psychology, University of Wisconsin-Milwaukee, Milwaukee, Wisconsin

JOSE A. YARYURA-TOBIAS, MD, Bio-Behavioral Institute, Great Neck, New York

CONTENTS

Over the years, different authors have emphasized the psychodynamic, cognitive-behavioral, and neurobiologic mechanisms thought to underlie overlapping conditions on the obsessive-compulsive spectrum of disorders. Advances in the cognitive-affective neuroscience of obsessive-compulsive disorder (OCD) suggest novel ways of delineating the obsessive-compulsive spectrum of disorders in terms of cortico-striatally mediated control and reward mechanisms. Some support for this approach to defining the obsessive-compulsive spectrum derives from empiric data on obsessive-compulsive spectrum disorders in patients who have OCD. These data suggest that the space defined by the obsessive-compulsive spectrum of disorders is best conceptualized as multidimensional in nature.

Obsessive-compulsive disorder (OCD) affecting children and adolescents is prevalent, and OCD has a childhood onset in about one third to one half of affected adults. Unlike adults, affected children are more often male. Mood and anxiety disorders are common in pediatric OCD; pediatric OCD also has a distinct association with disruptive behavior disorders, tic, and other specific and pervasive developmental disorders. Childhood-onset of OCD seems to be associated with a markedly increased risk for familial transmission of OCD, tic disorders, and ADHD. Both scientifically and clinically, the recognition of developmentally specific OCD phenotypes may be valuable.

Animal Models of Obsessive-Compulsive Disorder: Rationale to Understanding Psychobiology and Pharmacology

Schaun Korff and Brian H. Harvey

Obsessive-compulsive disorder (OCD) is a complex neuropsychiatric illness that presents with diverse neurologic manifestations together with severe anxiety. Animal models are increasingly being used to allow clinicians and researchers a better understanding of this disorder. Considering current theories for the neurobiology and treatment of OCD, this article reviews the rationale, validity, and application of putative animal models of OCD, particularly ethologic and pharmacologic models. The ever-increasing sophistication of animal models will play a vital role in extending current knowledge of the neurobiology and treatment of OCD and obsessive-compulsive spectrum disorders.

Common and Distinct Neural Correlates of Obsessive-Compulsive and Related Disorders

David Mataix-Cols and Odile A. van den Heuvel

Obsessive-compulsive disorder (OCD) often co-occurs with other anxiety disorders and a number of other disorders of similar phenomenology known as the "OCD spectrum" disorders. Neurobiologically, it is unclear how all these disorders relate to each other. The picture is further complicated by the clinical heterogeneity of OCD itself. This article reviews the literature on the common and distinct neural correlates of OCD, its symptom dimensions, and other anxiety and OCD spectrum disorders with the hope of providing a conceptual and heuristic framework to help understand the relationship between these phenomena.

The Current Status of Association Studies in Obsessive-Compulsive Disorder

Sîan M.J. Hemmings and Dan J. Stein

Evidence from family studies suggests that genetic factors play a role in mediating obsessive-compulsive disorder (OCD), although the pattern of inheritance is unclear. Case-control association analyses have yielded inconsistent results, making identification of predisposing alleles difficult. Clinical subtypes of the disorder have been proposed and may be more closely related to a particular genetic substrate than the higher-order construct of OCD. Furthermore, it is likely that the behavioral manifestations of OCD are mediated by a broad range of interconnected neurotransmitter and signaling pathways. This article reviews the current status of genetic studies in OCD and considers future directions.

This article reviews new developments of pharmacotherapy in obsessive-compulsive disorder (OCD) and OC spectrum disorders of the past five years. New developments primarily involved the extension of evidence of efficacy of serotonin reuptake inhibitors (SRIs), the use of atypical antipsychotics in addition to SRIs for treatment refractory patients, the combination of pharmacotherapy with behavior therapy, and studies assessing predictors of response. Today, frontline pharmacological treatment of OCD still consists of drugs with potent serotonin reuptake inhibition properties. In case of non-response, treatment options comprise adding another drug, increasing the dose, switching drugs, or changing the mode of delivery.

This article presents the learning theory model and its application to obsessive-compulsive disorder (OCD). It then reviews the various facets of OCD psychotherapy and reports on its efficacy. It looks at studies before 1995 and summarizes what had been established as therapeutic guidelines and extrapolates these guidelines to the spectrum disorders. Finally, it reviews studies conducted from 1995 to 2005, exploring what advances have been made and where further work is needed.

FORTHCOMING ISSUES

RECENT ISSUES

PSYCHIATRIC
CLINICS
OF NORTH AMERICA

Psychiatr Clin N Am 29 (2006) xiii–xv

Preface

Obsessive-Compulsive Spectrum Disorders: Current Advances, and Future Directions

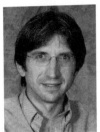

Dan J. Stein, MD, PhD
Guest Editor

This issue of the *Psychiatric Clinics of North America* is devoted to obsessive-compulsive disorder (OCD) and the obsessive-compulsive spectrum disorders (OCSDs). The current edition of the *Diagnostic and Statistical Manual of Mental Disorders* (DSM-IV-TR) classifies OCD as an anxiety disorder and does not include a category of obsessive-compulsive spectrum disorder [1]; an immediate question therefore concerns the definition of this spectrum of disorders. Different authors have taken different approaches to delineating the OCSDs, and the question remains open for debate.

One approach is to define the OCSDs as conditions in which there is overlapping phenomenology and psychobiology with OCD [2]. This approach requires an immediate focus on the phenomenology and psychobiology of OCD, and this issue therefore includes a number of articles addressing this. The issue begins with articles on OCD and OCSDs in adults and in children and then considers recent developments in animal models, neurocircuitry, neurogenetics, and neuroimmunology of OCD and OCSDs.

Tourette's disorder, body dysmorphic disorder, and hypochondriasis are arguably the obsessive-compulsive disorders par excellence. Patients with Tourette's disorder often have obsessive-compulsive symptoms, patients with OCD often have tics, and there seems to be considerable overlap in the genetics and neurocircuitry of the two conditions [3]. Body dysmorphic disorder and hypochondriasis have considerable overlap with OCD in the form and function of symptoms (with all these conditions characterized by anxiety-arousing concerns and anxiety-reducing rituals) [4]. There are separate articles on each of these conditions.

The relationship between compulsive and impulsive disorders is more complex. Some authors have suggested that compulsivity and impulsivity are orthogonal dimensions and that patients can have both compulsive and impulsive symptoms. Others have argued that compulsive and impulsive disorders lie at opposite ends of a unidimensional spectrum. This issue includes an article on trichotillomania, which, although classified in the DSM-IV-TR as an impulse-control disorder, has often been thought of as compulsive. There is also an article on other impulse-control disorders, such as pathologic gambling, in which suggestions of an overlap with OCD are more controversial.

For several reasons it may be of heuristic value to conceptualize two disorders as lying on a spectrum. Positing a spectrum may encourage clinicians to inquire about comorbidity and researchers to compare the psychobiology of different conditions. Further, a spectrum construct may encourage the adaptation of treatments found effective in one condition for use in another. For example, although serotonin-reuptake inhibitors are a first-line pharmacotherapy for OCD and dopamine receptor blockers are a first-line pharmacotherapy for Tourette's disorder, there may value in using antipsychotics as augmenting agents in treatment-refractory OCD and in using serotonin-reuptake inhibitors for comorbid OCD in Tourette's disorder. The current issue concludes with articles on pharmacotherapy and psychotherapy.

Contributions to the issue demonstrate that there have been considerable advances in the understanding of OCD and of OCSDs in recent years. There are now standardized diagnostic interviews and symptom measures for many of these conditions, a preliminary model of the neurocircuitry and neurochemistry of OCD has been developed, investigation of the psychobiology of the OCSDs has been initiated, and there is a considerable database of randomized, controlled trials of pharmacotherapy and psychotherapy for OCD and OCSDs.

At the same time, this issue indicates the limits of current knowledge and provides a number of directions for future work. There is growing awareness of the heterogeneity of OCD and of the multiple systems involved in its pathogenesis. Future work will need to delineate the complex psychobiology of OCD in greater detail. Additional studies of the OCSDs are needed to obtain sufficiently rich data on those conditions and allow careful comparison with the phenomenology and psychobiology of OCD. Given ongoing developments in psychometrics, imaging, and genetics, we can look forward to a better understanding of OCD and OCSDs, and ultimately to novel treatments.

I wish to thank all the contributors for being willing to participate in this project and for synthesizing current research in a way that addresses the practical demands of the busy clinician. Ongoing efforts to increase awareness of the high prevalence of OCD and OCSDs and to provide information about their optimal assessment and treatment are useful insofar as they ultimately contribute to better clinical care. The construct of OCSDs deserves a great deal of further exploration, but in the interim it has arguably helped many by usefully extending the adaptation of anti-OCD treatments to a range of previously neglected populations.

Dan J. Stein, MD, PhD
Department of Psychiatry, University of Cape Town
Cape Town, South Africa

E-mail address: dan.stein@curie.uct.ac.za

References

[1] American Psychiatric Association. Diagnostic and Statistical Manual for Mental Disorders. Fourth edition, text revision. Washington (DC): American Psychiatric Publishing, Inc.; 2000.

[2] Stein DJ, Hollander E. The spectrum of obsessive-compulsive related disorders. In: Hollander E, editor. Obsessive-compulsive related disorders. Washington (DC): American Psychiatric Press; 1993.

[3] Stein DJ. Neurobiology of the obsessive-compulsive spectrum disorders. Biol Psychiatry 2000;47:296–304.

[4] Abramowitz JS, Deacon BJ. The OC spectrum: a closer look at the arguments and the data. In: Abramowitz JS, Houts AC, editors. Concepts and controversies in obsessive-compulsive disorder. New York: Springer Science and Business Media; 2005.

PSYCHIATRIC
CLINICS
OF NORTH AMERICA

ELSEVIER
SAUNDERS

Psychiatr Clin N Am 29 (2006) 343–351

Obsessive-Compulsive Spectrum Disorders: a Multidimensional Approach

Dan J. Stein, MD, PhD[a,b,*], Christine Lochner, PhD[b]

[a]Department of Psychiatry, University of Cape Town, Cape Town, South Africa
[b]MRC Unit on Anxiety Disorders, University of Stellenbosch, Stellenbosch, South Africa

Over the years, a number of different approaches have been taken to defining the obsessive-compulsive spectrum of disorders. This article begins by reviewing these different approaches and then considers the implications of recent advances in the cognitive-affective neuroscience of obsessive-compulsive disorder (OCD) for the understanding of the spectrum disorders. It emphasizes the importance of cortico-striatally mediated control and reward systems in underpinning OCD symptoms and suggests that it may be useful to consider OCD spectrum disorders as falling along different dimensions (eg, impulse-related and reward-related conditions). The authors suggest that some support for this position is found in data on the comorbidity of obsessive-compulsive spectrum disorders in OCD and argue that the space defined by the obsessive-compulsive spectrum of disorders is multidimensional in nature.

Approaches to the obsessive-compulsive spectrum of disorders

An early approach to the obsessive-compulsive spectrum of disorders emphasized the importance of the psychodynamic defense mechanisms that produced obsessive-compulsive symptoms. Freud and other psychoanalytic authors argued that obsessive-compulsive character, obsessive-compulsive neurosis, and obsessive-compulsive psychosis lay on a spectrum and were all characterized by specific unconscious mechanisms (eg, heightened anal drive) [1]. If defenses against unconscious mechanisms are penetrated, a neurosis or even a psychosis may emerge. Although this work contributed

---

* Corresponding author. Groote Schur Hospital, Department of Psychiatry, J-Block, Anzio Rd, Observatory 7925, South Africa.
   E-mail address: dan.stein@curie.uct.ac.za (D.J. Stein).

0193-953X/06/$ - see front matter © 2006 Elsevier Inc. All rights reserved.
doi:10.1016/j.psc.2006.02.015

enormously to understanding the phenomenology of OCD, it has not received empiric support, and it has not led to effective treatments.

A subsequent approach to the obsessive-compulsive spectrum of disorders has highlighted the cognitive-behavioral mechanisms thought to underlie obsessive-compulsive symptoms. Obsessions are intrusive thoughts that increase levels of anxiety, and compulsions are mental acts or behaviors that neutralize obsessions and reduce anxiety. Obsessive-compulsive spectrum disorders, such as body dysmorphic disorder and hypochondriasis, similarly are characterized by intrusive thoughts that increase anxiety and by repetitive actions that reduce anxiety [2]. This work has been important in underpinning an effective set of psychotherapeutic interventions, but it does not necessarily address the broad range of empiric data that have emerged on the psychobiology of OCD.

A more recent approach has emphasized the neurobiology of obsessive-compulsive disorder. A serotonin hypothesis of OCD is based on data that serotonin-reuptake inhibitors are more effective than noradrenaline-reuptake inhibitors in OCD [3] and leads to a view that the OCD spectrum disorders comprise those conditions that respond selectively to serotonin-reuptake inhibitors [4]. A basal ganglia hypothesis of OCD is based on data that OCD is mediated by the striatum and leads to a concept of OCD spectrum disorders comprising those conditions in which psychopathology of the striatum leads to unwanted repetitive behavior [5].

Advances in cognitive-affective neuroscience have led to more integrated theories of OCD that incorporate data from a range of different studies, including neuropsychologic studies, functional brain imaging, and molecular research [6]. Two approaches in particular are discussed here. The first argues that OCD is characterized by disruption of control mechanisms, and the second argues that OCD is characterized by disruption of reward mechanisms. Each is supported by some empiric data and leads to a particular approach to the obsessive-compulsive spectrum of disorders.

Obsessive-compulsive disorder and the disruption of control mechanisms

Cortico-striatal neurocircuitry is thought to mediate the control of procedural strategies [7–9]. Certain habits may have a strong genetic component (eg, grooming in rats), and others may have a strong learned component (eg, bicycle riding in humans), but there is good evidence that cortico-striatal neurocircuitry plays an important role in encoding and releasing these sets of chunked actions [10]. A range of different neurochemicals, including the serotonin system, the dopamine system, and the glutamatergic system, may play a role in procedural strategies.

There are a number of reasons for conceptualizing OCD as a dysfunction in the control of procedural strategies with inappropriate release of symptoms ranging from simple motoric stereotypies to more complex behavioral programs. At a phenomenologic level, OCD is characterized by chronic intrusive symptoms, by inappropriate behavioral sequences, and by evidence of behavioral and cognitive disinhibition on neuropsychologic testing [11]. At a psychobiologic level, OCD is characterized by increased activity in prefrontal areas in functional imaging studies, arguably a compensatory mechanism that allows higher-order restraint over striatally mediated dyscontrol.

A good deal of data supports the hypothesis that OCD is characterized by disruption of cortico-striatally mediated procedural strategies [12]. First, neurologic disorders characterized by striatal lesions may be accompanied by obsessive-compulsive symptoms [13]. Second, functional imaging studies demonstrate that during implicit learning there is striatal activation in healthy controls but abnormal extra-striatal activity in OCD [14]. Third, successful treatment, whether using medication, cognitive-behavioral therapy, or neurosurgery, results in decreased symptoms and altered activity in cortico-striatal circuitry [15].

There is also good evidence that a number of the neurotransmitter systems involved in mediating procedural strategies also play a crucial role in OCD. In particular, there is evidence that the serotonin system is a key system in mediating both impulse dyscontrol and OCD symptoms [12]. Evidence for the role of the serotonergic system in OCD derives from data on concentrations of serotonin and 5-hydroxyindoleacetic acid in cerebrospinal fluid, on molecular imaging of serotonin receptors, on the role of variants in serotonergic genes in OCD, and on selective treatment response to serotonin-reuptake inhibitors.

What conditions other than OCD are potentially mediated by disruptions in cortico-striatally mediated procedural controls, with subtle forms of cognitive-affective dyscontrol or inappropriate execution of motoric sequences? It is notable that at least a subgroup of patients who have OCD displays evidence of increased impulsivity or aggression during childhood [16]. Furthermore, in patients with OCD, a cluster analysis of putative comorbid OCD spectrum disorders yields a cluster of impulsive disorders that comprises intermittent explosive disorder, kleptomania, eating disorders, and stereotypic self-injurious behaviors [17].

The existence of an impulse-control dimension within OCD means that compulsivity and impulsivity are not diametrically opposed but rather may lie on orthogonal planes. Also, it needs to be emphasized that the phenomenology of OCD is typically entirely different from that of conditions such as the impulse-control disorders. In OCD, there is a strong attempt to regulate symptoms; for example, obsessions with aggressive content are rarely enacted.

Perhaps different kinds of disturbances in control mechanisms result in various kinds of impulsive and compulsive phenomena. A schema that contrasts decreased cortico-striatal activity and serotonin hypofunction in impulsivity with increased cortico-striatal activity and serotonin hyperfunction in compulsivity provides an initial heuristic but is undoubtedly oversimplified. It is also possible that disruption in control processes is only a secondary phenomenon relevant to some subtypes of OCD and obsessive-compulsive spectrum disorders, with other striatally mediated psychobiologic processes more important in the majority of cases.

Obsessive-compulsive disorder and the disruption of reward mechanisms

Cortico-striatal circuitry is thought to mediate reward processes. In particular, the ventral striatum seems to play an important role in reward expectancy [18]. Furthermore, basic studies have demonstrated that reward mechanisms are mediated by the dopaminergic system with maximal dopamine release in the ventral striatum under conditions of maximal uncertainty about reward [19]. Such work has proved particularly relevant to understanding drug addiction in the clinic; patients who have substance-use disorders show abnormalities in the neurocircuitry and neurotransmitters that mediate reward processing and may respond to treatments that act on these pathways [20].

At first this work may not seem relevant to understanding OCD. Nevertheless, one way of conceptualizing OCD is in terms of the absence of a feeling of goal completion after an action is performed: people continue with their compulsions repetitively until there is finally the sense that things are now "just right." Although OCD and drug addiction have significant phenomenologic and psychobiologic differences, both conditions may be characterized by disruption of reward processes and consequent compulsive behavior.

A good deal of data on OCD supports the role of the dopamine system in OCD [21]. First, administration of dopamine agonists results in stereotypic movements in both healthy volunteers and OCD patients. Second, administration of dopamine receptor blockers as augmenting agents can result in decreased obsessive-compulsive symptoms. Third, there is evidence from molecular imaging studies that striatal dopaminergic receptor binding is abnormal in OCD. Fourth, there is evidence from genetic studies that dopaminergic candidate genes may play a role in at least some groups of OCD patients.

What conditions other than OCD are likely to involve cortico-striatally mediated disruption of reward circuitry? It is notable that dopaminergic agonists increase symptoms in a number of putative OCD spectrum disorders including Tourette's syndrome and trichotillomania [22]. Furthermore, dopamine receptor blockers are useful in the treatment of these conditions [23]. There is also evidence of dopaminergic involvement in molecular imaging and candidate gene studies of Tourette's syndrome, as well as evidence of familial relationships with OCD [24,25]. Finally, there is evidence that in patients with OCD a number of putative OCD spectrum disorders cluster together, including Tourette's syndrome, trichotillomania, pathologic gambling, and hypersexual disorder [17].

Tourette's, trichotillomania, pathologic gambling, and hypersexual disorder, even if sometimes called "compulsive," differ from OCD in key phenomenologic and functional ways. Trichotillomania, pathologic gambling, and hypersexual disorder may involve a sense of pleasure at the time of the behavior, whereas OCD typically is characterized by anxiety-inducing obsessions and anxiety-relieving compulsions. Such phenomenologic differences are not necessarily accompanied by psychobiologic distinctions [26]. At the same time, they are crucial for accurate diagnosis and evaluation.

Perhaps different kinds of disturbances in reward processing result in a spectrum of diverse reward-related disorders. In terms of underlying neurocircuitry, OCD is characterized by increased cortico-striatal activity, whereas pathologic gambling and substance-use disorders tend to be associated with reduced orbitofrontal activity [20,27]. On the other hand, substance-use disorders and OCD may both be characterized by low dopamine D2 receptor availability [20,28] and by glutamate dysfunction [29]. Significant additional research is needed to consolidate the preliminary ideas outlined here. It may be that disruption in processes signaling goal completion is only a secondary phenomenon relevant to some subtypes of OCD and obsessive-compulsive spectrum disorders.

Discussion

The hypothesis put forward here about the different dimensions of the OCD spectrum disorders is somewhat speculative. Nevertheless, it is in line with previous discussions on the cognitive-affective neuroscience of OCD. For example, previous work has suggested that OCD can be divided into a subtype characterized by abnormalities in control processes and a subtype characterized by abnormalities in goal attainment [30]. It is also consistent with some previous work suggesting that OCD lies on a compulsive-impulsive spectrum of disorders [31,32] or on a spectrum of reward-related affective disorders [33,34].

The hypothesis here has not yet addressed a number of other important putative OCD spectrum disorders, particularly hypochondriasis and body dysmorphic disorder. It is possible that these disorders can almost be considered a variant of OCD: they are fairly closely related to OCD in phenomenology and psychobiology. In a cluster analysis of putative obsessive-compulsive spectrum disorders in OCD, these body-focused disorders emerged as a third cluster of comorbid conditions [17]. Psychobiologic data on these disorders are relatively sparse but suggest at least some overlap with the neurocircuitry and neurochemistry of OCD [4,35].

Some authors have classified select obsessive-compulsive spectrum disorders as "neurologic." Nevertheless, given that all the obsessive-compulsive spectrum disorders are mediated by specific neurocircuitry, it may be preferable to use data on the relationship between neurologic disorders and obsessive-compulsive symptoms to try to shed light on the dimensions of the obsessive-compulsive spectrum disorders. For example, autoimmune responses seen after streptococcal infection result in striatal dysfunction and may therefore result in disruption of control mechanisms with the subsequent emergence of tics, compulsions, and emotional lability [36].

Similarly, it is possible that a range of environmental factors may affect the emergence of obsessive-compulsive spectrum disorders. Early exposure to trauma results in disruption of striatal architecture [37], sensitization of the dopaminergic system [38], and increased vulnerability to subsequent psychopathology [39]. The role of trauma in the pathogenesis of obsessive-compulsive disorder has been relatively little studied and may well deserve additional attention [40]. Furthermore, stressful conditions may exacerbate some of the obsessive-compulsive spectrum conditions.

The discussion here is similar to some of the debate on subtypes of OCD. It is possible that some subtypes of OCD are particularly related to control mechanisms (eg, repeated washing), whereas others involve a disruption of reward mechanisms (eg, symmetry concerns). Early-onset OCD seems to be characterized by symmetry concerns and by dopaminergic involvement [41]; nevertheless, it is not clear that there is an altogether straightforward relationship between subtypes of OCD and the particular dimensions on which OCD spectrums lie.

One approach to the cognitive-affective neuroscience of OCD emphasizes the emotion of disgust [42]. In particular, it has been suggested that whereas most of the anxiety disorders primarily involve fear and are mediated by the amygdala, obsessive-compulsive disorder primarily involves disgust and is mediated by the striatum and insula. This view undoubtedly deserves further exploration, but its implications for understanding the obsessive-compulsive spectrum disorders have not yet been well investigated.

Summary

One advantage of conceptualizing two disorders as related lies in the possibility that a similar treatment is effective for both conditions. The approach taken in this paper is somewhat different, however. The authors have argued that although a particular psychobiologic process may be relevant to OCD and obsessive-compulsive conditions, it may be disrupted in different ways in various conditions that fall along a spectrum. If so, different obsessive-compulsive spectrum disorders may well require different treatments. Thus, although OCD and trichotillomania can be conceptualized in terms of the pathologic release of motor programs, they may require rather different treatment approaches.

Furthermore, in the absence of a detailed understanding of the psychobiology of OCD and related disorders, conceptualizations of obsessive-compulsive spectrum disorders can remain only preliminary in nature. The involvement of cortico-striatal circuitry in OCD suggests that obsessive-compulsive spectrum disorders may be characterized by involvement of these paths. Striatal circuits mediate many different functions (including reward processes), however, and are involved in many disorders. Similarly, the involvement of serotonergic neurotransmitters in OCD suggests that these neurotransmitters are central to defining spectrum disorders. Again, however, serotonin plays a role in many functions (including impulse control) and mediates many different disorders.

Much work remains to be done to delineate optimally the obsessive-compulsive spectrum of disorders. Nevertheless, significant progress has been made. Empiric data demonstrate involvement of cortico-striatal circuitry in a number of putative obsessive-compulsive spectrum disorders [43]. Similarly, data demonstrate that a selective response to serotonin-reuptake inhibitors is seen in a range of these different spectrum disorders. As further progress is made in understanding the cognitive-affective neuroscience of OCD and related conditions, constructs about obsessive-compulsive spectrum disorders will become increasingly sharp.

References

[1] Stein DJ, Stone MH. Essential papers on obsessive-compulsive disorders. New York: New York University Press; 1997.
[2] Abramowitz JS, Deacon BJ. The OC spectrum: a closer look at the arguments and the data. In: Abramowitz JS, Houts AC, editors. Concepts and controversies in obsessive-compulsive disorder. New York: Springer Science and Business Media; 2005.
[3] Zohar J, Insel TR. Obsessive-compulsive disorder: psychobiological approaches to diagnosis, treatment, and pathophysiology. Biol Psychiatry 1987;22:667–87.
[4] Stein DJ. Neurobiology of the obsessive-compulsive spectrum disorders. Biol Psychiatry 2000;47:296–304.
[5] Palumbo D, Maugham A, Kurlan A. Hypothesis III: Tourette syndrome is only one of several causes of a developmental basal ganglia syndrome. Arch Gen Psychiatry 1997;54:475–83.
[6] Stein DJ, Goodman WK, Rauch SL. The cognitive-affective neuroscience of obsessive-compulsive disorder. Curr Psychiatry Rep 2000;2:341–6.
[7] Mishkin M, Petri H. Memories and habits: some implications for the analysis of learning and retention. In: Squire LR, Butters N, editors. Neuropsychology of memory. New York: Guilford Press; 1984.
[8] Robins TW, Brown VJ. The role of the striatum in the mental chronometry of action: a theoretical review. Rev Neurosci 1990;2:181–213.
[9] Saint-Cyr JA, Taylor AE, Nicholson K. Behavior and the basal ganglia. In: Weiner WJ, Lang AE, editors. Behavioral neurology of movement disorders. New York: Raven Press; 1995.
[10] Graybiel AM. The basal ganglia and chunking of action repertoires. Neurobiol Learn Mem 1998;70:119–36.
[11] Chamberlain SR, Blackwell AD, Fineberg NA, et al. The neuropsychology of obsessive compulsive disorder: the importance of failures in cognitive and behavioural inhibition as candidate endophenotypic markers. Neurosci Biobehav Rev 2005;29:399–419.
[12] Stein DJ. Seminar on obsessive-compulsive disorder. Lancet 2002;360:397–405.
[13] Cummings JL, Cunningham K. Obsessive-compulsive disorder in Huntington's disease. Biol Psychiatry 1992;31:263–70.

[14] Rauch SL, Savage CR, Alpert NM, et al. Probing striatal function in obsessive compulsive disorder: a PET study of implicit sequence learning. J Neurosci 1997;9:568–73.

[15] Whiteside SP, Port JD, Abramowitz JS. A meta-analysis of functional neuroimaging in obsessive-compulsive disorder. Psychiatry Res 2004;132:69–79.

[16] Stein DJ, Hollander E. Impulsive aggression and obsessive-compulsive disorder. Psych Annals 1993;23:389–95.

[17] Lochner C, Hemmings SMJ, Kinnear CJ, et al. Cluster analysis of obsessive-compulsive spectrum disorders in patients with obsessive-compulsive disorder: clinical and genetic correlates. Compr Psychiatry 2005;46:14–9.

[18] Knutson B, Fong GW, Adams CM, et al. Dissociation of reward anticipation and outcome with event-related fMRI. Neuroreport 2001;12:3683–7.

[19] Fiorillo CD, Tobler PN, Schultz W. Discrete coding of reward probability and uncertainty by dopamine neurons. Science 2003;299:1898–902.

[20] Volkow ND, Fowler JS, Wang GJ, et al. Dopamine in drug abuse and addiction: results from imaging studies and treatment implications. Mol Psychiatry 2004;9:557–69.

[21] Denys D, Zohar J, Westenberg HG. The role of dopamine in obsessive-compulsive disorder: preclinical and clinical evidence. J Clin Psychiatry 2004;65(Suppl)14:11–17.

[22] Goodman WK, McDougle CJ, Lawrence LP. Beyond the serotonin hypothesis: a role for dopamine in some forms of obsessive-compulsive disorder. J Clin Psychiatry 1990;51S: 36–43.

[23] O'Sullivan R, Christenson GA, Stein DJ. Pharmacotherapy of trichotillomania. In: Stein DJ, Christenson GA, Hollander E, editors. Trichotillomania. Washington (DC): American Psychiatric Press; 1999.

[24] Serra-Mestres J, Ring HA, Costa DC, et al. Dopamine transporter binding in Gilles de la Tourette syndrome: a [123I]FP-CIT/SPECT study. Acta Psychiatr Scand 2004; 109:140–6.

[25] Pauls DL, Towbin KE, Leckman JF, et al. Gilles de la Tourette's syndrome and obsessive compulsive disorder: evidence supporting a genetic relationship. Arch Gen Psychiatry 1986;43:1180–2.

[26] Moriarty J, Eapen V, Costa DC, et al. HMPAO SPET does not distinguish obsessive-compulsive and tic syndromes in families multiply affected with Gilles de la Tourette's syndrome. Psychol Med 1997;27:737–40.

[27] Stein DJ, Grant JE. Betting on dopamine. CNS Spectr 2005;10:268–70.

[28] Denys D, van der Wee N, Janssen J, et al. Low level of dopaminergic D2 receptor binding in obsessive-compulsive disorder. Biol Psychiatry 2004;55:1041–5.

[29] Carlsson ML. On the role of prefrontal cortex glutamate for the antithetical phenomenology of obsessive compulsive disorder and attention deficit hyperactivity disorder. Prog Neuropsychopharmacol Biol Psychiatry 2001;25:5–26.

[30] Stein DJ, Hollander E. Cognitive science and obsessive-compulsive disorder. In: Stein DJ, Young JE, editors. Cognitive science and clinical disorders. San Diego: Academic Press; 1992.

[31] Stein DJ, Hollander E. The spectrum of obsessive-compulsive related disorders. In: Hollander E, editor. Obsessive-compulsive related disorders. Washington (DC): American Psychiatric Press; 1993.

[32] Phillips KA. The obsessive-compulsive spectrums. Psychiatr Clin North Am 2002;25: 791–809.

[33] Hudson JI, Pope HG Jr. Affective spectrum disorder: does antidepressant response identify a family of disorders with a common pathophysiology? Am J Psychiatry 1990;147:552–64.

[34] Blum K, Sheridan PJ, Wood RC, et al. Dopamine D2 receptor gene variants: association and linkage studies in impulsive-addictive-compulsive behavior. Pharmacogenetics 1995;5: 121–41.

[35] Carey P, Seedat S, Warwick J, et al. SPECT imaging of body dysmorphic disorder. J Neuropsychiatry Clin Neurosci 2003.

[36] Swedo SE, Leonard HL, Garvey M, et al. Pediatric autoimmune neuropsychiatric disorders associated with streptococcal infections: clinical description of the first 50 cases. Am J Psychiatry 1998;155:264–71.

[37] Martin LJ, Spicer DM, Lewis MH, et al. Social deprivation of infant monkeys alters the chemoarchitecture of the brain: I. Subcortical regions. J Neurosci 1991;11:3344–58.

[38] Thierry AM, Tassin JP, Blanc G, et al. Selective activation of mesocortical DA system by stress. Nature 1976;263:242–4.

[39] Seedat S, Stein DJ. Trauma and post-traumatic stress disorder in women: a review. Int Clin Psychopharmacol 15S3, 25–34. 2000.

[40] Lochner C, du Toit PL, Zungu-Dirwayi N, et al. Childhood trauma in obsessive-compulsive disorder, trichotillomania, and controls. Depress Anxiety 2002;15:66–8.

[41] Hemmings SM, Kinnear CJ, Lochner C, et al. Early- versus late-onset obsessive-compulsive disorder: investigating genetic and clinical correlates. Psychiatry Res 2004;128:175–82.

[42] Stein DJ, Liu Y, Shapira NA, et al. The psychobiology of obsessive-compulsive disorder: how important is the role of disgust? Curr Psychiatry Rep 2001;3:281–7.

[43] Stein DJ. Neurobiology of the obsessive-compulsive spectrum of disorders. Biol Psychiatry 2001;47:296–304.

ELSEVIER
SAUNDERS

PSYCHIATRIC
CLINICS
OF NORTH AMERICA

Psychiatr Clin N Am 29 (2006) 353–370

Obsessive-Compulsive and Spectrum Disorders in Children and Adolescents

Daniel A. Geller, MBBS, FRACP[a,b,*]

[a]*Pediatric Obsessive Compulsive Disorder Program, Division of Pediatric Psychopharmacology, Massachusetts General Hospital, YAW 6A, Fruit Street, Boston, MA 02114, USA*
[b]*Department of Psychiatry Harvard Medical School, Boston, MA, USA*

Obsessive-compulsive disorder (OCD) is a prevalent neuropsychiatric disorder affecting children and adolescents as well as adults [1–9]. Early clinical descriptions of OCD noted a childhood onset of the disorder in a substantial proportion of adult cases [10], and in 1903 Janet [11] first described a case of pediatric OCD. Further clinical reports of pediatric OCD [12–15] appeared in the literature over the next few decades. Later reports of OCD suggested that about one third of adult cases had a childhood onset [16,17]. It was not until epidemiologic studies of both adults [7] and adolescents [1] were undertaken in the 1980s that the high prevalence of OCD in children and adolescents was recognized. Perhaps because the clinical phenotype of OCD is remarkably similar at all ages, there has been an assumption that the OCD that affects children and adults is the same disorder, but whether this is true is still unknown. This article highlights important differences between and similarities in pediatric and adult-onset OCD.

Although most of the literature regarding OCD pertains to adults, a burgeoning literature addressing the childhood form of the disorder has emerged during the last 15 years. In a recent review of the subject [18], a number of original articles with widely varying methodology and design were identified. Although the varying methodology and changing nosologic definition of OCD over time makes critical assessment of earlier reports [12–15] particularly difficult, these studies clearly illustrate that OCD in children and adolescents has long been recognized as a clinical concern.

* Correspondence. Pediatric Obsessive Compulsive Disorder Program, Massachusetts General Hospital, YAW 6A, Fruit Street, Boston, MA 02114.
E-mail address: dan@gellers.org

0193-953X/06/$ - see front matter © 2006 Elsevier Inc. All rights reserved.
doi:10.1016/j.psc.2006.02.012   *psych.theclinics.com*

Epidemiology

A number of epidemiologic studies have been conducted in adolescent populations, most using school surveys for sample ascertainment. These studies report prevalence rates of OCD ranging from 2% to 4% of the pediatric population in the United States and elsewhere. In the United States, Flament and colleagues [1] reported a lifetime prevalence rate of 1.9%, and Valleni-Basile and colleagues [19] reported a prevalence rate of 3%. International studies reported prevalence rates of OCD in juveniles of 2.3% in Israel [20], 3.9% in New Zealand [21], and 4.1% in Denmark [22].

These prevalence rates are not lower than those reported in adult population studies, suggesting a variable outcome for pediatric OCD. If all childhood-onset cases remained symptomatic over the lifespan, one would expect an increasing cumulative prevalence over time as new (adult-onset) cases are added. That the prevalence does not increase indicates that at least some cases of childhood- and adolescent-onset OCD become subclinical over time. In fact, prevalence rates in adult and pediatric studies are about the same, indicating that the incidence of new-onset cases is about the same as that of OCD cases leaving the affected population and no longer identified as clinical cases, presumably through remission.

Clinical features

Phenotype

In comparing specific OCD symptoms across different age groups, the author and colleagues [23] found several differences in children, adolescents, and adults in the frequency of particular obsessions and compulsions. For example, children and adolescents had much higher rates of aggressive/harm obsessions (including fears of catastrophic events, such as death or illness in self or loved ones) than adults (63% versus 69% versus 31%, $P < .001$). These fears were the most common obsessions in the pediatric age group. On the other hand, religious obsessions were over-represented in adolescents (36%) compared with children (15%) and adults (10%, $P < .001$), and sexual obsessions were under-represented in children (11%) compared with adolescents (36%) and adults (24%) ($P = .011$). For compulsions, only hoarding was seen more often in children and adolescents than in adults (30% and 36% versus 18%, respectively, $P = .001$). The high rates of obsessive fears of loss or harm to loved ones or self and the increased rates of hoarding/saving compulsions provide evidence of developmental variability in the phenotypic expression of the disorder and may be understood in the context of attachment theory in that the expected developmental stages of ambivalence and autonomy could affect the clinical picture of OCD in children and adolescents. As a corollary, rates of separation anxiety disorder seem to be inversely proportional to age and to be as high as 56% in childhood subjects [23]. Rituals involving parents (such as reassurance seeking, a form of verbal checking) are particularly common among children and adolescents. Religious/moral and sexual obsessions and their related compulsions are selectively over-represented in adolescents, a stage when these issues are prominent, sometimes conflicted, and frequently stressful (Figs. 1 and 2).

The mean Children's Yale–Brown Obsessive Compulsive Scale (CY-BOCS) score at ascertainment (23 ± 6.5) did not differ between the child and adolescent subjects who had OCD, indicating no difference in clinical severity. As did adults, pediatric subjects had multiple obsessions and compulsions (multiple obsessions ≥ 93%; multiple compulsions, 100%). Poor insight was noted more often in childhood cases (18%) than in adolescents (6%) and adults (6%) who had OCD ($P = .01$). It is possible, however, that this observation reflects a limited ability of children to articulate their obsessional ideation rather than true lack of self-awareness. In only 15% of pediatric subjects were clear precipitating factors or stressors identified, compared with 29% of adult subjects ($P = .015$). Examples of precipitating factors included maternal hemorrhage and sudden hospitalization, death of a grandparent, reading the book *Outbreak* (about a lethal virus), and watching a television program about AIDS. In such cases, the specific obsessions were closely related thematically to the precipitating event (eg, contamination obsessions and fear of blood related to information about AIDS). The notion of Group A beta-hemolytic streptococcus as a precipitant is discussed in more depth in another article and is a different (physiologic) stressor from those discussed here.

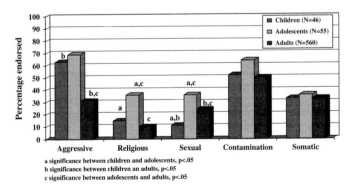

Fig. 1. Obsessions in child, adolescent, and adult subjects who have obsessive-compulsive disorder. a, significance between children and adolescents, $P < .05$; b, significance between children and adults, $P < .05$; c, significance between adolescents and adults, $P < .05$. (*Adapted from* Geller D, Biederman J, Agranat A, et al. Developmental aspects of obsessive compulsive disorder: findings in children, adolescents and adults. J Nerv Ment Dis 2001;189(7):471–7; with permission.)

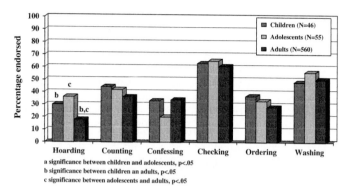

Fig. 2. Compulsions in child, adolescent, and adult subjects who have obsessive-compulsive disorder. a, significance between children and adolescents, $P < .05$; b, significance between children and adults, $P < .05$; c, significance between adolescents and adults, $P < .05$. (*Adapted from* Geller D, Biederman J, Agranat A, et al. Developmental aspects of obsessive compulsive disorder: findings in children, adolescents and adults. J Nerv Ment Dis 2001;189(7):471–7; with permission.)

OCD spectrum disorders such as trichotillomania, onychiophagia (nail biting), chronic skin picking, other impulse-control disorders, pathologic gambling, paraphilias, and body dysmorphic and eating disorders are less common in children and emerge more frequently in adolescence. Such behaviors often are not preceded by obsessions and are less clearly egodystonic, often produce gratification, and have less robust treatment response.

Age at onset

In a review of 11 studies that reported the clinical characteristics of children and adolescents who had OCD, the mean age of onset of OCD ranged from 7.5 to 12.5 years (mean, 10.3 years), and the mean age at ascertainment ranged from 12 to 15.2 years (mean, 13.2 years) [24]. Ten studies documented that, on average, age at assessment was 2.5 years after age at onset, a finding of considerable clinical importance and consistent with the secretive nature of the disorder. Two reports found that boys had an earlier age of onset of OCD than girls. In contrast, adult OCD studies have reported a mean age at onset of 21 years [7,25]. Taken together, these reports suggest a bimodal distribution of incidence with one peak in childhood and another peak in adulthood.

Gender

Most studies of pediatric OCD have reported a slight male predominance with an average 3:2 male-to-female ratio. In contrast, adult samples of OCD subjects report equal representation or a slight female preponderance [7]. Adult gender patterns appear in late adolescence.

Psychiatric comorbidity

The author and colleagues compared rates of comorbid psychiatric disorders in children, adolescents, and adults who had OCD (Fig. 3) [26].

Rates of lifetime comorbid major depression were significantly lower in children (39%) but increased markedly in adolescents (62%) and then were similar to adult rates (78%). In contrast, Tourette's disorder (TD) was more common in children who had OCD (25%) than in adolescents (9%) or adults (6%). This finding is consistent with recent reports that symptoms of TD frequently ameliorate in adolescence (mean age at remission is around 13 years) [27]. In any case, there is a substantial bidirectional overlap between OCD and TD, although the total pool of OCD-affected children is much larger than the total pool of TD-affected children. Comorbid TD showed associations with both chronologic age and age at onset as well as gender; earlier onset increases risk and greater chronologic age decreases risk of an associated TD diagnosis; male gender increases risk of TD. The presence of comorbid TD in youth who have OCD is important, because preliminary evidence suggests that treatment response and outcome may be adversely impacted. TD is discussed in more detail elsewhere in this issue.

Although disruptive behavior disorders are usually not reported in adult OCD samples, they are highly prevalent in both children and adolescents (51% and 36% for attention deficit hyperactivity disorder [ADHD]; 51% and 47% for oppositional defiant disorder). Boys are especially likely to have comorbid ADHD (53%, versus 24% in girls). Thus children who have OCD may be both compulsive as well as impulsive, a combination that is challenging to parents and clinicians. In seeking to clarify whether the symptoms of inattention and distractibility commonly seen in children and adolescents who have OCD represent true comorbidity with ADHD or a manifestation of obsessional anxiety, the author and colleagues [28,29] examined phenotypic features and functional correlates of ADHD-like symptoms in youth with and without OCD and OCD symptoms with and without ADHD from a large sample of consecutively referred pediatric

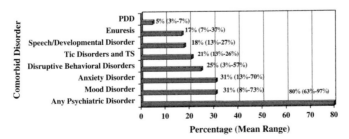

Fig. 3. Comorbidity in pediatric obsessive-compulsive disorder: review of clinical studies. (*Adapted from* Geller D, Biederman J, Jones J, et al. Is juvenile obsessive compulsive disorder a developmental subtype of the disorder? A review of the pediatric literature. J Am Acad Child Adolesc Psychiatry 1998;37(4):420–7; with permission.)

psychiatry patients. The number, frequency, and types of core ADHD symptoms as well as ADHD-associated functional indices were identical in all youth who had *Diagnostic and Statistical Manual of Mental Disorders,* fourth edition (DSM-IV)–diagnosed ADHD irrespective of the presence or absence of comorbid OCD. This finding suggests that ADHD-like symptoms youth who have OCD reflect a true comorbid state of OCD plus ADHD. The impact of comorbid ADHD in children who have OCD is not benign. Although comorbid ADHD has no meaningful impact on the phenotypic expression or clinical correlates of OCD, it was associated with higher rates of compromised global and educational functioning compared with youth who have OCD but not ADHD, so that both disorders contribute to morbid dysfunction and require independent treatment. The clinical triad of OCD, TD, and ADHD is common in affected preadolescent youth, especially boys, and represents a treatment challenge to mental health clinicians.

Unusually high rates of both specific and pervasive developmental disorders are seen in many clinically referred samples, but it is uncertain whether this prevalence reflects referral bias (Berkson's bias) [30] or is a correlate of associated comorbidity rather than being a correlate specific to childhood-onset OCD.

Non-OCD anxiety disorders are highly prevalent in all age groups, with only separation anxiety disorder showing significantly higher frequency in children (56%) and adolescents (35%) than in adults (17%). These disorders therefore are a nonspecific marker for a more severe anxiety diathesis. As expected, adults have higher rates of comorbid substance abuse/dependence (16%) than adolescents (2%) and children (0%). In addition adults (8%) had more comorbid eating disorders than either children (0%) or adolescents (2%).

One study examined possible referral bias affecting children and adolescents whose OCD was ascertained through specialized pediatric OCD clinics as opposed to general child psychiatry clinics [31]. OCD was identified in 8.6% of general pediatric psychiatry clinic subjects. Subjects whose OSD was ascertained from a specialty program tended to have longer duration of OCD and higher rates of OCD-specific treatment; otherwise no meaningful differences in the clinical or socio-demographic characteristics of the two groups were found.

Cognitive and neuropsychologic findings

Because of the potential involvement of frontal-striatal systems in OCD, several aspects of neuropsychologic performance (especially measures of visuospatial integration, short-term memory, attention, and executive functions) have been especially relevant to its study. Of these performance factors, executive functioning has received the greatest attention in the literature. Executive functions entail the ability to consider all aspects of a situation and use this knowledge to prioritize goals and plans, implement behavior strategically, and shift behavior as the environmental context changes [32]. A pattern of deficits has been observed among adults who have OCD, but far fewer studies have examined neuropsychologic processes among children who have the disorder [33]. A handful of neuropsychologic studies of OCD in children have yielded highly inconsistent results. Earlier studies found basal ganglia dysfunction, as evidenced by a pattern of executive functioning, visuospatial, and attentional deficits. A study of 42 adolescents who had OCD suggested frontal lobe and caudate nucleus dysfunction, as indicated by poorer performance on a stylus maze task and the Wisconsin Card Sorting Test, and more egocentric spatial judgment on a street map test in children who had OCD [34]. Similarly, in a study examining the neuropsychologic performance of children who had OCD, Behar and colleagues [35] compared 16 children (mean age, 13.7 years) with 16 matched controls. Participants were evaluated several neuropsychologic tests of frontal lobe functioning (eg, Money's Road Map Test). Compared with normal control participants, patients who had OCD demonstrated poorer performance on tasks assessing the ability to rotate themselves mentally in space and in maze learning. [35]. Finally, a neuropsychologic study of 92 children who had TD, with or without OCD and ADHD symptoms, found that children who had TD and OCD with or without ADHD symptoms were significantly more impaired on measures of verbal IQ, achievement, and executive functioning than the groups without OCD symptoms [36]. The group that had both OCD and ADHD symptoms was most impaired on these measures. There were no group differences in measures of attention, psychomotor performance, or sensory perception.

In a related line of research, Rosenberg and colleagues [37] examined cognitive functions associated with the prefrontal cortex, using an oculomotor paradigm. They examined the ability to suppress reflexive responses to external cues (eg, a target light), volitionally execute delayed responses, and anticipate predictable events and found that subjects who had pediatric OCD demonstrated higher rates of response-suppression failure than controls. These increased failure rates were correlated with impairments on other measures of frontostriatal functioning. Overall, controls developed the ability to suppress oculomotor responses (a function of prefrontal cortex development) approximately 5 years younger than OCD patients [37,38].

Executive-functioning impairments among children who have OCD would be consistent with those seen in other frontal lobe disorders, including Sydenham's chorea and brain injury [39,40]. Several studies have failed to find significant neuropsychologic deficits among youth who have OCD, however. The first of these, by Thomsen and Jensen [41], examined neurologic indicators of cerebral dysfunction in 61 patients who had OCD (age 8–17 years) and 117 age- and sex-matched psychiatric control subjects. Measures included hyperventilation, sleep, and photostimulation electroencephalograms and a neurodevelopmental assessment of motor and attentional functions. The authors assigned children to an "organic" versus "nonorganic" class based on the presence of moderate-to-severe encephalographic abnormality, specific developmental disorder, or attentional deficit. In this study fewer children in the OCD group than in the non-OCD group were assigned to the "organic" class. The authors concluded that childhood OCD did not depend on "major cerebral disturbance found by conventional neuropediatric methods" [41].

Douglass and colleagues [21] also observed no differences on cognitive and neuropsychologic measures between a group of 34 adolescents who had childhood onset of OCD symptoms and matched groups of psychiatric and normal controls [21]. Similarly, Beers and colleagues [40] examined cognitive functioning in 21 treatment-naive children who had OCD (mean age 12.3 years) and 21 matched-control participants. Children were assessed using a comprehensive neuropsychologic battery including multiple measures of frontal lobe functioning. Children in the OCD group did not evince cognitive impairment on any measures of frontal lobe functioning or executive functioning. Moreover, performance on neuropsychologic tests was not correlated with age of onset, duration of illness, or severity of OCD symptoms [42]. The authors offer several explanations for these results, including the possibilities that neuropsychologic tests may not be sensitive to dysfunction in the frontostriatal systems implicated in OCD or that children who have OCD may not display cognitive deficits early in their illness [42,43].

Family genetic factors

Although genetics of OCD are discussed in depth in a different article, some findings unique to childhood-onset OCD are reviewed here. Available family studies of children and adolescents find OCD to be highly familial. OCD and subclinical obsessive-compulsive symptoms may be found in 18% to 30% of relatives, but higher rates of both OCD and tics are found in the relatives of early-onset OCD probands [44–46]. Leonard and colleagues [45] also found an earlier age at onset of OCD in subjects who had comorbid TD. Lenane and colleagues [44] found that fathers were more likely than mothers to be affected with OCD and that father-son pairs were the most common familial pattern.

The contribution of genetic factors to the development of OCD has been explored in family genetic, twin, and segregation analysis studies [46–51]. In a cross-cultural sample of 4246 child twin pairs, Hudziak and colleagues [52] used structural equation modeling to examine the influence of both genetic (45%–58%) and unique environmental (42%–55%) factors and concluded that genetic and nongenetic factors are about equally important.

Although first-degree family members of adults who have OCD have significantly higher recurrence risk of OCD, an earlier age of onset of symptoms in adult probands is associated with still higher rates of OCD and subclinical OCD among first-degree family members [46,47]. Age of onset has been recognized as an important factor in the expression of both psychiatric and nonpsychiatric disorders and has been shown to influence results and power from linkage and associate tests [53]. The estimated familial risk for adults who have an affected relative is 11% to 12% [47], but recent studies suggest relative risk in family members of affected children to be around 25%, double that found in relatives of affected adult-onset cases.

In the author's family genetic study of pediatric-onset OCD [54], age-corrected recurrence risks to first-degree relatives of pediatric OCD probands estimated using Kaplan-Meier survival analyses of the time to onset of disorder showed a risk of 26% for OCD, of 9% for tics or TD, and of 18% for ADHD. These results concur with two recent studies suggesting an increased familial risk for relatives of children who have OCD compared with later adult-onset OCD and an increased genetic load for clinical expression in families that have an affected child [50,55]. These findings have relevance for further genetic studies of OCD and related disorders. In addition, relatives of males who had OCD showed higher rates of chronic tic disorders (including TD) (odds ratio [OR], 2.57; 95% confidence interval [CI], 1.03–6.41; $P = .043$) and ADHD (OR, 2.58; CI, 1.23–5.41; $P = .012$). Relatives of OCD probands who had ADHD showed an elevated risk for TD or tics (OR, 2.3; CI, 1.03–5.17; $P = .043$) as well as ADHD (OR, 2.18; CI, 1.13–4.19; $P = .02$).

Treatment

A separate article focuses on pharmacologic treatment of OCD. This discussion addresses the aspects of treatment that are especially relevant to children. This discussion recognizes the important role of cognitive behavior therapy (CBT) and family involvement in the management of child and adolescent patients who have OCD. Although the extant literature regarding CBT in young patients who have OCD does not achieve the scientific rigor of drug trials because of methodologic difficulties and small numbers, there is little doubt that CBT is an effective treatment for some children. This efficacy is reflected in the Expert Consensus Guidelines for treatment of OCD and the American Academy of Child and Adolescent Psychiatry Practice Parameters for OCD that recommend CBT, with or without medication, as a first-line intervention in youth [56].

Experience indicates that absence of comorbid disorders and good insight increase the chances for successful CBT in children, the latter permitting a subject to tolerate anxiety-provoking stimuli without ritualizing based on intact reality testing. In very young children, however, insight may not be necessary for a good outcome, because parents control so many of the contingencies of the CBT. In contrast, the presence of a concurrent major depressive disorder, other (multiple) anxiety disorders, or disruptive behavior disorders could severely limit the response to CBT in some children. Clinicians must be aware that a decision to treat with medication without a prior discussion of CBT with the parent or guardian is probably not made with a truly informed consent.

In the first meta-analysis of randomized, controlled pharmacologic trials of OCD or serotonin-reuptake inhibitors (SRIs) in children and adolescents, Geller and colleagues [57] found highly significant pooled effects of medication versus placebo as well as important similarities and differences between individual drugs and differential sensitivity of quantitative measures of severity to change (Table 1). The pooled studies found an overall effect size of 0.46, equaling a difference of 4 to 6 points in CY-BOCS score, between active and placebo treatments. Each drug examined individually was significantly better than placebo or comparator treatments. Translated into quantitative measures, analyses of randomized, controlled trials using an intent-to-treat model typically showed an absolute decrease in CY-BOCS scores of about 4 to 6 points, or a 30% to 38% decrement from baseline CY-BOCS scores [57]. This apparently limited effect size may actually reflect a dramatic clinical response because of the nonlinear properties of the CY-BOCS scale and its lack of sensitivity in the severe/extreme range. The results are similar to those observed in treatment studies of adults who have OCD. Therefore, even in the presence of a positive response, residual OCD symptoms frequently remain, because posttreatment scores of 15 to 20 indicate mild-to-moderate OCD. Thus, persistent low-grade

Table 1

Pair-wise comparison of standardized mean differences (SMD) of pooled drug and placebo effects in randomized, controlled trials of pediatric obsessive-compulsive disorder using meta-analysis

Comparator	Clomipramine	Sertraline	Fluvoxamine	Fluoxetine	Paroxetine
Placebo	$z = 6.23$ $P < .001$ $SMD = .693$	$z = 3.84$ $P < .001$ $SMD = .327$	$z = 3.52$ $P < .001$ $SMD = .375$	$z = 5.56$ $P < .001$ $SMD = .546$	$z = 3.95$ $P < .001$ $SMD = .405$
Paroxetine	$Z = 2.99$ $P = .003$	$z = -0.36$ $P = .72$	$z = -0.04$ $P = .97$	$z = 1.17$ $P = .24$	
Fluoxetine	$z = 2.24$ $P = .025$	$z = -1.86$ $P = 0.06$	$z = -1.33$ $P = .18$		
Fluvoxamine	$z = 3.24$ $P = .001$	$z = -0.36$ $P = .72$			
Sertraline	$z = 3.78$ $P < .001$				

The first row provides tests for each drug of the significance of its pooled SMD from placebo. Statistical significance indicates that the pooled observations find significant separation between drug and placebo. Rows two through four provide tests of the hypothesis that the SMD for the row drug is the same as the SMD for the column drugs. Significant findings indicate that the magnitude of separation between drug and placebo differs among the drugs. Meta-analysis used multiple regression to assess the degree to which the effect sizes varied with the methodological features of each study. Four covariates were used in this regression model: (1) type of dependent outcome measure, (2) type of drug, (3) type of design of study, and (4) type of outcome score used (change or posttreatment score). Where significant differences emerged in the omnibus analysis, pair-wise comparisons were undertaken controlling for other significant variables. Statistically significant findings in italics.

Adapted from Geller DA, Biederman J, Stewart ES, et al. Which SSRI? A meta-analysis of pharmacotherapy trials in pediatric obsessive compulsive disorder. Am J Psychiatry 2003;160(11):1919–28; with permission. © 2003 American Psychiatric Association.

symptoms and impairment are the norm for many children and adolescents who have OCD, even when treated.

Combined cognitive behavioral therapy and medication treatment in pediatric obsessive-compulsive disorder

The combination of medication treatment with CBT may be more efficient than either treatment alone. CBT may also reduce the relapse rate in patients withdrawn from medication. CBT seems to be a more durable form of intervention. The Pediatric OCD Treatment Study (POTS I) [58] was a 5-year treatment outcome study in three sites that used a balanced 1 × 4 design to compare placebo, sertraline, CBT, and combined CBT plus sertraline, using the CY–BOCS as the dependent measure. The POTS sample reflected a community clinical practice in that 80% of children had at least one comorbid disorder; 63% had an internalizing disorder, and 27% had an externalizing disorder. The magnitude of the effect for each treatment condition for combined treatment, CBT alone, and sertraline alone was 1.4, 0.97, and 0.67, respectively. Clinical remission rates (defined as a CY–BOCS score < 10) were 53.6% for combined treatment (95% CI, 36%–70%), 39.3% for CBT alone (95% CI, 24%–58%), 21.4% for sertraline alone (95% CI, 10%–40%), and 3.6% for placebo (95% CI, 0%–19%). The remission rate for combined treatment did not differ from that for CBT alone ($P = .42$) but did differ from sertraline alone ($P = .03$) and from placebo ($P = .002$). In summary, POTS found that combined treatment had an additive effect on outcome with the greatest overall effect size [59]. In general, therefore, children and adolescents who have OCD should start with either CBT or the combination of CBT and medication.

Impact of comorbid psychopathology and spectrum disorders on treatment of pediatric obsessive-compulsive disorder

Comorbid disorders, particularly those often seen in children who have OCD, may have a substantial impact on treatment decisions and response. For example, in children and adolescents who have OCD and comorbid tic or TD, selective serotonin-reuptake inhibitors (SSRIs) alone may have less anti-obsessional effect [60,61]. In addition, there are case reports suggesting that SSRIs, especially at higher doses, may exacerbate or even induce tics in some patients [62–64]. Specific anti-tic medications may be needed in addition to any treatment used for the primary OCD symptoms.

The presence of comorbid disruptive behavior disorders can limit the efficacy of behavioral and medication treatment for OCD [65] and lead to more severe impairment than OCD without disruptive behavior disorders [65,66], suggesting cumulative morbidity from each diagnosis. Stimulants have been the mainstay of treatment for ADHD with OCD but may increase primary obsessions and rituals or anxiety, and there is a lack of agreement on their benefits in anxiety disorders [67,68], for which they are relatively contraindicated (see package labels).

Obsessive-compulsive symptoms in children who have pervasive developmental disorders present diagnostic and nosologic dilemmas, and a small number of children may meet criteria for both diagnoses (eg, with typical contamination concerns and cleaning behavior). Fortunately, SRIs are effective in symptomatic management of both disorders, and good insight is not necessarily required for a drug response. Drug treatment of pervasive developmental disorders is similar to that for OCD, but low doses of SSRIs are advised because of the great sensitivity of such children to these agents.

Comorbid major depression may be more impairing than OCD symptoms in some children and may impact response to OCD treatments, whether pharmacologic or behavioral. Management of these patients does not differ markedly from adult practice, however, and mood symptoms should be treated aggressively with antidepressant augmentation or mood stabilizers as needed. Recently, several separate studies have reported a bidirectional overlap between bipolar disorder and OCD in children at rates greater than expected. Masi and colleagues [69] reported that fully 44% of their pediatric patients who had bipolar disorder had a lifetime diagnosis of OCD, which usually preceded the onset of mood symptoms. Similarly, Faedda and colleagues [70] found that 27% of children diagnosed as having bipolar disorder had comorbid OCD. The author and colleagues [71] also have identified higher-than-expected rates of comorbid bipolar disorder (approximately 5%–10%) in youth who have OCD. On the other hand, Reddy and colleagues [72] reported a much lower rate of bipolar disorder (1.9%) in their pediatric OCD population who were largely treatment naive and had OCD of only moderate severity. Although this inconsistency in the rate of co-occurrence of the two disorders could be attributed to selection or referral bias, it nevertheless suggests that a true comorbidity risk may have been overlooked in these patients. OCD with comorbid bipolar disorder clearly presents a therapeutic dilemma. Specifically, all agents (including SSRIs) documented to be helpful in treating OCD also have the risk of exacerbating mood symptoms and precipitating mania. Several reports have described the high risk of (hypo)manic switches in children and adolescents who have OCD and who are treated with tricyclics or SSRIs [73,74]. Further, antimanic agents, although effective in controlling manic symptoms, do not show any efficacy in treating OCD symptoms. Mood stabilizers or atypical neuroleptics may therefore be needed to counteract activating effects of SRIs required to treat OCD symptoms.

Outcome

The changing nosology of OCD in the DSM [75] and the ICD [76] during the last several decades and recent advances in pharmacologic and behavioral treatment modes mean that earlier studies of outcome may no longer be applicable to current patients who have pediatric OCD. In the first long-term outcome review of childhood- and adolescent-onset OCD, Stewart and colleagues [77] examined long-term outcome of childhood- and adolescent-onset OCD using a systematic search of medical databases. Meta-analysis regression was applied to evaluate predictors and persistence of OCD. Sixteen study samples (n = 6–132; total = 521 participants) in 22 studies had follow-up periods ranging between 1 and 15.6 years. Several important findings emerged that are relevant to both clinical practice and future research. This review showed that rates of persistence of OCD in childhood-onset cases are lower than previously believed and explicated in the DSM-IV. Two thirds of studies showed OCD did not persist as a full clinical syndrome in the majority of subjects. The pooled mean rate of persistence of OCD was 41% (95% CI, 32%–51%) across all samples and studies. Any OCD was persistent in a mean of 61% of the pooled samples (95% CI, 46%–76%), indicating an overall remission rate (not meeting criteria for full or subthreshold OCD) of 39%. Inpatient status, longer duration of illness, and an earlier age at onset of OCD were associated with a significantly increased rate of persistence over a mean of 5.7 years in these studies. In contrast, gender, age at assessment, length of follow-up, and year of publication were not reported as predictors of remission or persistence. The last finding suggests that rates of persistence have not lessened despite remarkable advances in the treatment of pediatric OCD during recent decades. This evidence is at odds with numerous reports of the therapeutic benefits of both SRI medication and CBT in affected youth [61,78,79]. This apparent contradiction may reflect the rather limited measures of outcome reported in these studies.

In a qualitative analysis of the extant literature, several reported findings in individual studies were noteworthy, although results of outcome predictor analyses often were inconsistent. For example, psychiatric comorbidity was reported to predict poorer outcome in a number of studies. The presence of a tic disorder or mood disorder was associated with increased OCD severity [5,80], and the presence of any comorbidity predicted worse global functioning at follow-up [81]. These findings align with recent reports of treatment resistance in comorbid youth who have OCD [82]. Few studies discussed psychosocial factors and outcomes despite their importance for global functioning and impairment. Those studies that did examine psychosocial function at follow-up reported high rates of social dysfunction, unmarried status, and unemployment, although educational achievement seemed to be relatively spared. These findings regarding psychosocial outcome suggest that multiple criteria are important when measuring outcome of OCD over time.

Summary

The available literature indicates that OCD affecting children and adolescents is highly prevalent. Pediatric-onset OCD seems to share important similarities with the adult disorder but also shows important differences. For example, the clinical phenotype of OCD is remarkably consistent at all ages with some allowances for developmental expression. Pediatric patients frequently demonstrate poor insight into the nature of their obsessions, which in association with their limited verbal expression may make the diagnosis more difficult. Obsessions involving fear of harm and separation, compulsions without obsessions, and rituals involving family members are more common in younger patients. Treatment response, including serotonergic specificity and the need for robust dosing, is another feature shared by early- and adult-onset OCD. Important differences across the life span can also be identified. Perhaps the clearest difference pertains to age of onset. Age-at-onset data have shown a bimodal distribution of age of onset of OCD, with one peak in preadolescent childhood and another peak in adulthood. Another distinction between child and adult OCD is gender representation. Whereas adult studies report equal gender representation or a slight female preponderance, pediatric clinical samples are clearly male predominant. Patterns of psychiatric comorbidity in pediatric OCD show high rates of tic and mood and anxiety disorders, similar to the patterns in adults, but also show a distinct association with disruptive behavior disorders (ADHD and oppositional defiant disorder) and other specific and pervasive developmental disorders. Family studies indicate that the disorder is highly familial and that a childhood onset of the disorder seems to be associated with a markedly increased risk for familial transmission of OCD, tic disorders, and ADHD.

Both scientifically and clinically, the recognition of developmentally specific OCD phenotypes may be valuable. For example, research efforts aimed at identifying OCD-associated genes are likely to be more successful if developmentally homogeneous samples are studied instead of combining data from children, adolescents, and adults, as has been common in OCD studies. Clinical management is also informed by an appreciation of the unique correlates of OCD affecting youth, especially comorbidity with chronic tic disorders and ADHD and their impact on treatment.

The so-called "spectrum disorders" related to OCD are less prominent in children and adolescents than in adults. Although sharing some features with typical OCD, these symptoms are less clearly ego-dystonic and less anxiety producing, frequently provide a measure of gratification, and are less responsive in general to SSRIs. Often cognitive antecedents to these behaviors are less well developed than in more typical OCD, and behavioral interventions are the mainstay of treatment but with more variable success.

References

[1] Flament M, Whitaker A, Rapoport J, et al. Obsessive compulsive disorder in adolescence: an epidemiological study. J Am Acad Child Adolesc Psychiatry 1988;27(6):764–71.
[2] Flament M, Whitaker A, Rapoport J, et al. An epidemiological study of obsessive-compulsive disorder in adolescence. In: Rapoport J, editor. Obsessive-compulsive disorder in children and adolescents. Washington (DC): American Psychiatric Press; 1989. p. 253–67.

[3] Rapoport JL. Obsessive-compulsive disorder in children and adolescents. Washington (D): American Psychiatric Press; 1989.

[4] Swedo S, Rapoport J, Leonard H, et al. Obsessive-compulsive disorder in children and adolescents: clinical phenomenology of 70 consecutive cases. Arch Gen Psychiatry 1989; 46:335–41.

[5] Leonard HL, Swedo SE, Lenane MC, et al. 2- to 7 year follow-up study of 54 obsessive-compulsive children and adolescents. Arch Gen Psychiatry 1993;50:429–39.

[6] Rasmussen SA, Eisen JL. The epidemiology and differential diagnosis of obsessive compulsive disorder. J Clin Psychiatry 1992;53(4 Suppl):4–10.

[7] Karno M, Golding J, Sorenson S, et al. The epidemiology of obsessive-compulsive disorder in five US communities. Arch Gen Psychiatry 1988;45:1094–9.

[8] Weissman M, Bland R, Canino G, et al. The cross national epidemiology of obsessive compulsive disorder. Am J Psychiatry 1994;55(Suppl):5–10.

[9] Jenike MA, Baer L, Minichiello WE. Obsessive-compulsive disorders: theory and management. Littleton (CO): Year Book Medical Publishers, Inc.; 1990.

[10] Pitres A, Regis E. Les obsessions et les impulsions. Paris: Doin; 1902.

[11] Janet P. Les obsessions et la psychasthenie. Paris: Felix Alcan; 1903.

[12] Berman L. The obsessive-compulsive neurosis in children. J Nerv Ment Dis 1942;95:26–39.

[13] Despert JL. Differential diagnosis between obsessive compulsive neurosis and schizophrenia in children. In: Hoch P, Zubin J, editors. Psychopathology in children. New York: Grune and Stratton, Inc.; 1955. p. 240–53.

[14] Judd L. Obsessive-compulsive neurosis in children. Arch Gen Psychiatry 1965;12:136–44.

[15] Adams P. Obsessive children. New York: Brunner Mazel, Inc.; 1973.

[16] Black A. The natural history of obsessional neurosis. In: Beech H, editor. Obsessional states. London: Methuen and Company, Ltd.; 1974. p. 1–23.

[17] Rachman SJ, Hodgson RJ. Obsessions and compulsions. Englewood Cliffs (NJ): Prentice Hall; 1980.

[18] Geller D, Biederman J, Jones J, et al. Obsessive compulsive disorder in children and adolescents: a review. Harv Rev Psychiatry 1998;5(5):260–73.

[19] Valleni-Basile L, Garrison C, Jackson K, et al. Frequency of obsessive-compulsive disorder in a community sample of young adolescents. J Am Acad Child Adolesc Psychiatry 1994; 33(6):782–91.

[20] Apter A, Fallon TJ Jr, King RA, et al. Obsessive-compulsive characteristics: from symptoms to syndrome. J Am Acad Child Adolesc Psychiatry 1996;35(7):907–12.

[21] Douglass HM, Moffitt TE, Dar R, et al. Obsessive-compulsive disorder in a birth cohort of 18-year-olds: prevalence and predictors. J Am Acad Child Adolesc Psychiatry 1995;34(11): 1424–31.

[22] Thomsen P. Obsessive-compulsive disorder in children and adolescents: self-reported obsessive-compulsive behaviour in pupils in Denmark. Acta Psychiatr Scand 1993;88: 212–7.

[23] Geller D, Biederman J, Agranat A, et al. Developmental aspects of obsessive compulsive disorder: findings in children, adolescents and adults. J Nerv Ment Dis 2001;189(7):471–7.

[24] Geller D, Biederman J, Jones J, et al. Is juvenile obsessive compulsive disorder a developmental subtype of the disorder? A review of the pediatric literature. J Am Acad Child Adolesc Psychiatry 1998;37(4):420–7.

[25] Rasmussen S, Eisen J. The epidemiology and clinical features of obsessive compulsive disorder. Psychiatr Clin North Am 1992;15(4):743–58.

[26] Geller D, Biederman J, Emslie G, et al. Comorbid psychiatric illness and response to treatment in pediatric OCD. In: Proceedings of the annual meeting of the American Psychiatric Association. New Orleans (LA): American Psychiatric Association; 2001.

[27] Coffey B, Biederman J, Geller D, et al. Re-examining tic persistence and tic-associated impairment in Tourette's disorder: findings from a naturalistic follow-up study. J Am Acad Child Adolesc Psychiatry 2004;192(11):776–80.

[28] Geller D, Biederman J, Faraone S, et al. Attention deficit hyperactivity disorder in children and adolescents with obsessive compulsive disorder: fact or artifact? J Am Acad Child Adolesc Psychiatry 2002;41(1):52–8.

[29] Geller DA, Coffey B, Faraone S, et al. Does comorbid attention-deficit/hyperactivity disorder impact the clinical expression of pediatric obsessive compulsive disorder? CNS Spectrums 2003;8(4):259–64.

[30] Berkson J. Limitations of the application of fourfold table analysis to hospital data. Biometrics Bulletin 1946;2:47–52.

[31] Geller D, Biederman J, Faraone SV, et al. Clinical correlates of obsessive compulsive disorder in children and adolescents referred to specialized and non-specialized clinical settings. Depress Anxiety 2000;11(4):163–8.

[32] Savage CR, Baer L, Keuthen NJ, et al. Organizational strategies mediate nonverbal memory impairment in obsessive-compulsive disorder. Biol Psychiatry 1998.

[33] Schultz RT, Evans DW, Wolff M. Neuropsychological models of childhood obsessive-compulsive disorder. Child Adolesc Psychiatr Clin N Am 1999;8(3):513–31.

[34] Cox C, Fedio P, Rapoport J. Neuropsychological testing of obsessive-compulsive adolescents. In: Rapoport J, editor. Obsessive-compulsive disorder in children and adolescents. Washington (DC): American Psychiatric Press; 1989. p. 73–85.

[35] Behar D, Rapoport J, Berg C, et al. Computerized tomography and neuropsychological test measures in adolescents with obsessive compulsive disorder. Am J Psychiatry 1984;141(3):363–9.

[36] DeGroot CM, Yeates KO, Baker GB, et al. Impaired neuropsychological functioning in Tourette's syndrome subjects with co-occurring obsessive-compulsive and attention deficit symptoms. J Neuropsychiatry Clin Neurosci 1997;9:267–72.

[37] Rosenberg D, Averbach D, O'Hearn K, et al. Oculomotor response inhibition abnormalities in pediatric obsessive-compulsive disorder. Arch Gen Psychiatry 1997;54(September):831–8.

[38] Rosenberg D, Keshavan M, O'Hearn K, et al. Frontostriatal measurement in treatment-naive children with obsessive compulsive disorder. Arch Gen Psychiatry 1997;54:824–30.

[39] Filley CM, Young DA, Reardon MS, et al. Frontal lobe lesions and executive dysfunction in children. Neuropsychiatry Neuropsychol Behav Neurol 1999;12(3):156–60.

[40] Casey BJ, Vauss Y, Chused A, et al. Executive functioning in Sydenham's chorea: a basal ganglia disorder: part II. Dev Neuropsychol 1994;10:89–96.

[41] Thomsen PH, Jensen J. Latent class analysis of organic aspects of obsessive-compulsive disorder in children and adolescents. Acta Psychiatr Scand 1991;84(4):391–5.

[42] Beers S, Rosenberg DR, Dick EL, et al. Neuropsychological study of frontal lobe function in psychotropic-naive children with obsessive-compulsive disorder. Am J Psychiatry 1999;156(5):777–9.

[43] Beers SR, Rosenberg DR, Ryan CM. Letter to the editor: Dr.Beers and colleagues reply. Am J Psychiatry 2000;157(7):1183.

[44] Lenane M, Swedo S, Leonard H, et al. Psychiatric disorders in first degree relatives of children and adolescents with obsessive compulsive disorder. J Am Acad Child Adolesc Psychiatry 1990;29(3):407–12.

[45] Leonard HL, Lenane MC, Swedo SE, et al. Tics and Tourette's disorder: a 2- to 7-year follow-up of 54 obsessive-compulsive children. Am J Psychiatry 1992;149:1244–51.

[46] Pauls D, Alsobrook J II, Goodman W, et al. A family study of obsessive-compulsive disorder. Am J Psychiatry 1995;152(1):76–84.

[47] Nestadt G, Samuels J, Bienvenu JO, et al. A family study of obsessive compulsive disorder. Arch Gen Psychiatry 2000;57(4):358–63.

[48] Grados M, Riddle M, Samuels J, et al. The familial phenotype of obsessive-compulsive disorder in relation to tic disorders: the Hopkins OCD family study. Biol Psychiatry 2001;50:559–65.

[49] Reddy P, Reddy J, Srinath S, et al. A family study of juvenile obsessive-compulsive disorder. Can J Psychiatry 2001;46:346–51.

[50] Hanna GL, Fischer DJ, Chadha KR, et al. Familial and sporadic subtypes of early-onset obsessive-compulsive disorder. Biol Psychiatry 2005;57:895–900.

[51] Alsobrook J II, Leckman J, Goodman W, et al. Segregation analysis of obsessive-compulsive disorder using symptom-based factor scores. Am J Med Genet 1999;88:669–75.

[52] Hudziak JJ, Van Beijsterveldt CE, Althoff RR, et al. Genetic and environmental contributions to the Child Behavior Checklist Obsessive-Compulsive Scale: a cross-cultural twin study. Arch Gen Psychiatry 2004;61(6):608–16.

[53] Li H, Hsu L. Effects of age at onset on the power of the affected sib pair and transmission/disequilibrium tests. Ann Hum Genet 2000;64(Pt 3):239–54.

[54] Geller D, Biederman J, Petty C, et al. Age-corrected risk of OCD in relatives of affected youth. In: Joint scientific proceedings of the American Academy of Child and Adolescent Psychiatry and the Canadian Academy of Child and Adolescent Psychiatry. Toronto (Ontario, Canada): American Academy of Child and Adolescent Psychiatry; 2005.

[55] Do Rosario-Campos MC, Leckman JF, Curi M, et al. A family study of early-onset obsessive-compulsive disorder. American Journal of Medical Genetics Part B: Neuropsychiatric Genetics 2005;136B(1):92–7.

[56] Action AO. Practice parameters for the assessment of treatment of children and adolescents with obsessive-compulsive disorder. Journal of the American Academy of Child and Adolescent Psychiatry 1998;37(10 Suppl):27S–45S.

[57] Geller DA, Biederman J, Stewart ES, et al. Which SSRI? A meta-analysis of pharmacotherapy trials in pediatric obsessive compulsive disorder. Am J Psychiatry 2003;160(11):1919–28.

[58] March J, Foa E, Gammon P, et al. Cognitive-behavior therapy, sertraline, and their combination for children and adolescents with obsessive-compulsive disorder: the Pediatric OCD Treatment Study (POTS) randomized controlled trial. JAMA 2004;292(16):1969–76.

[59] March JS. Pediatric OCD Treatment Study (POTS). In: Proceedings of the 156th annual meeting of the American Academy of Child and Adolescent Psychiatry. San Francisco: American Academy of Child and Adolescent Psychiatry; 2003.

[60] Kurlan R, Deeley C, McDermott M, et al. A pilot controlled study of fluoxetine for obsessive-compulsive symptoms in children with Tourette's syndrome. Clin Neuropharmacol 1993;16(2):167–72.

[61] Geller DA, Hoog SL, Heiligenstein JH, et al. Fluoxetine treatment for obsessive-compulsive disorder in children and adolescents: a placebo-controlled clinical trial. J Am Acad Child Adolesc Psychiatry 2001;40(7):773–9.

[62] Delgado P, Goodman W, Price L, et al. Fluvoxamine/pimozide treatment of concurrent Tourette's and obsessive-compulsive disorder. Br J Psychiatry 1990;157:762–5.

[63] Riddle M, Scahill L, King R, et al. Double-blind, crossover trial of fluoxetine and placebo in children and adolescents with obsessive-compulsive disorder. J Am Acad Child Adolesc Psychiatry 1992;31(6):1062–9.

[64] Fennig S, Fennig S, Pato M, et al. Emergence of symptoms of Tourette's syndrome during fluvoxamine treatment of obsessive-compulsive disorder. Br J Psychiatry 1994;164:839–41.

[65] Geller D, Biederman J, Wagner K, et al. Comorbid psychiatric illness and response to treatments, relapse rates, and behavioral adverse event incidents in pediatric OCD. J Child Adolesc Psychopharmacol 2001;11(4):331–2.

[66] Hanna GL, Yuwiler A, Coates JK. Whole blood serotonin and disruptive behaviors in juvenile obsessive-compulsive disorder. J Am Acad Child Adolesc Psychiatry 1995;34(1):28–35.

[67] Diamond IR, Tannock R, Schachar RJ. Response to methylphenidate in children with ADHD and comorbid anxiety. J Am Acad Child Adolesc Psychiatry 1999;38(4):402–9.

[68] Tannock R, Ickowicz A, Schachar R. Differential effects of methylphenidate on working memory in ADHD children with and without comorbid anxiety. J Am Acad Child Adolesc Psychiatry 1995;34(7):886–96.

[69] Masi G, Toni C, Perugi G, et al. Anxiety disorders in children and adolescents with bipolar disorder: a neglected comorbidity. Can J Psychiatry 2001;46(9):797–802.

[70] Faedda GL, Baldessarini RJ, Glovinsky IP, et al. Pediatric bipolar disorder: phenomenology and course of illness. Bipolar Disord 2004;6(4):305.

[71] Joshi G, Geller D,Wozniak J, et al. Clinical characteristics of comorbid obsessive-compulsive disorder and bipolar disorder in children and adolescents. In: Proceedings of the 52nd annual meeting of the American Academy of Child and Adolescent Psychiatry. Toronto (Ontario, Canada): the American Academy of Child and Adolescent Psychiatry; 2005.

[72] Reddy YC, Reddy PS, Srinath S, et al. Comorbidity in juvenile obsessive-compulsive disorder: a report from India. Can J Psychiatry 2000;45:274–8.

[73] Go FS, Malley EE, Birmaher B, et al. Manic behaviors associated with fluoxetine in three 12- to 18-year-olds with obsessive-compulsive disorder. J Child Adolesc Psychopharmacol 1998; 8(1):73–80.

[74] King R, Riddle M, Riddle M, et al. Emergence of self-destructive phenomena in children and adolescents during fluoxetine treatment. J Am Acad Child Adolesc Psychiatry 1991;30(2): 179–86.

[75] American Psychiatric Association. Diagnostic and Statistical Manual of Mental Disorders. Washington (DC): American Psychiatric Press; 1952.

[76] World Health Organization. ICD-10 classification of mental and behavioural disorders. Geneva (Switzerland): World Health Organization; 1992.

[77] Stewart SE, Geller DA, Jenike M, et al. Long term outcome of pediatric obsessive compulsive disorder: a meta-analysis and qualitative review of the literature. Acta Psychiatr Scand 2004;110(1):4–13.

[78] Flament MF, Rapoport JL, Berg CJ, et al. Clomipramine treatment of childhood obsessive-compulsive disorder: a double-blind controlled study. Arch Gen Psychiatry 1985;42(10): 977–83.

[79] March JS, Mulle K, Herbel B. Behavioral psychotherapy for children and adolescents with obsessive-compulsive disorder: an open trial of a new protocol-driven treatment package. J Am Acad Child Adolesc Psychiatry 1994;33(3):333–41.

[80] Wewetzer C, Jans T, Muller B, et al. Long-term outcome and prognosis of obsessive-compulsive disorder with onset in childhood or adolescence. Eur Child Adolesc Psychiatry 2001;10:37–46.

[81] Reddy YC, Srinath S, Prakash HM, et al. A follow-up study of juvenile obsessive-compuslive disorder from India. Acta Psychiatr Scand 2003;107:457–64.

[82] Geller DA, Biederman J, Stewart SE, et al. Impact of comorbidity on treatment response to paroxetine in pediatric obsessive compulsive disorder: is the use of exclusion criteria empirically supported in randomized clinical trials? J Child Adolesc Psychopharmacol 2003; 13(Suppl 1):S19–29.

ELSEVIER
SAUNDERS

PSYCHIATRIC
CLINICS
OF NORTH AMERICA

Psychiatr Clin N Am 29 (2006) 371–390

Animal Models of Obsessive-Compulsive Disorder: Rationale to Understanding Psychobiology and Pharmacology

Schaun Korff, MSc, Brian H. Harvey, BPharm, PhD*

*Division of Pharmacology, School of Pharmacy, North-West University,
Potchefstroom 2520, South Africa*

Animal models have proved extremely useful in assisting researchers to better understand a given clinical disorder. The difficulty in developing a suitable animal model lies in whether it can be assumed that an animal is truly exhibiting the behavioral and other manifestations of the human disorder it is designed to model. An animal model can never reflect fully the human situation that it is modeling, nor is there a model that is isomorphic with the symptomology in question (ie, the animal symptoms are similar but the cause of the symptoms differ between human and model) [1]. Consequently, the development of an animal model requires parallel development of measures that will allow meaningful comparisons.

Difficulties in setting up and identifying suitable animal models include the intrinsic problems in defining patient profiles and diagnostic criteria, variations between patients even when these are pathologically defined, and the possibility that the level of the disorder that the animal exhibits may not be equivalent in the human disorder. Even when it can be certain that the behaviors or signs are the same, humans are unusual in that they are verbal and so similar behaviors, signals, or signs may have different meanings. Furthermore, the observable changes in behavior that occur in animals, primarily rodents, are treated as secondary symptoms in humans [2], and little effort is made to characterize either human or animal behaviors in a manner that would allow assessment of analogy or homology. For example, hiding is normal behavior in many rodents but is considered

This work has been supported by the South African Medical Research Council (MRC).
* Corresponding author.
E-mail address: fklbhh@puk.ac.za (B.H. Harvey).

pathologic in humans; therefore the usefulness of the animal model in mimicking the human condition is limited [2].

In recent years, an understanding of obsessive-compulsive disorder (OCD) as a cognitive-behavioral disorder with a close functional relationship with other related disorders has emerged. Thus, OCD is characterized by intrusive thoughts or images (obsessions) that increase anxiety and by ritualistic actions (compulsions) that decrease anxiety. Most patients who have OCD are aware of the irrationality of their thoughts and behaviors and thus unwillingly partake in stereotyped behavior even though they recognize that the obsessions and impulses are the product of their own minds. These internal conflicts cause immeasurable anxiety in individuals suffering from OCD [3].

At a phenomenologic or psychologic level, OCD demonstrates a continuum with a broad range of other conditions (eg, on a spectrum of reward-related or affective disorders [4,5], on a spectrum of compulsive-impulsive disorders [6–9,10], or on a spectrum of stereotypic disorders [11]). Moreover, the behaviors associated with OCD have been linked to a wide variety of cognitive [12,13] and occasionally noncognitive deficits [14], including a fundamental impairment of executive function ability, deficits of immediate and secondary memory, and spatial information processing. The disorder therefore is extremely complex, with diverse neurologic manifestations, including neuropsychologic symptoms such as cognitive and noncognitive deficits, neuromotor symptoms such as stereotypy, and presentation with prominent symptoms of anxiety. Accordingly, OCD is a highly heterogeneous condition, and it has been suggested that it is actually composed of several distinct subtypes, as described in Table 1. Despite the apparent complexity of the disorder, its treatment reflects a direct paradox, with OCD responding with marked exclusivity to drugs that act selectively on the serotonergic system (eg, selective serotonin reuptake inhibitors [SRIs] such as fluoxetine [28]) and in more severe treatment resistant cases to the addition of an antidopaminergic agent [29,30].

Table 1
Proposed obsessive-compulsive disorder subtypes

Subtype	Selected references
Early versus later onset OCD	[15–17]
OCD with presence or absence of tics	[18,19]
OCD with presence or absence of disease, such as streptococci-related autoimmune disorder	[20,21]
OCD with presence or absence of psychotic or neurological features (ie, neuropsychologic and information processing differences)	[22–24]
OCD according to symptom presentation patterns (eg, washers versus checkers)	[25–27]

Abbreviation: OCD, obsessive-compulsive disorder.

The neurocircuitry of OCD is critical to an understanding of its pathophysiology and treatment [31]. Recent years have witnessed the rising importance of the orbitofrontal cortex (OFC), the anterior cingulate cortex (ACC), and in particular the prefrontal cortico-striatal-thalamic-cortico (CSTC) circuit (Fig. 1) in the neurobiology of OCD. The OFC and ACC seem to be overactive in OCD [32,33], whereas dysfunctional sensory gating in the CSTC circuit has become an important construct in explaining deficits in executing appropriate adaptive behaviors in OCD and a failure to switch to new behaviors [34–38]. The thalamic output of this circuit to the cortex regulates consciousness, perception, and integration of information (see Fig. 1) [39]. The OFC mediates the active expression of emotional response to significant biologic stimuli, the inhibition of behavioral response [40], and the motivational aspects of decision making. The ACC mediates cognitive processes such as attention, motivation, reward and error detection, working memory, problem solving, and action planning [41] and thus contributes to the emotional evaluation of the consequences of action (ie, error

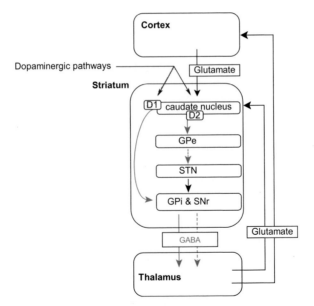

Fig. 1. Neurocircuits and neurochemicals underlying the cortico-striatal-thalamic-cortico (CSTC) circuit. The striatum receives both glutamatergic and dopaminergic afferents. Two loops arise in the striatum, one a direct pathway through the globus pallidus internal (GPi) or substantia nigra pars reticulla (SNr) to the thalamus, and the other an indirect pathway through the globus pallidus external segment (GPe) and subthalamic nucleus (STN). Cortical input to the striatum results in activation of the thalamus through the direct pathway and a GABAergic inhibition of the thalamus through the indirect pathway. The CSTC concludes with the thalamus sending glutamatergic afferents to the cortex. Broken lines indicate reduced neurochemical activity. Solid lines indicate increased neurochemical activity. Red lines indicate GABA, black lines indicate glutamate, and blue lines indicate dopamine signaling.

detection). Overactivity of the OFC leads to uncontrolled thoughts and behaviors [33,40] and the cognitive generation of inappropriate error-detection signals, whereas the ACC may link the cognitive and motor behavioral manifestations of OCD. The excessive, uncontrolled, and repetitive motor behaviors seen in patients who have OCD is thus propagated by regional cortical hyperexcitability and a failure of inhibitory mechanisms resulting in reduced ability to modulate sensory inputs [33,42,43]. Volumetric reductions in the striatum [44] and increased thalamic volume in patients who have OCD [45] may also originate in such aberrant circuitry. Because of its role in adapting to and controlling behavioral responses, decreased activity in the dorsolateral prefrontal cortex [34] also has been suggested as an explanation of the difficulty experienced in patients who have OCD in stopping compulsive behaviors such as reward-seeking and security motivation [46]. Finally, the expression of emotion (recognition of cues of threat/danger) and motivation that engenders the nonspecific anxiety symptoms in OCD is likely to involve fear circuitry, in particular the amygdala [34].

The response of OCD symptoms in most cases to the SRIs, and indeed the robust and reproducible findings describing the greater efficacy of SRIs over noradrenergic agents in this regard [29,47,48], has consolidated thinking that OCD involves aberrant central neurotransmitter systems, especially serotonin (5-HT) [47]. By enhancing serotonin release, SRIs evoke the gradual desensitization of terminal 5-HT autoreceptors in the previously described frontal-cortical brain regions, resulting in the reduction of symptoms [49]. Indeed, desensitization of the presynaptic $5-HT_{1D}$ autoreceptors is thought to mediate the anti-OCD effect of the antidepressants, whereas activation of 5-HT2-like receptors most likely mediates the enhanced 5-HT release postsynaptically [50].

Up to half of patients who have OCD do not respond to treatment with an SRI, however [28,30]. In fact, no definitive abnormality in the 5-HT system has been identified in OCD, although genetic linkage studies do suggest an involvement of the 5-HT transporter [51]. With the dominant role of 5HT in OCD in question, the importance of dopamine is becoming increasingly recognized. Dopamine agonists lead to stereotypic behavior in animals and can exacerbate the symptoms and tics of OCD [30]. Further, dopamine blockers are effective in treating Tourette's syndrome, one of the disorders on the OCD spectrum. The 5-HT and dopamine systems interact extensively, particularly in the basal ganglia [28], whereas 5-HT–dopamine cross-talk in subcortical regions may explain how serotonergic and dopaminergic drugs exert their therapeutic actions in OCD [52,53]. Clearly, many neurotransmitters and second/third messengers [53,54] need to be considered, particularly those acting within the CSTC circuit [42] (see Fig. 1) such as the second messenger precursor, myoinositol [53], glutamate [55], gamma aminobutyric acid (GABA) [56], and neuropeptides [57], especially cholecystokinin [58] which interacts closely with 5-HT [59], GABA [60], and dopamine [61] pathways. An imbalance between dopamine, GABA, and glutamate input into the striatal complex may be critical in determining the degree of CSTC activation and the eventual output to the cortex and thus may underlie the typical symptoms of OCD.

An effective animal model of OCD will need to focus on specific behavioral, neurochemical, and structural brain anomalies that are analogous to OCD. Validation of these illness-specific correlates in a model should allow meaningful and accurate interpretation of preclinical data with direct implications for understanding the neurobiology of OCD and to identify promising treatments for the disorder. Primary constructs of OCD that warrant consideration in a putative animal model would include the repetitive and compulsive behaviors evident in the disorder and the distinctive response of patients who have OCD to SRIs. Possibly secondary criteria would be the roles of reward and security motivation mechanisms. In addition, the model will benefit significantly if validated with respect to neurochemical and neurocircuitry findings in OCD. This article discusses putative animal models of OCD, highlighting how these models have validity in primary, and, where necessary, secondary constructs of OCD, including behavioral symptomology, neurocircuitry, neurobiology, and treatment.

Animal models of obsessive-compulsive disorder

In developing and assessing animal models for OCD, it is critical to consider the intended purpose of the model, because the anticipated function determines the criteria that the model must satisfy to establish its validity and further use in studying the neurobiologic and associated underpinnings of OCD. Validation therefore is critical if an animal model is to be taken seriously.

McKinney and Bunney [2] have specified certain requirements for an animal model system. In an animal model of OCD

1. The symptoms of the condition should be reasonably analogous to those seen in humans
2. There should be observable behavioral changes in both model and patients with OCD that can be objectively evaluated
3. Independent observers should agree on objective criteria for drawing conclusions about the subjective state
4. The treatment modalities effective in treating OCD should have the same effect on the animal condition
5. The system should be reproducible by other investigators

According to the criteria proposed by Wilner [62], an animal model of OCD therefore would require three types of validity: face validity (conditions 1–3); predictive validity in which the model shows the same effect for drugs used in treatment or induction of OCD (eg, response to an SRI; condition 4); and construct validity in which the model either relies on or elucidates the same underlying mechanism responsible for OCD [63]. Other validation criteria have been described and defined, including concurrent or convergent, discriminant, and ethologic validity [64–66]. Ultimately, the more types of validity a model is able satisfy, the greater is its usefulness and relevance to the human condition.

Many efforts have been made to produce animal models of OCD. These models can be divided broadly into ethologic and pharmacologic models. Because OCD probably has genetic underpinnings [51,67,68], the development of suitable genetic animal models that emphasize certain behavioral, neurochemical, and drug responses would be an additional valuable resource.

Ethologic models

Ethologic models may include naturally occurring repetitive or stereotypic behaviors, such as tail chasing, weaving, and fur chewing [69], and instinctive motor behaviors that occur during periods of conflict or stress, such as grooming, cleaning, and pecking [70]. These behaviors correlate with repetitive motor behaviors in humans, such as checking, washing, repetitive movements, face picking, hair pulling, and nail biting [3,71]. In addition, natural behaviors that occur after some behavioral manipulations are also valuable paradigms, such as food restriction–induced hyperactivity (FRIH) [72], rewarded alternation [73], and excessive lever pressing after devaluation [74]. Other ethologic behavior models include barbering, marble burying, acral lick dermatitis, and possibly feather picking. These models present with strong construct validity.

Models based on stereotypy and compulsivity

Stereotypy and compulsivity, inherent qualities of OCD, are invariably driven by obsessions, and this association represents a distinct drawback when attempting to model OCD. Obsessions are of a cognitive nature and as such cannot be observed directly in animals [75]. For example, OCD is strongly associated with low memory confidence and with memory biases toward threatening information. This association translates into an impaired ability to use strategies efficiently [76,77] and manifests in the patient as repetitive checking behavior. There is also some support for an attentional bias toward fear/threat-related stimuli in OCD [78,79], which could contribute to the development and maintenance of intrusive thoughts. The cognitive and motor behavioral manifestations of OCD are intimately linked, with distinct evidence that the disorder is a condition in which normal control of behavior is overridden by noncognitive-based systems. This evidence argues strongly that modeling compulsive behaviors is a meaningful surrogate endpoint for an OCD model. Thus, animal models of compulsive behaviors (eg, the genesis of compulsive and repetitive behaviors) can have credible face validity.

Marble burying. Pharmacologic evidence first suggested a possible relationship between the burying of glass marbles by laboratory rodents and OCD

[80]. In this model, burying begins as an appropriate, investigative activity but, after frustrated investigation of the nonreactive stimulus object (ie, the marble), begins to persist as a compulsive stereotypy. Marble burying can also be used as a model for hoarding, a subtype of compulsive behavior frequently encountered in OCD patients, and thus in line with the view that compulsive behaviors result from an inability to achieve a sense of task completion. SRIs suppress the compulsive behavior in this model [80–82]. The model therefore presents with good predictive as well as face validity.

Barbering. Hair pulling (trichotillomania) is a compulsive behavior often found in obsessive-compulsive spectrum disorders and OCD. Barbering, the plucking of fur or whiskers from cage mates or the animal itself, is a common form of abnormal, repetitive behavior in laboratory mice. Although barbering is probably an abnormal behavior, it is not a stereotypy. Although the drive to pluck hair from body locations is improperly repeated, the motor patterns involved are variable and goal directed [83], unlike stereotypies in which a motor pattern is repeated identically without any apparent goal. Barbering bears some strikingly similar phenomenological, etiological, and other characteristics with trichotillomania, including a idiosyncratic distribution of hair plucking, a strong female bias, onset in puberty, breeding status, and evidence for genetic underpinnings [84]. The phenomenology of trichotillomania and barbering are therefore similar, and consequently barbering has good face validity as an animal model for trichotillomania [85]. Furthermore, as pointed out by Garner and coworkers [85], barbering may represent a refined and noninvasive model for studies of the complex genetic and environmental etiologies of obsessive-compulsive spectrum disorders. Feather picking in birds overlaps somewhat with barbering and resembles compulsive skin picking and hair pulling in OCD, thus suggesting some predictive validity. There seem to be important differences between stereotypic behavior and feather picking, however [86], with the latter being classified as an abnormal compulsive behavior.

Models of exaggerated cleaning rituals. Acral-lick dermatitis and other models of excessive grooming present with symptoms similar to exaggerated cleaning rituals seen in OCD. Acral-lick dermatitis is a disorder of grooming seen in a variety of mammalian species, particularly in large-breed canines [87], and is characterized by excessive licking or biting of extremities. Its etiology has been considered environmental with a possible genetic predisposition [88]. The model has convergent face and predictive validity to OCD, because it responds to SRI treatment [89]. Transgenic mice have also been engineered to groom excessively, as discussed in more detail later.

Spontaneous stereotypy. Although stereotypy per se may not be equivalent to the stereotypy seen as part of the complex behavioral phenomenology of OCD, understanding the basis of stereotypy may reveal much about the neurobiology of OCD. Motor stereotypy is a common component of several genetic and neuropsychiatric disorders. In animals, these behaviors can be induced through pharmacologic manipulation, as discussed later, or may occur spontaneously.

The deer mouse, an animal that presents with spontaneous stereotypy as a consequence of changing environmental conditions, has been used as an animal model for stereotyped movement disorder [90]. These animals exhibit behaviors consisting of repetitive jumping, flipping, and patterned running and may offer excellent face validity as a putative animal model of OCD. Unfortunately, the model has not been evaluated for predictive validity with an SRI. The model also shows signs of construct validity by demonstrating the role of striatal glutamate in the mediation of spontaneous stereotypic behavior [91]. Other important findings using this model include the dissociation between spontaneously emitted and apomorphine-induced stereotypy [92], providing support for a limited involvement of the dopamine system in the mediation of these behaviors. Moreover, the model supports the hypothesis that stereotypy is expressed as a consequence of elevated feedback activity occurring along motor circuits of the basal ganglia [93].

Animals often develop spontaneous stereotypy in captivity [90,94]. In primates, the SRI fluoxetine has been found to decrease captivity-induced stereotypy gradually [95], thus paralleling the typical response observed in OCD and so presenting with some predictive validity. In a similar model, bank voles develop spontaneous stereotypic behavior when held in captivity, and a recent study has suggested that the female of this species may be a useful animal model for human anxiety disorders [96]. Additional studies describe the important role of 5-HT in stereotypies in these animals [97]. An interesting finding, however, is the paradoxical rate-dependent effect of fluoxetine on the stereotypic activity of these animals. Levels of stereotypy decrease in animals with high predrug rates but decrease in animals that have low predrug rates [97], showing interindividual variation in the effect of an SRI. Genetically manipulated animals have been developed that produce spontaneous stereotypic activity, as described later.

Food restriction–induced hyperactivity

In the FRIH paradigm, rats fed only once a day and given access to a running wheel begin to run excessively and eat less [72]. Here, excessive running can be viewed as a displacement or adjunctive behavior. In animals, stressors such as novelty, conflict, or frustration are known to cause inappropriate or displaced expression of normal behaviors [63]. Such displacement behaviors are seen in most species and include behaviors such as grooming, hoarding, and attack behavior. The spontaneous stereotypy seen in the stereotyped movement disorder model [90] can also be viewed as the expression of displacement or adjunctive behavior.

In the FRIH model, fluoxetine attenuates the development of FRIH syndrome, whereas imipramine, which is ineffective for treatment of OCD, does not affect the progress of the syndrome [72]. Thus the model demonstrates good predictive validity. Face validity is weakened, however, because compulsive running has not been defined as a variant of OCD.

Reward-based models

Many aspects of the phenomenology of OCD suggest a dysfunctional reward system. The compulsions of patients who have OCD can be seen as driven by a goal-directed reward-seeking mechanism that initiates appropriate cognitive and behavioral strategies. For patients who have OCD, the ability to generate the normal feeling of reward that would otherwise signal task completion and terminate the expression of goal-directed reward-seeking behavior is absent. The ensuing failure to attenuate reward-associated behavior would result in repetitive, stereotyped behavior that is typical of OCD. The content of most obsessional thoughts, ideas, or actions in OCD seems to revolve around the issue of security or safety, either of the self or others [98], suggesting that OCD constitutes the expression of a security motivational system [14]. The symptoms of OCD therefore stem from an inability to generate the normal "feeling of knowing" that would otherwise signal task completion and terminate the expression of a security motivation system.

The reward hypothesis and the concept of a dysfunctional security motivation system thus share similar neural underpinnings and can be seen as the inability to modulate goal-directed behavior and adapt to changing environmental demands. In other words, OCD represents deficient inhibitory control with respect to selected processes [99]. Animal models that attempt to model this complex neurocognitive behavior include schedule-induced behavior or adjunctive behavior, such as excessive lever pressing and rewarded alternation.

Excessive lever pressing. Excessive lever pressing [74] can be generated when reward presentation is regularly scheduled and dissociated from the animal behavior. Swedo [100] has proposed that OCD symptoms in humans, which are exacerbated by environmental stress, are analogous to displacement behaviors in animals. In the lever-press or signal attenuation model, rats are trained to press the lever for food with delivery that is signaled by the presentation of a stimulus [74]. The goal-directed behavior is to lever-press for food (the reward). Subsequently, the contingency between the stimulus and food is attenuated by repeatedly associating the stimulus with no food. The encounter of non-reward produces an increase in operant behavior. Excessive lever pressing and its association with uncompleted trials are attenuated by fluoxetine, but not by the anxiolytic drug diazepam [74] thus confirming the predictive validity of the model. These results suggest that attenuation of an external feedback of operant behavior may provide an animal analogue to a deficient response feedback mechanism that might be present in human patients and that has been suggested to underlie obsessions and compulsions in OCD. That "compulsive" lever pressing in rats is enhanced following lesions to the orbital cortex but not to the baso-lateral amygdala or dorsal medial prefrontal cortex [101] brings into sharper focus the role of the OFC in OCD. This model offers good predictive and face validity along with notable construct validity.

Rewarded spontaneous alternation model. Spontaneous alternation refers to the natural tendency of rats to sequentially explore novel places. Attenuated alternation has been proposed as a model of OCD [73], and is useful for modeling several aspects of human OCD particularly indecision. Yadin and co-workers [102] allowed food-deprived rats to run in a T-maze where goal-boxes were baited with flavored milk. Animals were placed in the start box and allowed to make a free choice. The mean number of choices made until alternation occurs was recorded, with spontaneous alternators scoring lower than perserverators. This model might have potential for assessment of the perservative symptoms and indecisiveness seen in people who have OCD. In addition the impairment does not seem to be the result of a general cognitive dysfunction, because animal performance during control studies was normal. Furthermore, 5HT-agonist-induced attenuation in spontaneous alternation and its inhibition by chronic pretreatment with fluoxetine has propogated the suggestion that 5HT-evoked behavior in this model may be analogous to indecision seen in OCD. Further evidence for good predictive validity is that, as with the human compulsive trait, fluoxetine offers protection against metachlorophenylpiperazine (mCPP)-induced increases in spontaneous persistence, whereas desipramine and diazepam (both with no specific anti-OCD action) do not block mCPP-induced symptom exacerbation [73]. Because of the 5-HT receptor–binding profile of mCPP, this model furthermore emphasizes the possible involvement of 5-HT_{2C} and 5-HT_{1D} receptors in the pathophysiology of OCD (ie, construct validity). Because motor perseveration is seen in other neuropsychiatric disorders, (eg, Parkinsons disease, schizophrenia), the choice of pharmacological manipulation becomes critical for its validity, thus also allowing its inclusion as a pharmacological model.

Pharmacologic models

The foremost criterion for a pharmacologic animal model of OCD is that the applied pharmacologic challenge should induce behavioral and neuro-chemical disturbances similar to those found in the disorder. Indeed, pharmacological isomorphism is an important factor in assessing validity. Animal models of OCD should therefore demonstrate both sensitivity to SRI's and insensitivity to other classes of psychotropics that are ineffective in OCD. Duration of treatment is also an important consideration, since response to drug treatment in OCD takes several weeks to become effective. Consequently, reponse to acute but not chronic treatment weakens the predictive validity of a model [62]. Nevertheless, acute treatment protocols remain a useful test in OCD research. An important consideration for the investigator is that pharmacologic studies often are not suited to long-term baseline studies because the animals need to be pharmacologically treated. Prudently selected drug-induced behaviors present with significant face, predictive, and construct validity, but even though these models may provide insight into the underlying pathophysiologic processes in disorders that include stereotypy or compulsivity, they may oversimplify complex neurologic disorders such as OCD. Clearly, the more primary and possibly secondary criteria used to validate a model, the more robust the animal model will be. Hence in many cases combining carefully selected ethologic and pharmacologic models would be the best choice for addressing certain research questions.

Compulsive checking models

Compulsive checking is one of the most distinctive behaviors evident in patients diagnosed as having OCD [103]. Checking is characterized by repeated rituals that are not caused by problems in memory recall but rather by an inability to achieve a sense of task completion [104]. This concept supports the interesting suggestion that patients who have OCD suffer from deficiencies in reward and security motivation systems. Although not a primary construct, these novel concepts of the illness open new avenues for investigating and validating a putative animal model of OCD.

Szechtman and colleagues [105] have proposed that checking can be pharmacologically induced by chronic treatment with the dopamine D_2/D_3 receptor agonist quinpirole. Using compulsive checking as its behavioral endpoint, this model provides substantial face validity, even though it would be presumptuous to assume that drug-induced repetitive behavior and the cognitive basis for checking in OCD are congruent. It demonstrates preoccupation with and hestitancy to leave items of interest, a ritual like motor activity, dependence on environment and can be suspended for a period of time, as in OCD. Nevertheless, the partial reversal of this behavior with the SRI clomipramine offers some evidence for good predictive validity.

Stereotypy models

Stereotypy, which represents a wide range of invariant and repetitive behaviors, can be provoked in otherwise nonstereotyping animals using specific drug treatment [92,106,107]. That stereotypy is a primary construct of OCD makes it a particularly useful endpoint for pharmacologic-challenge studies. Investigations have focused most frequently on the influence of the dopamine system in the expression of these behaviors, for example using psychostimulants or other dopamine agonists. Because dopamine agonists produce stereotypic activity, possibly through modulation of dopamine input into various stages of the CSTC circuit and specifically at the output level of the basal ganglia through the direct and indirect motor pathways (see Fig. 1), drugs with dopamine-selective actions will have great value in studying the underlying neurobiology of OCD.

Serotonergic agonists such as mCPP also evoke similar stereotypic responses [28], however, and highlight the complexity of motor function. This phenomenon opens the debate that stereotypy and other behavioral manifestations of OCD may represent a cross-talk between 5-HT and dopamine projections in the striatum [53]. Indeed, this 5-HT–dopamine interaction may be exploited therapeutically in especially refractory OCD by combining a serotonergic drug such as fluoxetine, which acts to decrease the expression of 5-HT receptors, and a dopamine D_2 receptor blocker such as risperidone [52].

Genetic animal models

Genetic models can be useful in identifying specific genes and neurobiologic pathways thought to be important in OCD, (eg, the involvement of 5-HT and GABA; see [108] for review). To date, a number of specific genetically engineered animal models of OCD have been developed, usually according to the research group's hypothesis concerning the underlying cause of OCD or OCD symptoms. However, there are no reports of the effects of SRI's or different pharmacological treatments in these models, which limits their predictive validity.

Compulsive behavior may have several features, including both perseverative tendencies and more rigid sequences of entire serial patterns. Some animal models of spontaneous compulsive behavior have successfully captured these perseverative features (eg, the $Hoxb8^{lox}$ mutant model, which shows increased persistence in grooming) [109]. Similarly, the D1CT models show persistence of grooming and other behaviors such as digging and climbing [110], and have demonstrated evidence for comorbid tic-like behaviors [111]. Greer and coworkers [109] engineered mice expressing two individual mutations in $Hoxb8^{lox}$, a gene expressed in the OFC and limbic system, areas implicated in OCD. Both mutant forms demonstrate excessive grooming, thus conferring face and construct validity. The altered behavior of the animals seems to have a genetic basis, because mutants backcrossed with normal, wild-type mice still display abnormal grooming behavior. It would be of great value to assess the predictive validity of this engineered model by examining whether excessive grooming can be inhibited with an SRI.

The D1CT-7 transgenic mouse model engages in episodes of perseverance or repetition of a range of normal and abnormal behaviors, for instance repeated biting and skin pulling of cage mates during grooming [110]. The mice are engineered to express a neuro-potentiating cholera toxin transgene in a subset of dopamine D_1 receptor–expressing neurons that induce cortical and amygdalar glutamate output. This model presents with good face validity. Construct validity is illustrated by the exacerbation by glutamatergic drugs of symptomatic behavior in these transgenic animals [55], thus linking to the prominent role of glutamate in basal ganglia circuitry, and the involvement of key neural systems such as the amygdala and cortex, in this behavior [110].

In sequential super-stereotypy, patients become trapped in overly rigid sequential patterns of action, language, or thought. Hyper-dopaminergic mutant mice [112] may elucidate some of the underlying causes of the stereotypy and compulsive behavior seen in these human subjects. It is not known, however, whether the two animal models discussed previously show excessively rigid sequences. To answer this question, mutant mice with a genetic knockout of the dopamine transporter (DAT) gene [113] have been developed. The result is an impaired synaptic reuptake of dopamine and elevated levels of extracellular dopamine in the neostriatum resulting in spontaneous, over-rigid, and serially complex behavior in the form of grooming. This model is yet to be tested for predictive validity, but good face and construct validity are present. The model differs from other genetic models in that the overly rigid and serially complex behavior allows highly predictable stereotyped patterns that can be easily quantified.

Mice with targeted gene disruption of the 5-HT$_{2C}$ receptor have been produced [114] that display strikingly organized compulsive-like behavior (as in OCD) such as clay and screen chewing and head dipping. Once again, the predictive validity of this engineered model with an SRI remains to be determined. The model presents with good face validity (compulsive behavior) and construct validity, the latter underscored by the fact that the 5-HT$_{2C}$ receptor is purported to play an important role in OCD [28,53,69].

Although transgenic models have great potential, an important question is whether the behavior is a direct result of the specific manipulated gene or caused by other targets lying downstream of the gene. Only when this question is addressed can the gene of interest be associated positively with the underlying pathology of OCD.

Summary

Animal models have shown progressive development and have undoubtedly proven their supportive value in OCD research. Thus, various animal models have confirmed the importance of the 5-HT [72–74] and dopamine systems [104,111] in the neurobiology and treatment of OCD. Given the neurochemical, emotional, and cognitive complexity of the disorder, however, animal models are being used to investigate more and more complicated neurochemical and behavioral theories purported to underlie OCD. The lever-press model, for example, has implicated deficient response feedback in a neural system that regulates operant behavior [74]. Studies on stereotypic movement disorder [89] have opened a new avenue of investigation into the neurobiology of stereotypy that may be applicable to more complex syndromes such as OCD. Models that have focused on specific neuropsychologic aspects of OCD such as reward [74], displacement behavior [63,101], perseveration and indecisiveness [73,102], and spontaneous stereotypy [90,94] are important in their attempt to unify the diverse behavioral manifestations of this disorder. It is clear that for a deeper, more holistic understanding of OCD, multiple animal models will be needed to allow investigation of the various aspects of the disorder and to provide convergent validation of the research findings.

The heterogeneous nature of OCD, the various subtypes that exist within the disorder, and the range of obsessive-compulsive spectrum disorders suggest that particular questions regarding OCD may be addressed best by using a particular ethologic model, whereas other questions might require a pharmacologic model or a combination of both for meaningful results [62,115]. Genetic models will be extremely useful for studying the genetics of pathologic behavior and for relating these findings to neuroanatomic and neurochemical changes in the model (eg, DICT-7 mice as a model for Tourette's syndrome and OCD). Neither ethologic nor pharmacologic models, however, can assess whether the "compulsive" behavior is a response to an "obsessive" anxiety or fear. Perhaps the symptoms seen in patients who have OCD, which may be exacerbated by everyday stress, are analogous to displacement behaviors in animals and also reflect some form of anxiety or stress [98]. In this regard, the bank vole model [116] has provided evidence that previously developed stereotypies increase markedly after acute stress and argues that healthy individuals "habituate" to everyday stress, whereas patients who have OCD do not.

Interindividual variation in behavioral response and attempts to replicate studies in different laboratories often is the nemesis of the behavioral scientist. Small within- and between-subject variability is usually desirable, however, because there are cases in which the study of the variability of the model could lead to a better understanding of the disorder. Variability cannot always be considered an error; it is possible that previously disregarded neuronal systems may have a place in the observed variation and, indeed, in the pathophysiology of OCD. In this regard, SRIs are not always effective for OCD [6,29,30] such that a lack of effect in a model may reflect an unknown neurobiological basis for compulsive behavior in a sub-group of SRI refractory patients. Similarly, separating the afflicted (ie, working with animals that show greater behavioral change in a model and/or after drug treatment) would have distinct benefits.

To increase successful implementation of an ethologic animal model, especially when reinforcement models or signal attenuation models are used, the laboratory must be equipped with the essential behavioral testing apparatus as well as the operant chambers/rooms in which to conduct the training and data collection. Quantification of certain stereotypy behaviors also requires experienced or trained observers. An illustration of the difficulty in measuring behavioral changes is that in the rewarded alternation model, a good response to behavioral treatment (alternation training) may lead to a floor effect [73] which, after successful drug treatment of the animal, produces no residual persistence (ie, measurable behavioral change) on which a drug treatment can be tested.

Clearly, the choice of ethologic, pharmacologic, or genetic models should be considered carefully. A well-validated model may quell many of the limitations and considerations described previously. Noninvasive neuroimaging (eg, the use of small-animal single-photon emission CT) to explore the neuroanatomic basis of OCD offers an exciting future challenge, especially if combined with pharmacologic or ethologic models, and could confirm or extend knowledge of the neuroanatomy of OCD. Although studies to investigate further the interactive role of 5-HT, dopamine, GABA, and glutamate are still needed, the role of neuroactive peptides such as cholecystokinin, corticotrophin-releasing factor, neuropeptide Y, tachykinins (ie, substance P), and natriuretic peptides in OCD should also be considered. Genetically engineered animal models will become increasingly valuable in combination with new technologies such as gene-chip microarrays, RNA interference, and advanced proteomics that will help further the understanding of OCD. Animal models of OCD are poised to play a vital role in extending the knowledge of the disorder now and in the future.

References

[1] Green S. Animal models in schizophrenia research. In: Davey GCL, editor. Animal models of human behavior. New York: John Wiley & Sons; 1983. p. 315–38.

[2] McKinney WT, Bunney WE. Animal models of depression. I. Review of the evidence: implications for research. Arch Gen Psychiatry 1969;21:240–8.

[3] American Psychiatric Association. Diagnostic and statistical manual of mental disorders. 4th edition. Washington (DC): American Psychiatric Press; 1994.

[4] Hudson JI, Pope HG Jr. Affective spectrum disorder: does antidepressant response identify a family of disorders with a common pathophysiology? Am J Psychiatry 1990;147:552–64.

[5] Blum K, Sheridan PJ, Wood RC, et al. Dopamine D2 receptor gene variants: association and linkage studies in impulsive-addictive-compulsive behavior. Pharmacogenetics 1995; 5:121–41.

[6] Stein DJ. Neurobiology of the obsessive-compulsive spectrum disorders. Biol Psychiatry 2000;47:296–304.

[7] Hollander E, Wang CM. Obsessive-compulsive spectrum disorders. J Clin Psychiatry 1995; 56:53–5.

[8] Baca-Garcia E, Salgado BR, Segal HD, et al. A pilot genetic study of the continuum between compulsivity and impulsivity in females: the serotonin transporter promoter polymorphism. Prog Neuropsychopharmacol Biol Psychiatry 2005;29:713–7.

[9] Stein DJ, Hollander E. The spectrum of obsessive compulsive related disorders. In: Hollander E, editor. Obsessive-compulsive related disorders. Washington (DC): American Psychiatric Press; 1993.

[10] Phillips KA. The obsessive-compulsive spectrums. Psychiatr Clin North Am 2002;25: 791–809.

[11] Ridley RM. The psychology of perseverative and stereotyped behavior. Prog Neurobiol 1994;44:221–31.

[12] Blashfield RK, Livesley WJ. Classification. In: Millon T, Blaney PH, Davis RD, editors. Oxford textbook of psychopathology. New York: Oxford University Press; 1999. p. 3–28.

[13] Tallis F. The neuropsychology of obsessive-compulsive disorder: a review and consideration of clinical implications. Br J Clin Psychol 1997;36:3–20.

[14] Szechtman H, Woody E. Obsessive-compulsive disorder as a disturbance of security motivation. Psychol Rev 2005;112:650–7.

[15] Hemmings SMJ, Kinnear CJ, Lochner C, et al. Early- versus late-onset obsessive-compulsive disorder: investigating genetic and clinical correlates. Psychiatry Res 2004;128: 175–82.

[16] Fontenelle LF, Mendlowitz MV, Marcques C, et al. Early- and late-onset obsessive-compulsive disorder in adult patients: an exploratory clinical and therapeutic study. J Psychiatr Res 2003;37:127–33.

[17] Schultz RT, Evans DW, Wolf M. Neuropsychological models of childhood obsessive-compulsive disorder. Child Adolesc Psychiatr Clin N Am 1999;8:523–31.

[18] Cath DC, Spinhoven P, Hoogduin CAL, et al. Repetitive behaviors in Tourette's syndrome and OCD with and without tics: what are the differences? Psychiatry Res 2001;101:171–85.

[19] Eichstedt JA, Arnold SL. Childhood-onset obsessive-compulsive disorder: a tic-related subtype of OCD? Clin Psychol Rev 2001;21:137–58.

[20] Allen AJ, Leonard HL, Swedo SE. Case study: a new infection-triggered, autoimmune subtype of pediatric OCD and Tourette's syndrome. J Amer Acad Child Adolesc Psychiatr 1995;34:307–11.

[21] Murphy TK, Sajid M, Soto O, et al. Detecting pediatric autoimmune neuropsychiatric disorders associated with streptococcus in children with obsessive-compulsive disorder and tics. Biol Pscychiatry 2004;55:61–8.

[22] Sobin C, Blundell ML, Weiller F, et al. Evidence of schizotypy subtype in OCD. J Psychiat Res 2000;34:15–24.

[23] Harbishettar V, Pal PK, Reddy YCJ, et al. Is there a relationship between Parkinson's disease and obsessive-compulsive disorder? Parkinsonism Relat Disord 2005;11:85–8.

[24] Gromb S, Lasseuguette K, Olivera A. Obsessive compulsive disorder secondary to head injury. J Clin Forensic Med 2002;9:89–91.

[25] Calamari JE, Wiegartz PS, Janeck AS. Obsessive-compulsive disorder subgroups: a symptom-based clustering approach. Behav Res Ther 1999;37:113–25.

[26] Fontenelle LF, Mendlowitz MV, Soares ID, et al. Patients with obsessive-compulsive disorder and hoarding symptoms: a distinctive clinical subtype. Compr Psychiatry 2004;45: 375–83.

[27] Horesh N, Dolberg OT, Kirchenbaum-Aviner N, et al. Personality differences between obsessive-compulsive subtypes: washers versus checkers. Psychiatry Res 1997;71:197–200.

[28] Goodman WK, Price LH, Woods SW. Pharmacologic challenges in obsessive-compulsive disorder. In: Zohar J, Insel T, Rasmussen SA, editors. The psychobiology of obsessive-compulsive disorder. New York: Springer; 1991. p. 162–86.

[29] Frenandez CE, Lopez-Ibor JJ. Monoclomipramine in the treatment of psychiatric patients resistant to other therapies. Actas Luso Esp Neurol Psiquiatr Cienc Afines 1967; 26:119–47.

[30] Goodman WK, McDougle CL, Lawrence LP. Beyond the serotonin hypothesis: a role for dopamine in some forms of obsessive-compulsive disorder. J Clin Psychiatry 1990;51: 36–43.

[31] Insel TR. Towards a neuroanatomy of obsessive-compulsive disorder. Arch Gen Psychiatry 1992;49:739–44.

[32] Lacerda AL, Dalgalarrondo P, Caetano DC, et al. Elevated thalamic and prefrontal regional cerebral blood flow in obsessive-compulsive disorder: a SPECT study. Psychiatric Res 2003;123:125–34.

[33] Alptekin K, Degirmenci B, Kivircik B, et al. Tc-99m HMPAO brain perfusion SPECT in drug-free obsessive-compulsive patients without depression. Psychiatry Res 2001;107:51–6.

[34] Baxter LR. Functional imaging of brain systems mediating obsessive-compulsive disorder: clinical studies. In: Charney DS, Nestler EJ, Bunney BS, editors. Neurobiology of mental illness. New York: Oxford University Press; 1999. p. 534–47.

[35] Rauch SL, Whalen PJ, Dougherty DD. Neurobiological models of obsessive-compulsive disorders. In: Rauch SL, editor. Obsessive-compulsive disorders: practical management. Boston: Mosby; 1998. p. 222–53.

[36] Rossi S, Bartalini S, Ulivelli M, et al. Hypofunctioning of sensory gating mechanisms in patients with obsessive-compulsive disorder. Biol Psychiatry 2005;57:16–20.

[37] Van den Heuvel O, Veltman DJ, Groenewegen HJ, et al. Frontal-striatal dysfunction during planning in obsessive-compulsive disorder. Arch Gen Psychiatry 2005;62: 301–10.

[38] Kathman N, Rupertseder C, Hauke W, et al. Implicit sequence learning in obsessive-compulsive disorder: further support for the fronto-striatal dysfunction model. Biol Psychiatry 2005;58:239–44.

[39] Rosenberg DR, MacMillan SN. Imaging and neurocircuitry of OCD. In: Davis KL, Charney D, Coyle JT, et al, editors. Psychopharmacology: the fifth generation of progress. Philadelphia: Lippincott Williams & Wilkins; 2002. p. 1621–45.

[40] Rolls ET. The neural basis of emotion. In: Rolls ET, editor. The brain and emotion. New York: Oxford University Press; 1999. p. 112–38.

[41] Devinsky O, Morrell MJ, Vogt BA. Contributions of anterior cingulated cortex to behaviour. Brain 1995;(Pt 1):279–309.

[42] Cummings JL. Obsessive-compulsive disorder in basal ganglia disorders. J Clin Psychiatry 1996;57:1180.

[43] Greenberg BD, Ziemann U, Cora-Locatella G, et al. Altered cortical excitability in obsessive-compulsive disorder. Neurology 2000;54:142–7.

[44] Rosenberg DR, Keshavan MS, O'Hearn KM, et al. Frontal-striatal measurement of treatment-naïve pediatric obsessive-compulsive disorder. Arch Gen Psychiatry 1997;54: 824–30.

[45] Gilbert AR, Moore GJ, Keshavan MS, et al. Decrease in thalamic volumes of pediatric obsessive-compulsive disorder patients taking paroxetine. Arch Gen Psychiatry 2000;57: 449–56.

[46] Dubois B, Verin M, Teixeira-Ferreira C, et al. How to study frontal lobe functions in humans. In: Theirry A-M, Glowinski J, Goldman-Rakic PS, et al, editors. Motor and cognitive functions of the prefrontal cortex. Berlin: Springer-Verlag; 1994. p. 1–16.

[47] Zohar J, Insel TR. Obsessive-compulsive disorder: psychobiological approaches to diagnosis, treatment and pathophysiology. Biol Psychiatry 1987;2:667–87.

[48] Stein DJ. Obsessive-compulsive disorder. Lancet 2002;360:397–405.

[49] El Mansari M, Bouchard C, Blier P. Alteration of serotonin release in the guinea pig orbitofrontal cortex by selective serotonin reuptake inhibitors. Relevance to treatment of obsessive-compulsive disorder. Neuropsychopharmacol 1995;13:117–27.

[50] El Mansari M, Blier P. Responsiveness of postsynaptic 5-HT$_{1A}$ and 5-HT$_2$ receptors in rat OFC following long-term serotonin reuptake inhibition. J Psychiatry Neurosci 2005;30: 268–74.

[51] Grados MA, Walkup J, Walford S. Genetics of obsessive-compulsive disorders: new findings and challenges. Brain Dev 2003;25(Suppl):55–61.

[52] Li X, May RS, Tolbert LC, Jackson WT, et al. Risperidone and haloperidol augmentation of serotonin reuptake inhibition in refractory obsessive-compulsive disorder: a crossover study. J Clin Psychiatry 2005;66:736–43.

[53] Harvey BH, Brink CB, Seedat S, et al. Defining the neuromolecular action of myo-inositol: application to obsessive-compulsive disorder. Prog Neuropsychopharmacol Biol Psychiatry 2002;26:21–32.

[54] Marazziti D, Masala I, Rossi A, et al. Increased inhibitory activity of protein kinase C on the serotonin transporter in OCD. Neuropsychobiology 2000;41:171–7.

[55] McGrath MJ, Campbell KM, Parks CR, et al. Glutamatergic drugs exacerbate symptomatic behavior in a transgenic model of comorbid Tourette's syndrome and obsessive-compulsive disorder. Brain Res 2000;877:23–30.

[56] Zai G, Arnold P, Burroughs E, et al. Evidence for the gamma-amino-butyric acid type B receptor 1 (GABBAR1) gene as a susceptibility factor in obsessive-compulsive disorder. Am J Med Genet B Neuropsychiatry Gen 2005;134:25–9.

[57] McDougle CL, Barr LC, Goodman WK, et al. Possible role of neuropeptides in obsessive compulsive disorder. Psychoneuroendocrinology 1999;24:1–24.

[58] Fekete M, Szabo A, Balazs M, et al. Effects of intraventricular administration of cholecystokinin octapeptide sulfate ester and unsulfated cholecystokinin octapeptide on active avoidance and conditioned feeding behavior of rats. Acta Physiol Acad Sci Hung 1981;58:39–45.

[59] Rex A, Fink H, Marsden CA. Effects of BOC-CCK-4 and L 365.260 on cortical 5-HT release in Guinea-pigs on exposure to the elevated plus maze. Neuropharmacology 1994;33: 559–65.

[60] Siniscalchi A, Rodi D, Cavallini S, et al. Effects of cholecystokinin tetrapeptide (CCK(4)) and anxiolytic drugs on GABA outflow from the cerebral cortex of freely moving rats. Neurochem Int 2003;42:87–92.

[61] Vaccarino FJ. Nucleus accumbens dopamine-CCK interactions in psychostimulant reward and related behaviours. Neurosci Biobehav Rev 1994;18:207–14.

[62] Wilner P. Behavioral models in psycopharmacology. In: Wilner P, editor. Behavioral models in psychopharmacology: theoretical, industrial and clinical perspectives. Cambridge: Cambridge University Press; 1991. p. 3–18.

[63] Overall KL. Natural animal models of human psychiatric conditions: assessment of mechanisms and validity. Prog Neuropsychopharmacol Biol Psychiatry 2000;24:727–76.

[64] Cambell DT, Fiske DW. Convergent and discriminant validation by the multitrait-multimethod matrix. Psychol Bull 1959;56:81–105.

[65] Cronbach LJ, Mehl PE. Construct validity in psychological test. Psychol Bull 1955;52: 281–302.

[66] Mosier CI. A critical examination of the concepts of face validity. Educ Psychol Meas 1947; 7:191–205.

[67] Black DW, Goldstein RB, Noyes R, et al. Psychiatric disorders in relatives of probands with obsessive-compulsive disorder and co-morbid major depression or generalized anxiety. Psychiatr Genet 1995;5:37–41.

[68] Tot S, Erdal ME, Yazici K, et al. T102C and -1438G/A polymorphisms of 5–HT2A receptor gene in Turkish patients with obsessive-compulsive disorder. Eur Psychiatry 2003;18: 249–54.

[69] Stein DJ, Dodman NH, Borhelt P, et al. Behavioral disorders in veterinary practice: relevance to psychiatry. Compr Psychiatry 1994;35:275–85.

[70] Ricciardi JN, Hurley J. Development of animal models of obsessive-compulsive disorders. In: Jenike MA, Baer L, Minichiello WE, editors. Obsessive-compulsive disorders: theory and management. Chicago: Year Book Medical Publishers; 1990. p. 189–99.

[71] Rasmussen SA, Eisen JL. The epidemiology and clinical features of obsessive compulsive disorder. Psychiatr Clin North Am 1992;15:743–58.

[72] Altemus M, Glowa JR, Galliven E, et al. Effects of serotonergic agents on food-restriction-induced hyperactivity. Pharmacol Biochem Behav 1996;53:123–31.

[73] Tsaltas E, Kontis D, Chryskakou S, et al. Reinforced spatial alternation as an animal model of obsessive-compulsive disorder (OCD): investigation of 5-HT$_{2C}$ and 5-HT$_{1D}$ receptor involvement in OCD pathophysiology. Biol Psychiatry 2005;57:1176–85.

[74] Joel D, Avisar A. Excessive level pressing following post-training signal attenuation in rats: a possible animal model of obsessive compulsive disorder? Behav Brain Res 2001;123: 77–87.

[75] Man J, Hudson AL, Ashton D, et al. Animal models for obsessive-compulsive disorder. Current Neuropharmacology 2004;2:169–81.

[76] Savage CR, Baer L, Keuthen NJ, et al. Organizational strategies mediate nonverbal memory impairment on obsessive-compulsive disorder. Biol Psychiatry 1999;45:905–16.

[77] Deckersbach T, Otto MW, Savage CR, et al. The relationship between semantic organization and memory in obsessive-compulsive disorder. Psychother Psychosom 2000;69:101–7.

[78] Direnfeld DM, Pato MT, Roberts JE. Attentional biases in obsessive compulsive disorder: relationship to symptomatology and treatment. Poster presented at the 2001 Meeting of the Association for the Advancement of Behavior Therapy. Philadelphia, PA. November 2001.

[79] Kampman M, Keijsers GPJ, Verbraak MJPM, et al. The emotional Stroop: a comparison of panic disorder patients, obsessive-compulsive patients, and normal controls, in two experiments. J Anxiety Disord 2002;16:425–41.

[80] Broekamp CL, Jenck F. The relationship between various animal models of anxiety, fear-related psychiatric symptoms and response to serotonergic drugs. In: Bevan P, Cools R, Archer T, editors. Behavioural pharmacology of 5-HT. Hillsdale (NJ): Erlbaum; 1989. p. 321–35.

[81] Li X, Morrow D, Witkin M. Decreases in nestlet shredding of mice by serotonin uptake inhibitors: comparison with marble burying. Life Sci 2005 In press.

[82] Ichimaru Y, Egawa T, Sawa A. 5-HT-1A-receptor subtype mediates the effect of fluvoxamine, a selective serotonin reuptake inhibitor, on marble burying behavior in mice. Jpn J Pharmacol 1995;68:65–70.

[83] Sarna JR, Dyck RH, Whishaw IQ. The Delilah effect: C57BL6 mice barber whiskers by plucking. Behav Brain Res 2000;108:39–45.

[84] Garner JP, Dufour B, Gregg LE, et al. Social and husbandry factors affecting the prevalence and severity of barbering (whisker trimming) by laboratory mice. Appl Anim Behav Sci 2004;89:263–82.

[85] Garner JP, Weiker SM, Dufour B, et al. Barbering (fur and whisker trimming) by laboratory mice as a model of human trichotillomania and obsessive compulsive spectrum disorder. Comp Med 2004;54:216–24.

[86] Garner JP, Meehan CL, Famula TR, et al. Genetic, environmental, and neighbor effects on the severity of stereotypies and feather picking in orange-winged Amazon parrots (Amazona amazonica): an epidemiological study. Appl Anim Behav Sci 2006;96:153–68.

[87] Veith L. Acral lick dermatitis in the dog. Canine Pract 1985;13:15–22.

[88] Voith VL. Behavioral disorder. In: Davis LE, editor. Handbook of small animal therapeutics. New York: Churchill Livingstone; 1985.

[89] Moon-Fanelli AA, Dodman NH, O'Sullivan RL. Veterinary models of compulsive self-grooming: parallels with trichotillomania. In: Stein DJ, Christenson GA, Hollander E, editors. Trichotillomania. Washington (DC): American Psychiatric Press; 1999. p. 63–92.

[90] Powell SB, Newman HA, Pendergast J, et al. A rodent model of spontaneous stereotypy: initial characterization of developmental, environmental, and neurobiological factors. Physiol Behav 1999;66:355–63.

[91] Presti MF, Watson CJ, Kennedy RT, et al. Behavior-related alterations of striatal neurochemistry in a mouse model of stereotyped movement disorder. Pharmacol Biochem Behav 2004;77:501–7.

[92] Presti MF, Powell SB, Lewis MH. Dissociation between spontaneously emitted and apomorphine-induced stereotypy in Peromyscus maniculatus bairdii. Physiol Behav 2002;75: 347–53.

[93] Presti MF, Mikes HM, Lewis MH. Selective blockade of spontaneous motor stereotypy via intrastriatal pharmacological manipulation. Pharmacol Biochem Behav 2003;74:833–9.

[94] Ödberg FO, Meers L. The influence of cage size and environmental enrichment on the development of stereotypies in bank voles. Behav Processes 1987;14:155–73.

[95] Hugo C, Seier J, Mdhluli C, et al. Fluoxetine decreases stereotypic behavior in primates. Prog Neuropsychopharmacol Biol Psychiatry 2003;27:639–43.

[96] Schoenecker B, Heller KE. Stimulation of serotonin (5-HT) activity reduces spontaneous stereotypies in female but not in male bank voles (Clethrionomys glareolus). Stereotyping

female voles as a new animal model for human anxiety and mood disorders. Appl Anim Behav Sci 2003;80:161–70.

[97] Meers L, Ödberg FO. Paradoxical rate-dependent effect of fluoxetine on captivity-induced stereotypies in bank voles. Prog Neuropsychopharmacol Biol Psychiatry 2005;29:964–71.

[98] Salkovskis PM. Obsessional-compulsive problems: a cognitive-behavioral analysis. Behav Res Ther 1985;23:571–83.

[99] Krikorian R, Zimmerman ME, Fleck DE. Inhibitory control in obsessive-compulsive disorder. Brain Cogn 2004;54:257–9.

[100] Swedo S. Rituals and releasers: an ethological model of obsessive-compulsive disorder. In: Rapoport J, editor. Obsessive-compulsive disorder in children and adolescents. Washington (DC): American Psychiatric Association Press; 1989. p. 269–88.

[101] Joel D, Doljansky J, Schiller D. "Compulsive" lever pressing in rats is enhanced following lesions to the orbital cortex, but not to the basolateral nucleus of the amygdale or to the dorsal medial prefrontal cortex. Eur J Neurosci 2005;21:2252–62.

[102] Yadin E, Friedman E, Bridger WH. Spontaneous alternation behavior: an animal model for obsessive-compulsive disorder? Pharmacol Biochem Behav 1991;40:311–5.

[103] Henderson JG Jr, Polland CA. Three types of obsessive compulsive disorder in a community. J Clin Psychol 1988;44:747–52.

[104] Savage CR, Keuthen NJ, Jenike MA. Recall and recognition memory in obsessive-compulsive disorder. J Neuropsychiatry Clin Neurosci 1996;8:99–103.

[105] Szechtman H, Sulis W, Eilam D. Quinpirole induces compulsive checking behavior in rats: a potential animal model of obsessive-compulsive disorder (OCD). Behav Neurosci 1998; 112:1475–85.

[106] Roffman J, Raskin LA. Stereotyped behavior: effects of D-amphetamine and methylphenidate in the young rat. Pharmacol Biochem Behav 1997;58:1095–102.

[107] Harvey BH, Scheepers AS, Brand L, et al. Chronic inositol increases striatal D_2 receptors but does not modify dexamphetamine-induced motor behavior: relevance to obsessive compulsive disorder. Pharmacol Biochem Behav 2001;68:245–53.

[108] Finn DA, Rutledge-Gorman MT, Crabbe JC. Genetic animal models. Neurogenetics 2003; 4:109–35.

[109] Greer JM, Capecchi MR. Hoxb8 is required for normal grooming in mice. Neuron 2002;33: 23–34.

[110] Campbell KM, de Lecca L, Severynse DM, et al. OCD-like behaviours caused by a neuro-potentiating transgene targeted to cortical and limbic D1 + neurons. J Neurosci 1999;19: 5044–53.

[111] Nordstrom EJ, Burton FH. A transgenic model of comorbid Tourette's syndrome and obsessive-compulsive disorder circuitry. Mol Psychiatry 2002;7:617–25.

[112] Berridge KC, Aldrige JW, Houchard KR, et al. Sequential super-stereotypy of an instinctive fixed pattern in hyper-dopaminergic mutant mice: a model of obsessive compulsive disorder and Tourette's. BMC Biol 2005;3:1–32.

[113] Zhuang X, Oosting RS, Jones SR, et al. Hyperactivity and impaired behaviors in mutant mice with a dysregulated dopamine system. Proc Natl Acad Sci U S A 2001;98:1982–7.

[114] Chou-Green JM, Holscher TD, Dallman MF, et al. Compulsive behavior in the 5–HT2C receptor knockout mouse. Phys Behav 2003;78:641–9.

[115] Geyer MA, Markou A. The role of preclinical models in the development of psychotropic drugs. In: Davis KL, Charney D, Coyle JT, et al, editors. Psychopharmacology: the 5th generation of progress. Philadelphia: Lippincott Williams & Wilkins; 2002. p. 445–55.

[116] Schoenecker B, Heller KE. The involvement of dopamine (DA) and serotonin (5-HT) in stress-induced stereotypies in bank voles (Clethrionomys glareolus). Appl Anim Behav Sci 2001;73:311–9.

PSYCHIATRIC
CLINICS
OF NORTH AMERICA

ELSEVIER
SAUNDERS

Psychiatr Clin N Am 29 (2006) 391–410

Common and Distinct Neural Correlates of Obsessive-Compulsive and Related Disorders

David Mataix-Cols, PhD[a],*,
Odile A. van den Heuvel, MD, PhD[b]

[a]Departments of Psychological Medicine and Psychology, King's College London,
Institute of Psychiatry, London SE5 8AF, UK
[b]Department of Psychiatry, VU University Medical Center, GGZ Buitenamstel,
p/a Oldenaller 1, 1081 HJ, Amsterdam, The Netherlands

Neurobiological theories of obsessive-compulsive disorder (OCD) suggest that specific frontal-subcortical circuits are involved in the symptoms and cognitive deficits associated with the disorder. These theories arose from various sources of evidence: the presence of OCD symptoms in some neurological conditions (Tourette's syndrome, Huntington's disease, Sydenham's chorea, and other basal ganglia disorders), the emergence of OCD-like behaviors in patients who have focal brain injury, and the improvement in mood and OCD symptoms when frontal-subcortical circuits are interrupted by surgical interventions. However, the strongest support for these models came from modern neuroimaging techniques, which provide a direct window into the OCD brain in vivo. These technological advances were combined with various study designs or paradigms including volumetric measurements, resting-state studies, symptom provocation, cognitive probes, pre- and posttreatment designs, and ligand studies. Several excellent recent reviews of this literature exist and are not duplicated here [1–3]. Briefly, although the replicability among these studies has been imperfect, they strongly link OCD symptoms with activation of the orbitofrontal cortex, with less consistent involvement of the anterior cingulate gyrus, striatum, thalamus, lateral frontal and temporal cortices, amygdala, and insula [1–3]. This literature has led to the development of a widely accepted neurobiological model of OCD.

---

* Corresponding author. King's College London, Institute of Psychiatry. P.O. Box 69, De Crespigny Park, London SE5 8AF, UK.
E-mail address: d.mataix@iop.kcl.ac.uk (D. Mataix-Cols).

0193-953X/06/$ - see front matter © 2006 Elsevier Inc. All rights reserved.
doi:10.1016/j.psc.2006.02.006

Current neuroanatomical model of obsessive-compulsive disorder

Currently, the most widely accepted neuroanatomical model of OCD pro-poses the involvement of a direct and an indirect cortico-striato-thalamic pathway [4–6]. In the direct pathway, an excitatory glutamatergic signal pro-jects to the striatum, sending an inhibitory gamma-aminobutyric acid (GABA)-ergic signal to the internal part of the globus pallidus. This signal re-sults in a decreased inhibition (disinhibition) of the thalamus and thus an in-creased excitatory effect on the prefrontal cortex. In the indirect pathway, the striatum projects an inhibitory signal to the external part of the globus pal-lidus and the subthalamic nucleus, sending an excitatory signal to the internal part of the globus pallidus. The net effect is an increased inhibition of the thal-amus and decreased excitation on the prefrontal cortex. It is hypothesized that the direct pathway functions as a self-reinforcing positive feedback loop and contributes to the initiation and continuation of behaviors, whereas the indirect pathway provides a mechanism of negative feedback which is im-portant for the inhibition of behaviors and in switching between behaviors. Based on functional neuroimaging results, Saxena and Rauch [1] described how an imbalance between these frontal-striatal circuits might mediate OCD symptomatology. Focusing on the ventromedial frontal-striatal circuit, they hypothesized an excess tone in the direct relative to the indirect frontal-striatal circuit, resulting in enhanced activation of the orbitofrontal cortex, ventral striatum, and medial-dorsal thalamus. Based on the positive thera-peutic effects of selective serotonergic re-uptake inhibitors on OCD symptom-atology and the inhibitory effect of serotonin on dopamine, it is suggested that failure of the serotonergic system results in decreased compensation of the do-paminergic influence on the frontal-striatal circuits. Dopamine (D) has a dual role on the balance between the direct and indirect frontal-striatal pathways. In the human brain D_1 receptor expression is prominent in the ventromedial (relative to dorsolateral) prefrontal cortex and ventral (relative to dorsal) striatum [7]. Functionally, this dopaminergic differentiation implies a stronger D_1 influence on the direct pathway of the ventromedial frontal-striatal circuit and a stronger D_2 influence on the indirect pathway of the dorsolateral frontal-striatal circuit, resulting in a hyperactivated ventral and an inhibited dorsal frontal-striatal system (Fig. 1). This differentiation corresponds with the results of functional neuroimaging studies in OCD, showing increased activation of limbic and ventral frontal-striatal regions at rest and in response to disease-relevant information and decreased responsiveness of dorsal frontal-striatal regions during executive performance [3,8].

Myths about the brain in obsessive-compulsive disorder

Appealing as it may be, this model is likely to be overly simplistic because it is based on several assumptions or myths about the OCD brain and OCD itself:

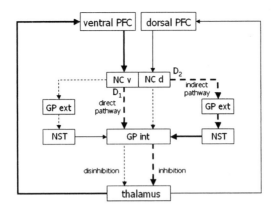

Fig. 1. A widely accepted frontal-striatal model of OCD, based on the work of Alexander and colleagues [4], Cummings [5], Saxena and Rauch [1], and Groenewegen and Uylings [6]. The direct connections function as a self-reinforcing positive feedback loop and contribute to the initiation and continuation of behaviors, whereas the indirect connections provide a mechanism of negative feedback that is important for the inhibition of behaviors and in switching between behaviors. It is hypothesized that an imbalance between these pathways results in a hyperactivated ventral and an inhibited dorsal frontal-striatal system. D_1, dopamine type 1; D_2, dopamine type 2; GP ext, external part of globus pallidus; GP int, internal part of globus pallidus; NC d, dorsal part of caudate nucleus; NC v, ventral part of caudate nucleus; NST, subthalamic nucleus; PFC, prefrontal cortex. Dotted lines indicate inhibitory GABA-ergic projections; solid lines indicate excitatory glutamatergic projections.

1. That these brain structures mediate all types of OCD symptoms (ie, OCD is a unitary nosologic entity)
2. That these circuits represent the unique neural signature of OCD (ie, they are not implicated in other disorders)
3. That there are *qualitative* differences between the OCD and the healthy brain
4. That dysfunction in these brain regions *causes* OCD

The available literature clearly challenges these views. Each of these points is discussed briefly below.

Myth 1: obsessive-compulsive disorder is a unitary nosologic entity

Psychiatric classification systems (*Diagnostic and Statistical Manual of Mental Disorders*, fourth edition, text revised [DSM-IV-TR] and International Classification of Diseases [ICD-10]) view OCD as a unitary nosologic entity, but researchers are currently disputing this view. Factor and cluster analytical studies have identified at least four robust and temporally stable symptom dimensions (ie, contamination/washing, obsessions/checking, symmetry/ordering and hoarding) [9,10]. Each symptom dimension is associated with specific patterns of comorbidity, genetic transmission, treatment response, neuropsychological function, and neural response (for recent reviews, see references [9–12]). Therefore any revised neurobiological model of OCD will need to take this heterogeneity into account.

Myth 2: these circuits represent the unique neural signature of obsessive-compulsive disorder

The picture is further complicated because OCD (currently classified as an anxiety disorder) often co-occurs with other anxiety disorders and depression. OCD has also been associated with other non–anxiety disorders, known as "OCD spectrum disorders," that share phenomenological features, family aggregation, and (in some cases) treatment response with OCD. This elevated comorbidity is also reflected in a substantial degree of overlap in their neural substrates.

Myth 3: there are qualitative differences between the obsessive-compulsive brain and the healthy brain

Another assumption that remains untested is that there are qualitative differences between the OCD brain and healthy brain. The few symptom-provocation studies that included healthy control groups seem to suggest that the differences could be more quantitative than qualitative. Mataix-Cols and colleagues [13,14] presented symptom-related material to patients who had OCD and to healthy controls. The results revealed similar patterns of brain activation in both groups, although the degree of activation was, for the most part, significantly higher in the patient group. Clearly more research on this topic is needed, but the neuroimaging findings in OCD could reflect exaggerations of normal emotional responses to biologically relevant stimuli rather than fundamentally abnormal neuronal responses.

Myth 4: dysfunction in these brain regions causes obsessive-compulsive disorder

Differences in brain function between patients and controls do not necessarily indicate that dysfunction in these regions causes OCD. Neuroimaging tools should be regarded as correlational techniques that allow researchers to understand the neurophysiological bases of the behaviors under study but not necessarily their cause. At least three interpretations of the neuroimaging data are possible: (1) dysfunction in certain brain regions causes OCD; (2) dysfunction in certain brain regions is a consequence of OCD; and (3) another spurious variable causes both phenomena [2].

Aim of this article

Keeping these conundrums in mind, this article reviews the literature on the common and distinct neural correlates of OCD, its symptom dimensions, and other anxiety and OCD spectrum disorders. This is not an exhaustive review because other excellent reviews and meta-analyses of the neuroanatomy of OCD already exist. Instead, the authors aim to provide a conceptual and heuristic framework to help understand the relationship between these phenomena from the neurobiological point of view. They hope this article will contribute to the current debate surrounding the classification of OCD and related disorders.

The article first touches briefly on the phenomenological relationship between specific OCD symptom dimensions and other anxiety and spectrum disorders. Next it summarizes the literature on the common and unique neural substrates of several of these limbic and frontal-striatal disorders. This summary is followed by a review of the specific neural correlates of the symptom dimensions within OCD. Finally, the discussion integrates these findings and offers suggestions for future research in the field.

Phenomenological relationship between obsessive-compulsive disorder symptom dimensions and anxiety and spectrum disorders

Phenomenologically, the different OCD symptom dimensions are more likely to be associated with certain comorbid conditions (for recent reviews see references [9–12]). This association is represented graphically in Fig. 2. Symmetry/ordering symptoms have been strongly associated with comorbid chronic tics and Tourette's syndrome [9,12]. These patients also are more likely to be male, to have a relative who has OCD, and to have had an earlier onset of the disorder [9,12]. Harm obsessions and checking rituals have also been associated with Tourette's syndrome [9] and, more recently, with

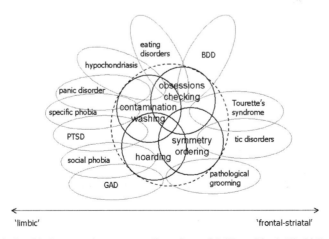

Fig. 2. Relationship between the symptom dimensions of OCD and both "limbic" and "frontal-striatal" Axis I disorders. BDD, body dysmorphic disorder; GAD, generalized anxiety disorder; pathological grooming, pathologic grooming behaviors such as trichotillomania, nail biting, skin picking; PTSD, posttraumatic stress disorder.

a variety of anxiety and mood disorders [15,16]. Excessive checking behavior is also a prominent symptom of hypochondriasis and body dysmorphic disorder (BDD), two of the OCD spectrum disorders. Hoarding symptoms have been associated with social phobia, depression, posttraumatic stress disorder (PTSD), BDD, and pathologic grooming behaviors (eg, trichotillomania, nail biting, skin picking) [17–19]. In addition, hoarding has been associated with cluster C (anxious-fearful) personality disorders and traits [20–22]. Patients who have OCD with contamination fears and washing rituals resemble specific animal phobics, although methodologically sound studies examining the association of the two phenomena are still lacking. Both are characterized by strong avoidance and elevated disgust sensitivity [23–26].

Although the evidence is still patchy, these phenomenological studies led the authors to hypothesize that patients who have OCD with prominent contamination/washing and hoarding symptoms are phenomenologically and neurobiologically closer to the "limbic" spectrum of disorders, whereas patients who have symmetry/order and checking symptoms are closer to the "frontal-striatal" spectrum of disorders (see Fig. 2).

"Limbic" disorders

"Limbic" disorders are a group of disorders that share several phenomenological characteristics: anticipatory anxiety, inadequate or enhanced anxiety responses with accompanying arousal, subsequent avoidance behavior, comorbid depressive symptoms, or generalized anxiety. Also, similarities in personality traits seem to be present across anxiety categories (eg, neuroticism, uncertainty, inhibited temperament). Because of the clinical overlap among these disorders, it seems reasonable to suggest common underlying neural substrates, that is, predominant involvement of limbic (most notably the amygdala) and paralimbic brain regions. Important contributions to the understanding of normal and pathologic emotional responses in humans came from animal learning studies. Fear-conditioning studies elicited how a conditioned stimulus (or learned cue) can induce a fear response (conditional reflex or learned response) after a few pairings with an unconditioned stimulus (or natural cue). The amygdala plays a central role in fear learning. LeDoux [27] described two parallel pathways, the direct pathway and the indirect pathway (Fig. 3). In the direct pathway, information about external stimuli reaches the lateral nucleus of the amygdala by direct connections from the thalamus ('thalamic pathway'), bypassing the cortical regions. Because of the lack of cortical processing, it can provide the amygdala only with a crude representation of the external stimulus (LeDoux called it the "quick and dirty" processing pathway). It allows the organism to respond to potential danger before it is conscious that it is in danger. The indirect pathway provides the amygdala with more detailed information and is able to modify the initial effect of the direct pathway. The conditioned

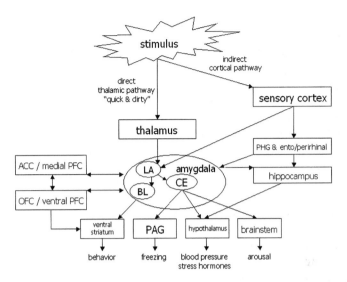

Fig. 3. The direct and indirect pathways involved in fear responses. ACC, anterior cingulate cortex; BL, basolateral nucleus of amygdala; CE, central nucleus of amygdala; ento/perirhinal, entorhinal and perirhinal cortex; OFC, orbitofrontal cortex; PAG, periaquaductal gray; PFC, prefrontal cortex; PHG, parahippocampal gyrus. (*Adapted from* LeDoux J. The emotional brain, the mysterious underpinnings of emotional life. 1st edition. New York: Touchstone; 1996.)

stimulus can also be a context. In contextual learning, the hippocampus plays an important role. Fear conditioning is a fast process, with a long-lasting effect, but repeated exposure to the conditioned stimulus in the absence of the unconditioned stimulus can lead to extinction. Extinction reduces the likelihood that the conditioned stimulus will elicit the fear response. The medial prefrontal and anterior cingulate cortices have been implicated in extinction learning [28–30]. Understanding how learned fears are diminished and how extinction learning is changed in patients who have anxiety disorders might be an important step in translating neurobiological research to diagnosis and treatment of these patients. Perhaps the best example of an anxiety disorder that seems to follow the classical fear-conditioning model is PTSD. Using the Ekman and Friesen [31] face series (a standard set of emotional facial expressions), PTSD patients demonstrated greater amygdala activations than healthy controls. Furthermore, activations in the amygdala correlated with attenuated activation of the medial prefrontal cortex and hippocampus [32,33].

The amygdala and the hippocampus also seem to play a crucial role in the pathophysiology of social phobia. Abnormal activation of these regions has been reported in social phobics both during symptom provocation (ie, public speaking) [34,35] and while viewing emotional facial expressions [36–38].

These brain regions may play a smaller or more indirect role in other anxiety disorders such specific phobias and OCD, however [39]. Symptom-provocation and emotional face-processing studies in animal phobics often have failed to find amygdala activation [40,41], although there are some exceptions [42]. Taken together, the specific phobia literature suggests a more primary involvement of somatosensory and anterior paralimbic regions, especially the insular cortex. The insular cortex and its adjacent regions have been strongly linked with disgust perception in healthy volunteers [43,44]. These findings are in agreement with the psychological literature linking animal phobias to disgust sensitivity [26].

Similarly, most resting-state and symptom-provocation studies in OCD found no amygdala activation (see [1] for a review), although there were some exceptions [45–47]. A recent face-perception study also failed to report amygdala activation [48]. It is possible that the amygdala is hyperresponsive in OCD only when patients are presented with symptom-specific emotional information, whereas other anxiety disorders, such as panic disorder and generalized anxiety disorder, may be responsive to a broader range of emotional stimuli [47]. Finally, it is also possible that some, but not all, OCD symptom dimensions are associated with exaggerated amygdala responses.

There is a conspicuous lack of studies directly comparing the neural substrates of all these disorders. Differences in historical background partly explain the limited overlap in the functional imaging paradigms used. Neuroimaging research in OCD has long been dominated by a limited, or at least a predominant, focus on the basal ganglia and the ventral prefrontal-striatal circuits. In contrast, neuroimaging work in panic disorder consisted largely of pharmacologic-challenge studies to induce panic attacks and ligand studies, most of which addressed the functioning of the GABA-benzodiazepine-receptor complex. In PTSD research most experiments followed the classical fear-conditioning model, focusing on the amygdala, hippocampus, and medial prefrontal cortex. One study combined data from various symptom-provocation studies (OCD, PTSD, and specific phobia) and found that the right inferior frontal cortex, right posterior medial orbitofrontal cortex, bilateral insular cortex, bilateral lenticulate nuclei, and bilateral brain stem may mediate symptoms across the different anxiety disorders, including OCD [49]. Using the emotional Stroop task, van den Heuvel and colleagues [47] investigated the disorder specificity of the neural response to disease-specific emotional information in OCD, panic disorder, and hypochondriasis. All patients showed increased distractibility for emotional information associated with frontal-striatal and limbic involvement, but clear differences were found between patients who had OCD, on the one hand, and patients who had panic disorder or hypochondriasis, on the other. In patients who had OCD the response was specific to disease-relevant information (OCD-related words) and correlated mainly with ventral brain regions, mostly the bilateral amygdala (Fig. 4) and the ventrolateral prefrontal cortex. Patients who had panic disorder showed a generalized response to negative stimuli (both OCD- and panic-related words), correlating with both ventral and dorsal regions. Also in patients who had panic disorder the amygdala response was specific to disease-relevant information

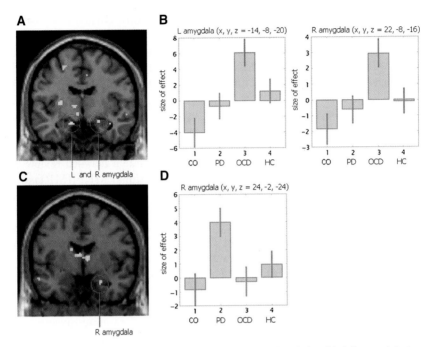

Fig. 4. (*A*) Increased blood oxygenation level–dependant (BOLD) signal in left amygdala (x, y, z = −14, −8, −20; z-score = 3.68; *P* < .05 corrected) and right amygdala (x, y, z = 22, −8, −16; z-score = 3.80; *P* < .05 corrected) in response to OCD-related words during the emotional Stroop task in patients who have OCD compared with healthy controls. (*B*) Plot of size of effect in the right and left amygdalae in patients who have OCD in comparison with patients who have panic disorder or hypochondriasis and healthy controls. (*C*) Increased BOLD signal in right amygdala (x, y, z = 24, −2, −24; z-score = 3.23; *P* < .05 corrected) to panic-related words during the emotional Stroop task in patients who have panic disorder compared with healthy controls. (*D*) Plot of size of effect in the right amygdala in patients who have panic disorder in comparison with patients who have OCD or hypochondriasis and healthy controls. Co, healthy controls, HC, hypochondriasis; OCD, obsessive-compulsive disorder; PD, panic disorder. (*Adapted from* van den Heuvel OA, Veltman DJ, Groenewegen HJ, et al. Disorder-specific neuroanatomical correlates of attentional bias in obsessive-compulsive disorder, panic disorder and hypochondriasis. Arch Gen Psychiatry 2005;62:922–33.)

(panic-words). The activation patterns of the hypochondriasis group were more similar to those of the panic disorder group than the OCD group.

"Frontal-striatal" disorders

The "frontal-striatal" disorders include a variety of neurological conditions that have been associated with OCD (eg, Tourette's syndrome, tics) and other spectrum disorders classified in different sections of the DSM-IV-TR, such as BDD (somatoform disorders) and trichotillomania (impulse-control disorders). It is hypothesized that the predominant neural systems underlying these disorders are the sensorimotor cortico-striato-thalamic loops [4–6]. Unfortunately, there are relatively few neuroimaging studies in these disorders, with the exception of Tourette's syndrome. Structural MRI studies in Tourette's syndrome have reported volumetric abnormalities in the basal ganglia [50] and related cortical structures [51]. In the study by Peterson and colleagues [50], basal ganglia volumes did not correlate with the severity of tics at the time of the scanning, but the volumes of the caudate nucleus in childhood predicted the severity of tic and OCD symptoms 7.5 years later [52]. These results were supported further by functional neuroimaging studies, although space limitations preclude a detailed review of this literature. One important study [53] used functional MRI (fMRI) and a tic-suppression paradigm in 22 patients who had Tourette's syndrome and found significant changes in the basal ganglia (increases in caudate nucleus, decreases in putamen/globus pallidus), thalamus (decreases), and related cortical regions (increases in prefrontal and temporal regions) during tic suppression (compared with spontaneous expression of tics).

The neuroimaging literature in trichotillomania is limited. In a morphometric MRI study of 10 female patients and 10 matched controls, O'Sullivan and colleagues [54] reported smaller left putamen volumes in the patient group. Stein and colleagues [55], however, compared caudate nucleus volumes and ventricular-brain ratios in 13 women who had OCD, 17 women who had trichotillomania, and 12 healthy controls and found no significant differences among the groups on either variable. Using a semiautomated cortical morphometric method, Grachev [56] reported volumetric reductions in the right inferior frontal gyrus and increases in the right cuneus in 10 female patients who had trichotillomania, compared with controls. Using fluorodeoxyglucose positron-emission tomography, Swedo and colleagues [57] found that 10 women who had trichotillomania showed increased metabolic rates in bilateral cerebellar and superior parietal cortex compared with 20 healthy controls. They also found that clomipramine-induced improvement was negatively correlated with anterior cingulate and orbitofrontal metabolism, findings that resemble methodologically comparable studies in OCD. In a single-photon emission CT study, Stein and colleagues [58] found that the severity of hair pulling correlated with decreased perfusion in the left mid-posterior frontal, parietal, and striatum and that this pattern of correlations was reversed after treatment with citalopram in 10 patients.

There have been even fewer neuroimaging studies in BDD. In one morphometric study of eight women who had BDD and eight matched controls, Rauch and colleagues [59] reported overall increased white (but not gray) matter volume in BDD compared with controls. They did not find any differences in regional volumes in the two groups. The BDD group did show a significantly different asymmetry of the caudate nucleus, with a leftward shift in the laterality quotient. In a recent single-photon emission CT study of six patients, Carey and colleagues [60] found widespread perfusion deficits in parieto-occipital, temporal, and frontal regions. The authors speculated that the involvement of the parieto-occipital cortex might reflect the core feature of disturbed perception of body appearance in BDD.

In short, the literature on Tourette's syndrome strongly suggests a more prominent involvement of the sensorimotor circuits and a less obvious involvement of limbic/paralimbic regions. The neuroimaging literature in other spectrum disorders such as BDD and trichotillomania is sparse and plagued with methodological problems (mainly small sample sizes). It therefore is difficult at this stage to draw any firm conclusions about the common and distinct neurobiological substrates of these disorders and how they relate to OCD.

Specific neural correlates of the symptom dimensions of obsessive-compulsive disorder

A limited number of studies have recently begun examining the neural correlates of the symptom dimensions of OCD. In the first such study, using positron-emission tomography, Rauch and colleagues [61] found that checking symptoms correlated with increased, and symmetry/ordering with reduced, regional cerebral blood flow in the striatum, whereas washing symptoms correlated with increased regional cerebral blood flow in bilateral anterior cingulate and left orbitofrontal cortex. Phillips and colleagues [62] compared patients who had OCD with mainly washing (n = 7) or checking (n = 7) symptoms while viewing pictures of either normally disgusting scenes or washer-relevant pictures using fMRI. When viewing washing-related pictures, only washers demonstrated activations in regions implicated in emotion and disgust perception (ie, visual regions and insular cortex), whereas checkers demonstrated activations in frontal-striatal regions and the thalamus. In a similar study, eight patients who had OCD with predominantly washing symptoms demonstrated greater activation than controls in the right insula, ventrolateral prefrontal cortex, and parahippocampal gyrus when viewing disgust-inducing pictures [63]. Another study found increased amygdala activation in a group of 11 washers during the presentation of contamination-related pictures [46]. Saxena and colleagues [64] found that 12 patients who had predominantly hoarding symptoms showed reduced glucose metabolism in the posterior cingulate gyrus (versus controls) and the dorsal anterior cingulate cortex (versus nonhoarding OCD) and that severity of hoarding in the whole patient group (n = 45) correlated negatively with metabolism in the latter region. Limitations of these studies included the artificial division between washers, checkers, and hoarders and, in the symptom-provocation studies, the exclusive use of washing-related or disgust-related material. One recent fMRI study used a symptom-provocation paradigm to examine, within the same patients, the neural correlates of the washing, checking, and hoarding symptom dimensions of OCD [14]. Each of these dimensions was mediated by distinct but partially overlapping neural systems. Although both patients and controls activated similar brain

regions in response to symptom provocation, patients showed greater activations in bilateral ventromedial prefrontal regions (washing experiment),
putamen/globus pallidus, thalamus, and dorsal cortical areas (checking experiment), and left precentral gyrus and right orbitofrontal cortex (hoarding
experiment). These results were further supported by correlation analyses
within the patient group, which revealed highly specific positive associations
between subjective anxiety, questionnaire scores, and neural response in
each experiment (Fig. 5).

Structural neuroimaging OCD studies have been remarkably inconsistent. Only one recent study examined the correlations between symptom
scores and gray matter volumes. Pujol and colleagues [65] found that patients who had high scores on the aggressive/checking dimension had

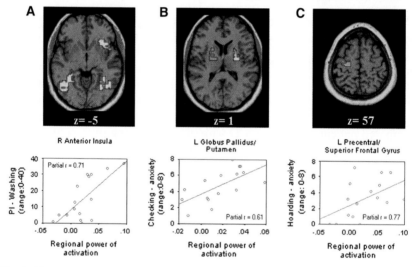

Fig. 5. Significant correlations between (A) washing scores of the Padua Inventory (PI) and activation in the washing experiment, (B) checking scores of the PI and activation in the checking
experiment, and (C) subjective anxiety scores and activation in the hoarding experiment. All
partial correlations controlled for Beck Depression Inventory scores. (A) Positive correlations
were found in bilateral fusiform gyrus (BA19; left: −36, −67, −7; voxels: 32; partial r =
0.69; right: 29, −63, −7; partial r = 0.68), right superior temporal gyrus (BA38;
47, 11, −7; voxels: 16; partial r = 0.75), right ventrolateral prefrontal cortex (BA47; 25,
11, −18; voxels: 15; partial r = 0.71); bilateral lingual gyrus (BA19/18; left: −25, −67, −2; voxels: 14; partial r = 0.61; right: 25, −74, −2; voxels: 11; partial r = 0.64), and right anterior insula
[32,7,4] (voxels: 7; partial r = 0.71). (B) Positive correlations were found in left precentral/
superior frontal gyrus (BA6; −11, −15, 59; voxels: 13; partial r = 0.62), left inferior frontal gyrus (BA45; −43, 19, 20; voxels:12; partial r = 0.57), bilateral globus pallidus/putamen (left: −14,
−7, −2; voxels: 7; partial r = 0.61; right: 25, −4, 9; voxels: 8; partial r = 0.43), and left thalamus
(−11, −4, 9; voxels: 6; partial r = 0.64). (C) A significant positive correlation was found in the
left precentral/superior frontal gyrus (BA4/6; −18, −15, 59; voxels: 9; partial r = 0.77). (Adapted
from Mataix-Cols D, Wooderson S, Lawrence N, et al. Distinct neural correlates of washing,
checking and hoarding symptom dimensions in obsessive-compulsive disorder. Arch Gen Psychiatry 2004;164:564–76.)

reduced gray matter volume in the right amygdala. The significance of this finding is unclear, especially because the convergent validity of the aggressive/checking factor of the Yale–Brown Obsessive-Compulsive Scale-Symptom Checklist is poor [66].

Although preliminary, these studies suggest that different symptoms may be mediated by distinct, albeit partially overlapping, neural systems. Previous discrepant findings may have resulted in part from phenotypic variations in the studied samples. These results also provide preliminary support for the hypothesis that the contamination/washing and hoarding symptom dimensions are predominantly mediated by limbic regions and that the checking and symmetry/ordering dimensions are predominantly frontal-striatal regions.

Discussion and future directions

The most widely accepted neurobiological model of OCD suggests that an imbalance between a direct and an indirect fronto-striato-thalamic circuit underlies the symptoms and specific cognitive and emotional deficits of these patients. Although this model has esthetic appeal, the authors believe that it may be a gross oversimplification. First, OCD is a compendium of multiple overlapping syndromes rather than a unitary nosologic entity. Any viable neurobiological model would need to take into account this heterogeneity. Second, OCD co-occurs with other anxiety/mood disorders as well as with the OCD spectrum disorders. If one adopts a "lumping" perspective, these high levels of comorbidity could be seen as indicative of core etiologic processes underlying all of these disorders. If one adopts a "splitting" perspective, each of these disorders (and indeed each of the OCD symptom dimensions) would have a different etiology and pathophysiology and simply co-occur with one another. This situation poses a formidable dilemma for psychiatry research in general [67] and OCD research in particular. The authors have recently proposed a multidimensional model of OCD [9,10] that suggests a middle ground between the "splitting" and "lumping" extremes: OCD might be better understood as multiple potentially overlapping syndromes that share etiologic factors but also have unique etiologic factors. In evolutionary terms, general anxiety, which is common to patients who have OCD and indeed other anxiety disorders, may have evolved to deal with nonspecific threats (eg, increased vigilance, physiological arousal), whereas specific types of anxiety evolved to protect against specific threats [68]. This model could be extended easily to the symptom dimensions of OCD; for instance, cleanliness is important for protection against infections; harming obsessions and checking rituals to keep people safe; and hoarding to help people survive periods of scarcity [9,10].

From a heuristic point of view, the most fruitful research strategy therefore would be to investigate the common and specific etiologic factors implicated in each syndrome. The different symptom dimensions of OCD (and indeed of other anxiety and spectrum disorders) are likely to share common neural substrates dedicated to general threat detection and emotional arousal because these reactions are adaptive and useful to deal with different kinds of threat. Likewise, preliminary research suggests syndrome-specific neural substrates that may have evolved to deal with specific threats.

Clearly, much research is still needed on the common and distinct neural correlates of the various OCD symptom dimensions and related disorders. The field will benefit from using identical imaging paradigms across these syndromes to facilitate direct comparisons. The authors also recommend that researchers systematically gather comprehensive information about their patients' symptom scores, which they can correlate with their neuroimaging results. Several comprehensive measures of OCD symptom dimensions now exist, notably the Dimensional Yale–Brown Obsessive-Compulsive Scale [16].

Third, the current neurobiological model of OCD assumes that there are fundamental qualitative differences between the OCD brain and healthy brain, but recent research raises the question of whether the differences between OCD patients and controls are more quantitative than qualitative [13]. Furthermore, the brain areas implicated in the model are also implicated in the mediation of normal emotional responses in healthy individuals. The multidimensional model of OCD proposes that OCD symptoms are distributed normally in the general population [9]. Research shows that many individuals in the general population experience normal obsessive and compulsive symptoms at some time that resemble the form and content of abnormal, pathologic phenomena [69,70]. Furthermore, studies involving nonclinical samples have demonstrated that normal individuals who have high scores on self-administered scales of obsessions and compulsions show striking similarities to patients who have OCD in clinical and personality characteristics and in performance on neuropsychological tests [71–73]. Neuroimaging studies comparing healthy individuals with high and low levels of OCD symptoms would provide a more definitive answer to this fundamental question. Eventually, such studies would shed some light on the categorical versus dimensional nature of OCD and obsessive-compulsive–related phenomena.

Fourth, the widely accepted frontal-striatal model minimizes the role of (para)limbic regions in the pathophysiology of OCD and related disorders. This model may be inadequate, at least for some OCD subtypes. It will be important to understand more fully the complex interactions between the limbic and the frontal-striatal systems and their relative contributions to all these syndromes. Based on imaging results in OCD, one might hypothesize that altered dorsal frontal-striatal function is responsible for decreased inhibition of ventral frontal-striatal and limbic recruitment in response to disease-relevant emotional cues. This hypothesis implies a primary failure (hypofunction) of the dorsal frontal-striatal circuit. This dorsal failure could explain the executive dysfunctions displayed by some patients who have OCD. The opposite hypothesis, of a primary deficit (hypersensitivity) of the limbic or ventral frontal-striatal circuits, might be defended as well. Even in this case, executive impairment may be the consequence, resulting from anxiety-related amygdala influence on the dorsal frontal-striatal circuitry. Moreover, it might even be possible that the etiology differs across symptom dimensions, with a primary limbic hypersensitivity in patients who have OCD with contamination fear and hoarding behaviors and a primary dorsal frontal-striatal failure in patients who have OCD with mainly symmetry and ordering behaviors.

Although both hypotheses imply direct connections between the amygdala and dorsal frontal-striatal regions, little is known about these complex interactions (Fig. 6). Whereas connections of the amygdala with the medial prefrontal and orbitofrontal cortex are robust and bidirectional, connections with lateral prefrontal areas are sparse, unidirectional, and primarily ascending [74]. There seem to be two important questions with regard to the communication between the limbic and dorsal frontal-striatal regions: (1) which direct and indirect descending connections from the dorsolateral prefrontal cortex to the amygdala play a role in the presumed top-down control of the amygdala response, and (2) how can activation of the amygdala directly or indirectly influence executive functioning by the dorsolateral prefrontala acortex? One possible way in which diverse streams of information could guide behavior would be through the rich interconnections between prefrontal areas [75,76] involving cortico-cortical and cortico-thalamo-cortical connections. So far, research in functional connectivity has depended mainly on tracing studies in animals. An important problem with the interpretation of neuroanatomical tracing studies is that these are

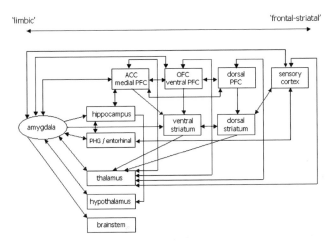

Fig. 6. Possible interactions between the various regions of the limbic and frontal-striatal circuits, explaining the overlap between the various disorders. ACC, anterior cingulate cortex; entorhinal, entorhinal cortex; OFC, orbitofrontal cortex; PFC, prefrontal cortex; PHG, parahippocampal gyrus.

performed in rodents and nonhuman primates, necessitating the extrapolation of the results to the more complex human brain. It is assumed that humans differ from animals in the way cognition is used to modify instinct-driven behavior. Possibly, humans differ from nonhuman primates in the complexity of the neuroanatomical connections between dorsolateral prefrontal areas and limbic structures. Recent developments in noninvasive neuroimaging techniques (eg, diffusion tension imaging) might contribute to the understanding of functional connectivity within the human brain and altered connections within patients who have psychiatric disorders. Another way to investigate the interactions between limbic and frontal-striatal circuits is by using transcranial magnetic stimulation (TMS). The effect of cortical modulation by TMS, both inhibition and stimulation, on the subcortical and limbic structures can be measured with resting-state MRI and fMRI during cognitive and emotional paradigms directly after single or repeated treatment with TMS.

Useful neuropsychological paradigms to investigate the functional interactions between limbic and frontal-striatal circuits are based on the various strategies for reducing or modulating emotional responses. Ochsner and Gross [77] described a hypothetical continuum of strategies for (1) controlling attention to and (2) cognitively changing the meaning of emotionally evocative stimuli. These processes of attentional control (eg, attentional bias and attentional distraction) and cognitive modulation (eg, reappraisal) might be dysfunctional in patients who have OCD and related disorders.

Future research in this field may benefit from a longitudinal and multimodal approach. Longitudinal studies with appropriate untreated controls are needed to establish which abnormalities are related to the symptomatic state and which (if any) are trait markers of OCD. These techniques have great potential as clinical tools (eg, in predicting treatment outcome), but these applications are still in their infancy. Probably the most interesting population for study are young children with and without obsessive-compulsive and related disorders. Longitudinal follow-up of these children into adolescence and adulthood would enable visualization of the natural history of these disorders as well as the evaluation of long-term effects of environmental influences and treatment strategies. Multimodal designs combining volumetric, resting state, functional, and chemical measurements may contribute to a better differentiation between cause and effect. For instance, altered morphology may be related to an imbalance of interacting neurotransmitter systems, and differences in task-related blood oxygenation level–dependant responses may be confounded by early maturation deficits.

To conclude, the authors propose that the most fruitful research strategy will be to examine the common and distinct neural correlates of the various OCD syndromes and related disorders using well-validated methods and paradigms. More insight on the interactions between the limbic and frontal-striatal circuits might contribute to a better understanding of the clinical overlap and differentiation between specific disorders. This ambitious endeavor will require large patient samples and a multimodal, multidisciplinary, and longitudinal approach.

References

[1] Saxena S, Rauch SL. Functional neuroimaging and the neuroanatomy of obsessive-compulsive behavior. Psychiatr Clin North Am 2000;23:563–86.

[2] Whiteside SP, Port JD, Abramowitz JS. A meta-analysis of functional neuroimaging in obsessive-compulsive disorder. Psychiatry Res 2004;132(1):69–79.

[3] Remijnse PL, van den Heuvel OA, Veltman DJ. Neuroimaging in obsessive-compulsive disorder. Current Medical Imaging Reviews 2005;1:331–51.

[4] Alexander GE. Parallel organization of functionally segregated circuits linking basal ganglia and cortex. Annu Rev Neurosci 1986;9:357–81.

[5] Cummings JL. Frontal-subcortical circuits and human behavior. Arch Neurol 1993;50:873–80.

[6] Groenewegen HJ, Uylings HBM. The prefrontal cortex and the integration of sensory, limbic and autonomic information. Prog Brain Res 2001;126:3–28.

[7] Hurd YL, Suzuki M, Sedvall GC. D1 and D2 dopamine receptor mRNA expression in whole hemisphere sections of the human brain. J Chem Neuroanat 2001;22:127–37.

[8] van den Heuvel OA, Veltman DJ, Groenewegen HJ, et al. Frontal-striatal dysfunction during planning in obsessive-compulsive disorder. Arch Gen Psychiatry 2005;62:301–10.

[9] Mataix-Cols D, Rosario-Campos MC, Leckman JF. A multidimensional model of obsessive-compulsive disorder. Am J Psychiatry 2005;162:228–38.

[10] Mataix-Cols D. Deconstructing obsessive-compulsive disorder: a multidimensional perspective. Curr Opin Psychiatry 2006;19:84–9.

[11] McKay D, Abramowitz JS, Calamari JE, et al. A critical evaluation of obsessive-compulsive disorder subtypes: symptoms versus mechanisms. Clin Psychol Rev 2004;24(3):283–313.

[12] Miguel EC, Leckman JF, Rauch S, et al. Obsessive-compulsive disorder phenotypes: implications for genetic studies. Mol Psychiatry 2005;10(3):258–75.

[13] Mataix-Cols D, Cullen S, Lange K, et al. Neural correlates of anxiety associated with obsessive-compulsive symptom dimensions in normal volunteers. Biol Psychiatry 2003;53:482–93.

[14] Mataix-Cols D, Wooderson S, Lawrence N, et al. Distinct neural correlates of washing, checking and hoarding symptom dimensions in obsessive-compulsive disorder. Arch Gen Psychiatry 2004;164:564–72.

[15] Hasler G, LaSalle-Ricci VH, Ronquillo JG, et al. Obsessive-compulsive disorder symptom dimensions show specific relationships to psychiatric comorbidity. Psychiatry Res 2005;135(2):121–32.

[16] Rosario-Campos MC, Miguel EC, Quatrano S, et al. The Dimensional Yale-Brown Obsessive Compulsive Scale (DY-BOCS): an instrument for assessing obsessive-compulsive symptom dimensions. Mol Psychiatry. 2006 Jan 24; [Epub ahead of print].

[17] Steketee G, Frost R. Compulsive hoarding: current status of the research. Clin Psychol Rev 2003;23(7):905–27.

[18] Samuels J, Bienvenu OJ III, Riddle MA, et al. Hoarding in obsessive compulsive disorder: results from a case-control study. Behav Res Ther 2002;40(5):517–28.

[19] Lasalle-Ricci VH, Arnkoff DB, Glass CR, et al. The hoarding dimension of OCD: psychological comorbidity and the five-factor personality model. Behav Res Ther. 2005 Dec 28; [Epub ahead of print].

[20] Frost RO, Steketee G, Williams LF, et al. Mood, personality disorder symptoms and disability in obsessive compulsive hoarders: a comparison with clinical and nonclinical controls. Behav Res Ther 2000;38(11):1071–81.

[21] Mataix-Cols D, Baer L, Rauch SL, et al. Relation of factor-analyzed symptom dimensions of obsessive-compulsive disorder to personality disorders. Acta Psychiatr Scand 2000;102(3): 199–202.

[22] Fullana MA, Mataix-Cols D, Caseras X, et al. High sensitivity to punishment and low impulsivity in obsessive-compulsive patients with hoarding symptoms. Psychiatry Res 2004; 129(1):21–7.

[23] Mancini F, Gragnani A, D'Olimpio F. The connection between disgust and obsessions and compulsions in a non-clinical sample. Pers Indiv Dif 2001;31:1173–80.

[24] Olatunji BO, Sawchuk CN, Lohr JM, et al. Disgust domains in the prediction of contamination fear. Behav Res Ther 2004;42(1):93–104.

[25] Woody SR, Tolin DF. The relationship between disgust sensitivity and avoidant behavior: studies of clinical and nonclinical samples. J Anxiety Disord 2002;16(5):543–59.

[26] Woody SR, McLean C, Klassen T. Disgust as a motivator of avoidance of spiders. J Anxiety Disord 2005;19(4):461–75.

[27] LeDoux J. The emotional brain, the mysterious underpinnings of emotional life. 1st edition. New York: Touchstone; 1996.

[28] Quirck GJ, Russo GK, Barron JL, et al. The role of ventromedial prefrontal cortex in the recovery of extinguished fear. J Neurosci 2000;20:6225–31.

[29] Quirck GJ, Likhtik E, Pelletier JG, et al. Stimulation of medial prefrontal cortex decreases the responsiveness of central amygdala output neurons. J Neurosci 2003;23:8800–7.

[30] Phelps EA, Delgado MR, Nearing KI, et al. Extinction learning in humans: role of the amygdala and vmPFC. Neuron 2004;43:897–905.

[31] Ekman P, Friesen WV. Pictures of facial affect. Palo Alto (CA): Consulting Psychologists Press; 1976.

[32] Rauch SL, Whalen PJ, Shin LM, et al. Exaggerated amygdala response to masked facial stimuli in posttraumatic stress disorder: a functional MRI study. Biol Psychiatry 2000;47: 769–76.

[33] Shin LM, Wright CI, Cannistraro PA, et al. A functional magnetic resonance imaging study of the amygdala and medial prefrontal cortex responses to overtly presented fearful faces in posttraumatic stress disorder. Arch Gen Psychiatry 2005;62:273–81.

[34] Tillfors M, Furmark T, Marteinsdottir I, et al. Cerebral blood flow during anticipation of public speaking in social phobia: a PET study. Biol Psychiatry 2002;52(11):1113–9.

[35] Furmark T, Tillfors M, Marteinsdottir I, et al. Common changes in cerebral blood flow in patients with social phobia treated with citalopram or cognitive-behavioral therapy. Arch Gen Psychiatry 2002;59(5):425–33.

[36] Birbaumer N, Grodd W, Diedrich O, et al. fMRI reveals amygdala activation to human faces in social phobics. Neuroreport 1998;9(6):1223–6.

[37] Schneider F, Weiss U, Kessler C, et al. Subcortical correlates of differential classical conditioning of aversive emotional reactions in social phobia. Biol Psychiatry 1999;45(7): 863–71.

[38] Stein MB, Goldin PR, Sareen J, et al. Increased amygdala activation to angry and contemptuous faces in generalized social phobia. Arch Gen Psychiatry 2002;59(11):1027–34.

[39] Cannistraro PA, Rauch SL. Neural circuitry of anxiety: evidence form structural and functional neuroimaging studies. Psychopharmacol Bull 2003;37:8–25.

[40] Rauch SL, Savage CR, Alpert NM, et al. A positron emission tomographic study of simple phobic symptom provocation. Arch Gen Psychiatry 1995;52(1):20–8.

[41] Wright CI, Martis B, McMullin K, et al. Amygdala and insular responses to emotionally valenced human faces in small animal specific phobia. Biol Psychiatry 2003;54:1067–76.

[42] Dilger S, Straube T, Mentzel H-J, et al. Brain activation to phobia-related pictures in spider phobic humans: an event-related functional magnetic resonance imaging study. Neurosci Lett 2003;348:29–32.

[43] Phillips ML, Young AW, Senior C, et al. A specific neural substrate for perceiving facial expressions of disgust. Nature 1997;389(6650):495–8.

[44] Wicker B, Keysers C, Plailly J, et al. Both of us disgusted in My insula: the common neural basis of seeing and feeling disgust. Neuron 2003;40(3):655–64.

[45] Breiter HC, Rauch SL, Kwong KK, et al. Functional magnetic resonance imaging of symptom provocation in obsessive-compulsive disorder. Arch Gen Psychiatry 1996;53: 595–606.

[46] van den Heuvel OA, Veltman DJ, Groenewegen HJ, et al. Amygdala activity in obsessive-compulsive disorder with contamination fear: a study with oxygen-15 water positron emission tomography. Psychiatry Research Neuroimaging 2004;132:225–37.

[47] van den Heuvel OA, Veltman DJ, Groenewegen HJ, et al. Disorder-specific neuroanatomical correlates of attentional bias in obsessive-compulsive disorder, panic disorder and hypochondriasis. Arch Gen Psychiatry 2005;62:922–33.

[48] Cannistraro PA, Wright CI, Wedig MM, et al. Amygdala responses to human faces in obsessive-compulsive disorder. Biol Psychiatry 2004;56:916–20.

[49] Rauch SL, Savage CR, Alpert NM, et al. The functional neuroanatomy of anxiety: a study of three disorders using positron emission tomography and symptom provocation. Biol Psychiatry 1997;42(6):446–52.

[50] Peterson BS, Thomas P, Kane MJ, et al. Basal ganglia volumes in patients with Gilles de la Tourette syndrome. Arch Gen Psychiatry 2003;60(4):415–24.

[51] Peterson BS, Staib L, Scahill L, et al. Regional brain and ventricular volumes in Tourette syndrome. Arch Gen Psychiatry 2001;58(5):427–40.

[52] Bloch MH, Leckman JF, Zhu H, et al. Caudate volumes in childhood predict symptom severity in adults with Tourette syndrome. Neurology 2005;65(8):1253–8.

[53] Peterson BS, Skudlarski P, Anderson AW, et al. A functional magnetic resonance imaging study of tic suppression in Tourette syndrome. Arch Gen Psychiatry 1998;54:326–33.

[54] O'Sullivan RL, Rauch SL, Breiter HC, et al. Reduced basal ganglia volumes in trichotillomania measured via morphometric magnetic resonance imaging. Biol Psychiatry 1997; 42(1):39–45.

[55] Stein DJ, Coetzer R, Lee M, et al. Magnetic resonance brain imaging in women with obsessive-compulsive disorder and trichotillomania. Psychiatry Res 1997;74(3):177–82.

[56] Grachev ID. MRI-based morphometric topographic parcellation of human neocortex in trichotillomania. Psychiatry Clin Neurosci 1997;51(5):315–21.

[57] Swedo SE, Rapoport JL, Leonard HL, et al. Regional cerebral glucose metabolism of women with trichotillomania. Arch Gen Psychiatry 1991;48(9):828–33.

[58] Stein DJ, van Heerden B, Hugo C, et al. Functional brain imaging and pharmacotherapy in trichotillomania. Single photon emission computed tomography before and after treatment with the selective serotonin reuptake inhibitor citalopram. Prog Neuropsychopharmacol Biol Psychiatry 2002;26(5):885–90.

[59] Rauch SL, Phillips KA, Segal E, et al. A preliminary morphometric magnetic resonance imaging study of regional brain volumes in body dysmorphic disorder. Psychiatry Res 2003; 122(1):13–9.

[60] Carey P, Seedat S, Warwick J, et al. SPECT imaging of body dysmorphic disorder. J Neuropsychiatry Clin Neurosci 2004;16(3):357–9.

[61] Rauch SL, Dougherty DD, Shin LM, et al. Neural correlates of factor-analyzed OCD symptom dimensions: PET study. CNS Spectr 1998;3:37–43.

[62] Phillips ML, Marks IM, Senior C, et al. A differential neural response in obsessive-compulsive disorder patients with washing compared with checking symptoms to disgust. Psychol Med 2000;30:1037–50.

[63] Shapira NA, Liu Y, He AG, et al. Brain activation by disgust-inducing pictures in obsessive-compulsive disorder. Biol Psychiatry 2003;54:751–6.

[64] Saxena S, Brody AL, Maidment KM, et al. Cerebral glucose metabolism in obsessive-compulsive hoarding. Am J Psychiatry 2004;161(6):1038–48.

[65] Pujol J, Soriano-Mas C, Alonso P, et al. Mapping structural brain alterations in obsessive-compulsive disorder. Arch Gen Psychiatry 2004;61:720–30.

[66] Mataix-Cols D, Fullana MA, Alonso P, et al. Convergent and discriminant validity of the Yale-Brown Obsessive Compulsive Symptom Checklist. Psychother Psychosom 2004;73: 190–6.

[67] Krueger RF, Piasecki TM. Toward a dimensional and psychometrically-informed approach to conceptualizing psychopathology. Behav Res Ther 2002;40(5):485–99.

[68] Marks IM, Nesse RM. Fear and fitness: an evolutionary analysis of anxiety disorders. Ethol Sociobiol 1994;15:247–61.

[69] Rachman S, de Silva P. Abnormal and normal obsessions. Behav Res Ther 1978;16:233–48.

[70] Muris P, Merckelbach H, Clavan M. Abnormal and normal compulsions. Behav Res Ther 1997;35:249–52.

[71] Gibbs NA. Nonclinical populations in research on obsessive-compulsive disorder: a critical review. Clin Psychol Rev 1996;16:729–73.

[72] Mataix-Cols D, Junqué C, Sánchez-Turet M, et al. Neuropsychological functioning in a sub-clinical obsessive sample. Biol Psychiatry 1999;45:898–904.

[73] Mataix-Cols D, Barrios M, Sánchez-Turet M, et al. Reduced design fluency in sub-clinical obsessive-compulsive subjects. J Neuropsychiatr Clin Neurosci 1999;11:395–7.

[74] Amaral DG, Price JL. Amygdalo-cortical projections in the monkey (*Macaca fascicularis*). J Comp Neurol 1984;230:465–96.

[75] Barbas H. Connections underlying the synthesis of cognition, memory, and emotion in primate prefrontal cortices. Brain Res Bull 2000;52:319–30.

[76] Haber SN. The primate basal ganglia: parallel and integrative networks. J Chem Neuroanat 2003;26:317–30.

[77] Ochsner KN, Gross JJ. The cognitive control of emotion. Trends Cogn Sci 2005;9(5):242–9.

ELSEVIER
SAUNDERS

PSYCHIATRIC
CLINICS
OF NORTH AMERICA

Psychiatr Clin N Am 29 (2006) 411–444

The Current Status of Association Studies in Obsessive-Compulsive Disorder

Sîan M.J. Hemmings, PhD[a],*, Dan J. Stein, MD, PhD[b]

[a]Department of Medical Biochemistry, Faculty of Health Sciences,
University of Stellenbosch, Tygerberg, South Africa
[b]Department of Psychiatry and Mental Health, University of Cape Town,
Cape Town, South Africa

The genetic epidemiology of obsessive-compulsive disorder

Although once conceptualized as a psychogenic disorder, there is growing evidence that obsessive-compulsive disorder (OCD) is mediated by specific neurobiologic dysfunctions that may, in turn, comprise a genetic component. Indeed, a large body of evidence for a genetic contribution to the etiology of OCD exists. A recent meta-analysis performed by Hettema and colleagues [1] to estimate summary statistics associated with aggregate familial risk and heritability for a number of anxiety disorders, including OCD, provided substantial evidence for familial aggregation of the disorder.

It has also been observed that OCD morbidity rates are significantly higher among relatives of OCD probands whose age at onset is below 14 years [2]. These findings are consistent with those by Nestadt and colleagues [3], who found that no cases were reported in relatives of probands whose age at onset exceeded 18 years. In addition, results from a more recent controlled family study indicated that early-onset OCD is highly familial, with significantly higher rates of definite OCD in first-degree relatives of early-onset OCD probands than in first-degree relatives of late-onset probands [4]. The cumulative results suggest that an earlier age at onset is likely to be valuable in characterizing a familial subtype of the disorder.

Familial transmission has also been found to extend beyond the domain of OCD and into that of disorders occurring within the so-called "OCD spectrum," indicating the likelihood of a common physiologic, genetic, and

---

* Corresponding author. PhD Department of Medical Biochemistry, Faculty of Health Sciences, University of Stellenbosch, P.O. Box 19063, Tygerberg 7505, South Africa.
 E-mail address: smjh@sun.ac.za (S.M.J. Hemmings).

psychologic etiology for some of these disorders. Evidence from family studies indicates a putative common genetic basis for OCD and Tourette's syndrome [5–7]. Pauls and colleagues [5] also reported on an increased familiality of OCD among probands who presented with comorbid tics (OCD plus tics).

Twin studies pertaining to OCD are capable of delimiting the genetic and environmental influences on the variation in liability to the disorder, although they have been somewhat limited by the paucity of the subjects. Nonetheless, the few twin studies that have been conducted suggest the involvement of hereditary components, with monozygotic concordance rates of between 53% and 87% and dizygotic concordance rates between 22% and 47% [5,8–10].

In a larger study of twin samples, a higher rate of concordance for OCD and subclinical OCD was found in monozygotic twins than in dizygotic twins [8,11], and the specific nature of the symptoms and response to therapeutic agents has been found to be more similar for monozygotic than for dizygotic twins [12,13]. It also has been shown that monozygotic twins have a higher concordance for obsessive-compulsive spectrum disorders than dizygotic twins [14], with heritability calculated at between 26% and 33% [14,15]. Although all the results found higher concordance rates for monozygotic twins than for dizygotic twins, the transmission in monozygotic twins has been shown to be incomplete, indicating that environmental factors such as birth complications and other physiologic vulnerabilities may have significance in the development of OCD.

The genetics of obsessive-compulsive disorder

Once sufficient evidence for the familial transmission of OCD has been obtained, the next step is to determine whether genetic factors are responsible for the observed familiality, and, if so, the mode of genetic transmission. Using complex segregation analysis in a sample of individuals diagnosed as having OCD, chronic motor tics, or Tourette's syndrome, Nicolini and colleagues [16] found that the autosomal-dominant model was most compatible with the observed levels of segregation. Because of the small numbers of probands included in the study, neither the autosomal-dominant nor autosomal-recessive model could be rejected, indicating that OCD cannot be explained by a simple mode of transmission.

Cavallini and colleagues [17] confirmed the presence of a major locus with Mendelian properties accounting for most of the genetic liability to OCD. They could not, however, exclude the possibility of potential heterogeneity in their model when the phenotypic boundaries were widened to include OCD, Tourette's syndrome, and chronic motor tics. They also noted differential penetrance values for OCD phenotypes between males and females, with females exhibiting slightly higher penetrance values. In an attempt to limit the phenotypic heterogeneity of OCD, Alsobrook and colleagues [18] categorized families in the sample according to four factor analytic symptom dimensions of OCD. Segregation analysis of 96 families allowed rejection only of the no-transmission model, providing evidence that OCD is genetically transmitted, although no specific mode of transmission could be specified. When only the families of probands with high symmetry/ordering scores were analyzed, only the polygenic mode of inheritance was rejected, indicating the involvement of a major locus.

Nestadt and colleagues [19] found that neither Mendelian dominant nor codominant models could be rejected, indicating the involvement of a major locus. Unexplained familial factors were also observed to be important in the expression of OCD, however. For example, significant heterogeneity on the basis of gender of the proband was detected. This finding prompted separate segregation analyses of families with male and female probands. The transmission of OCD in female-proband families was compatible with the Mendelian major locus (either dominant or codominant) model; although a Mendelian mode of transmission also was found to be the most compatible in the male-proband families, the details of this model were less evident than for the female group.

In the most recent complex segregation analysis conducted, Hanna and colleagues [4] found evidence for a major susceptibility locus in families ascertained through probands with early-onset OCD. As with the previously mentioned complex segregation analysis by Nestadt and colleagues [19], however, Mendelian models were found to explain the observed familial aggregation only partially, with residual familial effects also playing a role in the expression of the disorder. Families ascertained through female probands allowed the rejection of the recessive Mendelian model, whereas those ascertained through male probands did not. Moreover, under the dominant model, females were found to have a higher penetrance than males, in line with previous results obtained by Nestadt and colleagues [19].

Thus, collective evidence from the segregation analyses indicates that the familial transmission of OCD is caused, in part at least, by genetic factors, and that this mode of inheritance is not simple. The genetic contribution to the disorder is probably complex, representing a mixed mode of transmission, involving genes of major effect with appreciable impact operating against a milieu of polygenic inheritance. Once it has been proven that genetic transmission accounts for at least some of the familiality of a disorder, the next logical step is to locate the susceptibility genes.

Linkage studies in obsessive-compulsive disorder

Genetic linkage analysis provides a powerful approach with which to elucidate the underlying genetic factors in inherited disorders. The objective of linkage analysis is to establish the co-segregation of polymorphic genetic markers of known chromosomal location with the disease phenotype within a family unit or pedigree (ie, the nonrandom sharing of marker alleles between affected members of each family).

To date, one genome-wide linkage study involving OCD has been published [20]. This study used seven probands whose age at onset was between 3 and 14 years. Fifty-six individuals from seven families were initially genotyped with 349 microsatellite markers spaced at an average of 11.3 centi-Morgan. A region on the telomere of chromosome 9p met the criterion for suggestive linkage, and weak evidence for linkage was observed on chromosomes 2q, 6q, 16q, 17q, and 19q. The investigators followed up their initial findings on chromosomes 2q, 9p, and 16q by genotyping 24 additional markers in the original 56 subjects and in 10 additional family members from one of the families. They found the region that displayed the strongest evidence for linkage was 9p24.

Recently, the evidence for linkage on 9p24 has been replicated [21] using 50 pedigrees from the John Hopkins OCD family study [3]. The 9p24 chromosomal region spans approximately 75 megabases and thus contains numerous potential candidate genes that could be investigated for a possible role in the development of OCD. Veenstra-vanderWeele and colleagues [22] conducted a mutation screen on one such candidate, the gene encoding the neuronal and epithelial glutamate transporter, *EAAC1*. They reported two exonic synonymous single nucleotide polymorphisms and six intronic polymorphisms that did not seem to alter the functioning of the gene. Using a family-based association study, however, the investigators observed no statistically significant association between two of the intronic polymorphisms and OCD. In an attempt to improve the power of the previous studies and to replicate the results [21], a collaborative effort is underway to collect almost 300 sib-pair and multiplex families.

Association studies in obsessive-compulsive disorder

Association studies offer an alternative strategy for studying genetic factors involved in complex psychiatric disorders. The aim of the association study is to demonstrate a significantly different distribution of allelic variants in affected (case) and unaffected (control) individuals. To date, no genome-wide association study of OCD has been completed, and most of the genetic analyses have been based on candidate gene analyses in the context of population- or family-based association studies. A candidate gene is one that, on the basis of prior physiologic, genetic, or biochemical characterization, is suspected to contribute to the etiology of the disorder under investigation.

The probability that a candidate gene is involved in the etiology of OCD is increased if it is found to be transcribed at fairly high levels in the tissue affected by the pathologic process. It thus is imperative to take the neurobiologic and neurochemical etiology of OCD into account when choosing candidates for investigation in genetic association studies. Results from cumulative functional and structural neuroimaging studies have converged to form a relatively cohesive picture implicating a dysfunction in the cortico-striato-thalamo-cortical (CSTC) network (a neuronal loop linking the basal ganglia and frontal association areas [23]) in the pathology of OCD [24–35].

Obviously, from a genetics point of view, the main interest would be to identify the neurotransmitter systems that play a role in the proposed CSTC dysfunction in OCD. The CSTC circuitry is innervated by a variety of neurotransmitter pathways. Serotonin (5-HT) and dopamine serve to modulate the activity of efferents from the basal ganglia, whereas glutamate has been found to moderate excitatory inputs to the network [36]. These neurotransmitter systems thus play a pivotal role in maintaining physiologic and psychological processes in the brain and represent a particularly rich area for research into the biologic basis of OCD.

The serotonergic hypothesis of obsessive-compulsive disorder

At present, one of the main neurobiologic hypotheses regarding the pathophysiology of OCD is that OCD results from an abnormality in the brain 5-HT system, mainly because serotonin-reuptake inhibitors (SRIs) demonstrate better clinical efficacy than other pharmacotherapeutic agents in treating the disorder [37–39]. A number of genetic association studies (both case-control and family-based) have been conducted in various populations to investigate the possible contribution of genes encoding components within the 5-HT system to the etiology of OCD and related subtypes (Tables 1A, 1B, and 1C).

Serotonin transporter

The serotonin transporter (5-HTT) is expressed both peripherally and in the brain and may be important in the pathogenesis of OCD because it represents the primary target on which SRIs act. A common insertion/deletion polymorphism (creating either long (L) and short (S) alleles) (5-$HTTLPR$) in the promoter region of the 5-HTT gene (5-HTT) has been shown to affect basal transcriptional activity, with the S-allele reported to result in lower levels and activity of 5-HTT [40,41].

In a transmission disequilibrium test (TDT) association study between 5-HTT and OCD, McDougle and colleagues [42] found that the L-allele of 5-$HTTLPR$ was significantly more commonly transmitted by heterozygous parents to their OCD-affected offspring. Similarly, in a population-based association study, Bengel and colleagues [43] found that patients who had OCD were more likely than controls to carry two copies of the 5-$HTTLPR$ L-allele. These statistically significant results were not confirmed in recently conducted genetic association studies performed by Frisch and colleagues [44], Camarena and colleagues [45], Cavallini and colleagues [46], Walitza and colleagues [47], Meira-Lima and colleagues [48], Chabane and colleagues [49], or Kinnear and colleagues [50], who subsequently performed a meta-analysis using results obtained from population-based studies by Bengel and colleagues [43] and McDougle and colleagues [42] and found that the results remained

Table 1A
Published population and family-based genetic association studies in OCD: serotonergic candidate genes

Gene/Variant	Population	Study design	Phenotype investigated	Sample number			Result (p-values, and implicated risk allele)	Reference
				Affected				
				Unrelated	Families	Control		
5-HTT								
	European-American	FB	OCD		35		P < .03 (L^a-allele)	[42]
	White American	CC	OCD	75		397	P = .023 (LL-genotype)	[43]
	Jewish (Ashkenazi [A] and non-A)	CC	OCD	75 (39 A)		172 (112 A)	NS	[44]
5-HTTLPR	South African Afrikaner	CC	OCD	54		82	NS	[50]
	Meta-analysis^b	CC	OCD	129		479	NS	[50]
	Mexican	CC/FB	OCD	115	43	136	NS	[45]
	Italian	CC	OCD	180		112	NS	[46]
	German	FB	OCD		63		NS	[47]
	Brazilian	CC	OCD	79		202	NS	[48]
	French/German	CC/FB	OCD	106	86	171	NS	[49]

Abbreviations: CC, population-based case-control association; FB, family-based association; NS, non-significant finding (*P* > .05); L, long allele, OCD, obsessive-compulsive disorder; *5-HT*, serotonin transporter; *5-HTTLPR*, variable number of tandem repeat polymorphism in the promoter region of 5-HTT, producing either long (*L*) or short (*S*) alleles.

[a] *L* refers to the "long" allele.

[b] Studies included in meta-analysis [50] are references 42, 43 and 50.

nonsignificant, even in a larger, more statistically powerful cohort. These results are summarized in Table 1A.

Serotonin receptor type 2A

A wide range of pharmacologic and genetic evidence implicates the serotonin receptor type 2A ($5-HT_{2A}$) in the pathophysiology of OCD. Recent case reports indicate that the chronic use of hallucinogenic drugs, which are potent stimulators of the $5-HT_{2A}$ receptor, may have beneficial effects in individuals who have OCD and related obsessive-compulsive spectrum disorders [51–53], suggesting a beneficial role of $5-HT_{2A}$ receptor activation. Supporting this notion is the increasing number of reports that describe the tendency of clozapine, a $5-HT_{2A}$ receptor antagonist, to unmask obsessive-compulsive symptoms in schizophrenic subjects [54–56].

The gene encoding the $5-HT_{2A}$ receptor has been widely investigated for its potential role in the etiology of OCD. Two variants in particular, one occurring near the promoter region (*-1438 A/G*) and a silent variation reported to be in linkage disequilibrium with it in exon 1 (*T102C*), have been widely investigated for a possible role in mediating the development of the disorder (Table 1B). Although the function of these two polymorphisms is presently under debate [57–61], OCD has been found to be associated with the *A* allele of the *-1438 G/A* promoter polymorphism [62,63] (see Table 1B). This association, however, was observed only in female subjects, perhaps indicating differential 5-HT effects operating in men and women who have OCD. These results were replicated in a study by Walitza and colleagues [64], who found that the *A*-allele was associated with OCD in German children and adolescents. These results were not replicated in a subsequent population-based association study, however [65].

A number of studies have also investigated the *T102C* polymorphism for association with OCD, although none have yielded significant findings in Mexican [66], Jewish [44], Afrikaner [67,68], Turkish [65], or Brazilian [48] populations (see Table 1B). Tot and colleagues [65] found that although neither the *T102C* or the *-1438A/G* polymorphisms were associated with OCD per se, the *T102T* genotype from the *T102C* variant and the *AA* genotype from the *-1438A/G* variant were associated with increased severity of OCD, as measured by scores on the Yale–Brown Obsessive Compulsive Scale (Y–BOCS). Moreover, although Meira-Lima and colleagues [48] observed no association between the *T102C* polymorphism and OCD, they did observe an association between the silent *C516T* variant and OCD. No function has been ascribed to this variant, indicating that a variant in linkage disequilibrium with *C516T* may be associated with OCD, although this hypothesis requires empiric investigation.

Serotonin receptor type 2C

Numerous animal and pharmacologic studies have suggested the possible involvement of serotonin receptor type 2C ($5-HT_{2C}$) in the etiology of OCD

Table 1B
Published population and family-based genetic association studies in obsessive-disorder: serotonergic candidate genes

Gene/Variant	Population	Study design	Phenotype investigated	Sample number		Result (p-values, and implicated risk allele)	Reference
				Affected	Control		
5-HT$_{2A}$	North American white	CC	OCD	62	144	A-allele increased in OCD patients $P < .05$	[62]
-1438A/G	North American white	CC	OCD	101	138	$P = .015$ and $P = .023$ (allele and genotype); A-allele in females	[63]
	German	CC	OCD	55	223	$P = .046$ (genotype) A-allele	[64]
	Mexican	CC	OCD	67	54	NS	[66]
	Jewish (Ashkenazi [A] and non-Ashkenazi)	CC	OCD	75 (39 A)	172 (112 A)	NS	[44]
	Afrikaners	CC	OCD	71	129	NS	[67]
T102C	South African whites, stratified into Afrikaner	CC	Early-onset[a] OCD versus late-onset OCD	Early-onset = 95 (45 Afrikaner) Late-onset = 85 (35 Afrikaner)		NS	[68]

	Population	CC	Comparison	Cases	Controls	Result	Ref
			OCD	58	83	NS	
			OCD + tics versus OCD − tics	OCD + tics = 8		NS	
T102C & -1438A/G	Turkish	CC	FH OCD versus no FH OCD	FH OCD = 27		NS	[65]
			SRI response versus no SRI response	SRI response = 35		NS	
C561T 5-HT$_{2C}$ ser23cys	Brazilian	CC	OCD	79	202	$P = 7 \times 10^{-5}$ (C-allele)	[48]
			OCD	109	107	NS	
	Italian	CC	OCD + tics versus OCD − tics	OCD + tics = 23		NS	[77]
	Jewish (Ashkenazi [A] and non-Ashkenazi)	CC	OCD	75 (39 A)	172 (112 A)	NS	[44]

Abbreviations: CC, population-based case-control association; FH, family history; NS, non-significant finding ($P > .05$); OCD, Obsessive-compulsive disorder; SRI, serotonin-reuptake inhibitor; 5-HT$_{2A}$, serotonin receptor 2A; 5-HT$_{2C}$, serotonin receptor 2C.

[a] EO OCD ≤ 15 years.

or OCD-related disorders. $5-HT_{2C}$-knockout mice have been found to exhibit compulsive-like syndromes [69], and pharmacologic studies have indicated an acute worsening of obsessive-compulsive symptoms after the administration of the selective $5-HT_{2C}/5-HT_{1A}/5-HT_{1D}$ agonist, m-CPP. In addition, a recent study using an animal model of OCD suggests that the $5-HT_{2C}$ receptors are probably involved in the exacerbation of obsessive-compulsive symptoms after m-CPP administration [70]. It has also been suggested that chronic treatment with selective serotonin-reuptake inhibitors (SSRIs) could result in the reduction of mesocorticolimbic dopaminergically mediated transmission by $5-HT_{2C}$ activation, representing an important step in therapeutic efficacy of SSRIs [71,72].

A structural variant in the extracellular N-terminal region of the receptor, resulting in a cysteine-to-serine amino acid substitution at position 23 (cys23ser), has been described [73], but its functional significance is not yet clear [74–76]. In a case-control genetic association study to assess the relationship between the $5-HT_{2C}$ receptor and OCD, Cavallini and colleagues [77] found no significant association between the $5-HT_{2C}$ cys23ser variant and OCD in an Italian population or between the variant and a subgroup of subjects who had OCD stratified according to the presence or absence of tics. Likewise, Frisch and colleagues [44] observed no statistically significant differences in genotypic or allelic distribution between patients who had OCD and controls drawn from both an Ashkenazi Jewish population and a non-Ashkenazi Jewish population (see Table 1B).

Serotonin receptor type 1Dβ

Preclinical evidence of the role that the serotonin type 1Dβ ($5-HT_{1Dβ}$) autoreceptor may play in OCD has been obtained from animal studies, where it was found that the enhanced release of 5-HT in the orbito-frontal cortex brought about by SRIs was attributable to the desensitization of the $5-HT_{1Dβ}$ auto-receptor [78]. The putative role that the $5-HT_{1Dβ}$ auto-receptor may play in the mediation of OCD in humans has been investigated using pharmacologic challenge with 5-HT probes, namely m-CPP and sumatriptan, both of which have been found to exacerbate obsessive-compulsive symptoms [79–82].

Evidence from two genetic studies using TDT analysis has implicated the possible involvement of the $5-HT_{1Dβ}$ auto-receptor in the etiology of OCD (Table 1C) [83,84]. In these studies, a significant association was observed between the distribution of the silent polymorphic G861C allelic variant of the $5-HT_{1Dβ}$ and OCD, with preferential transmission of the G-allele to the affected subjects. These results have not been replicated in subsequent family [47,85,86] and population-based [67,68] association studies, however (see Table 1C). Although Camarena and colleagues [86] observed no significant association between G861C and the *Diagnostic and Statistical Manual of Mental Disorders*, fourth edition diagnosis of OCD, they did observe that subjects who had a preferential transmission of *G861* exhibited higher Y–BOCS obsession scores than those who had the *C861* allele. Mundo and colleagues [84] observed no such association in their sample.

Tryptophan hydroxylase

Tryptophan hydroxylase (TPH) represents the rate-limiting step in the synthesis of 5-HT and therefore represents an important candidate gene. Recently, TPH has been found to occur in two differentially expressed forms: *TPH1* has been detected only in the periphery (mainly the blood and duodenum) and not in the brain, whereas *TPH2* has been identified exclusively in the brain [87,88].

Two association studies, both investigating genetic variants in *TPH1*, have yielded no significant association between the gene and OCD (see Table 1C) [44,47]. Results from a more recent investigation focusing on two variants in *TPH2* indicate that the gene may be involved in the etiology of early-onset OCD [89] (see Table 1C).

The dopaminergic hypothesis of obsessive-compulsive disorder

Dopaminergic dysregulation is thought to contribute to the pathophysiology of OCD based on neurobiologic and pharmacologic data obtained from humans and animals. In animal models, agents that increase synaptic dopamine levels produce stereotypies and repetitive behavior that resemble some of the symptomatology manifested by individuals who have OCD [90–92]. In addition, a novel transgenic mouse expressing a neuropotentiating transgene in a subset of neurons expressing dopamine receptor (DRD)-1 in regions of the amygdala and cortical areas that project to the orbitofrontal cortex and striatum has recently been characterized. Chronic potentiation of these neurons (known to induce efferent glutamatergic neurotransmission to the striatum) resulted in the transgenic mice exhibiting Tourette's syndrome/OCD-like behaviors, including repeated leaping, OCD-like persistent grooming, nonaggressive OCD-like repeated biting of cage mates, episodes of repetition or perseverance of normal behaviors, and repeated climbing or leaping and tics [93–96]. More recently, results from a dopamine transporter (DAT)-knockdown mouse model indicate that hyperdopaminergic mice exhibit excessively strong and rigid manifestations of a complex, fixed action pattern (thought to characterize a number of human disorders involving the basal ganglia, including OCD and Tourette's syndrome), in comparison with wild-type mice [97].

In pharmacologic-challenge studies, the function of the dopaminergic system in a group of individuals who had OCD was investigated by measuring growth hormone [98] and cortisol [99] responses to stimulation with apomorphine. Inconsistent results in the two studies suggest heterogeneity in the dopaminergic system functions in OCD, with dopamine neurotransmission

Table 1C
Published population and family-based genetic association studies in obsessive-compulsive disorder: serotonergic candidate genes

Gene/ Variant	Population	Study design	Phenotype investigated	Sample number Affected Unrelated	Families	Control	Result (p-values, and implicated risk allele)	Reference
5-HT$_{1D\beta}$								
G861C	Italian	FB	OCD		32		$P < .006$ (*G*-allele)	[83]
			OCD		121		$P = .023$ (*G*-allele)	
			Age at onset (quantitative)		30		NS	
	Italian	FB	Y–BOCS obsession score		37		NS	[84]
			Y–BOCS compulsion score		37		NS	
			Y–BOCS total score		37		NS	
			OCD		48		NS	
			Y–BOCS compulsion score		48		NS	
			Y–BOCS obsession score		48		NS	
	Italian	FB	Y–BOCS total score		48		NS	[85]
			FH OCD versus no FH OCD		FH OCD = 18		NS	
			FH (tics) versus no FH (tics)		FH tics = 5		NS	
			OCD + tics versus OCD – tics		OCD + tics = 9		NS	
	Afrikaners	CC	OCD	71		129	NS	[67]
	Mexican	FB	OCD		47		NS	[86]

Gene/SNP	Population	Type	Phenotype	Sample	Result	Ref
	German	FB	Y–BOCS compulsion score	29	NS	
	South African whites, stratified into Afrikaner	CC	Y–BOCS obsession score	29	$P = .034$ (G-allele)	
	German	FB	OCD	64	NS	[47]
		CC	Early-onset[a] OCD versus Late-onset OCD	Early-onset = 95 (45 Afrikaner) Late-nser = 85 (35 Afrikaner)	NS	[68]
TPH rs1800532 (*TPH1*)	Jewish (Ashkenazi [A] and non-Ashkenazi)	CC	OCD	75 (39 A), 172 (112 A)	NS	[44]
rs4570625 and rs4565946 (*TPH2*)	German	FB	OCD	59	NS	[47]
	German	FB	Early-onset OCD[b]	71	the rs4570625-rs4565946 G-C haplotype was transmitted more frequently to OCD patients ($P = .035$)	[89]

Abbreviations: CC, population-based case-control association; FB, family-based association; NS, nonsignificant finding ($P > .05$); OCD, obsessive-compulsive disorder; *TPH*, tryptophan hydroxylase; Y–BOCS, Yale Brown Obsessive-Compulsive Scale; 5-$HT_{1D\beta}$, serotonin receptor 1Dβ.

[a] Early-onset OCD age ≤15 years.

[b] OCD patient sample of children and adolescents had a mean age at onset of OCD of 11.73 years.

being impaired in brain regions related to obsessive-compulsive pathology and normal in other brain regions [99]. Finally, a significant improvement has been noted in patients who have OCD and do not respond to SSRIs when neuroleptics, which are primarily dopamine antagonists, are added to the ongoing SRI monotherapy [100–102].

Dopamine receptor 4

DRD4 is of interest in molecular studies of psychiatric disorders because of its involvement in higher brain functions and its modulatory role in dopamine synthesis and turnover in the brain [103]. Indeed, it has been widely investigated to determine its role in the development of OCD (see Table 2A). In the gene encoding DRD4, a variable number of tandem repeats (VNTR) polymorphisms, occurring within the third cytoplasmic loop (situated in the third exon), has been of great interest in psychiatric genetic investigations. This polymorphism consists of a variable number of imperfect 48–base pair (bp) motifs that may be repeated between 2 and 10 times [104,105].

At present, no major functional consequences of the polymorphism have been elucidated, although small effects on signaling efficiency have been reported. Studies have indicated that the seven-repeat allele (*A7*) possesses the ability to blunt the receptor's response for the reduction of cyclic AMP, requiring at least threefold more dopamine to induce responses similar in magnitude to receptors containing *A4* alleles [104,106]. One of the earliest published studies reported on the significantly higher frequency of *A7* among Mexican individuals who had OCD and who presented with comorbid tics, compared with patients who had OCD who did not have comorbid tics [107]. Moreover, Billet and colleagues [108] observed statistically significant differences in overall allele distribution between Canadian subjects who had OCD and controls, although this association did not remain significant after correcting for multiple testing (see Table 2A).

On the other hand, Frisch and colleagues [44] observed a reduced number of *A7* alleles among patients who had OCD compared with healthy controls, although the authors concede that this significant finding may be as a result of a type I error resulting from multiple testing. This result was not replicated in a larger French study, which used both family- and population-based designs [109]. This same investigation did however, report a significantly lower frequency of *A2* among patients who had OCD than in a control cohort and replicated this result in a subsequent family study. Their results remain significant even after correction for multiple testing. These results were not replicated in a study published by the authors' group [67], however, which found no statistically significant differences in either allele or genotype distribution between Afrikaner subjects who had and Afrikaner controls. In a more recent study, when a South African group of white patients who had OCD was stratified categorically according to age at onset of the disorder, a statistically significant difference was noted in the allelic distribution between

Table 2A
Published population and family-based genetic association studies in obsessive-compulsive disorder: dopaminergic candidate genes

Gene/Variant	Population	Study design	Phenotype investigated	Sample number			Results (p-value and allele implicated)	Reference
				Affected				
				Case	Families	Control		
DRD4								
48 bp VNTR	Mexican	CC	OCD + tics versus OCD – tics	61 (OCD + tics = 12)			$P = .018$	[107]
	North American white	CC	OCD	118		118	$P = .021$; NS for genotype (overall allele frequency)	[108]
	Jewish (Ashkenazi [A] and non-Ashkenazi)	CC	OCD	75 (39 A)		172 (112 A)	non-Ashkenazi: *A7* less frequent in OCD ($P = .04$) CC: $P < 1 \times 10^{-4}$ (genotype); $P = 1 \times 10^{-4}$ (allele)	[44]
	French	CC/FB	OCD	49	34	63	FB: $P = .03$ for genotype and allele analyses Both implicated *A2* as protective allele	[109]
			OCD + tics versus OCD – tics	OCD + tics = 16			NS	
	Afrikaner	CC	OCD	71		129	NS	[67]
	South African whites, stratified into Afrikaner	CC	Early-onset[a] OCD versus late-onset OCD	Early-onset = 95 (45 Afrikaner) Late-onset = 85 (35 Afrikaner)			South African whites: $P = .0128$ (overall allele frequency); NS for Afrikaners	[68]

Abbreviations: *A7*, *DRD4* 48bp VNTR 7-repeat allele; *A2*, *DRD4* 48bp VNTR 2-repeat allele; CC, case-control; *DRD4*, dopamine receptor 4; FB, family-based; OCD, obsessive-compulsive disorder; NS, nonsignificant ($P > .05$); VNTR: variable number of tandem repeats polymorphism.

[a] Early-onset OCD age ≤ 15 years.

early- and late-onset OCD, although no significant differences were noted in the genotypic distribution [68]. These results are summarized in Table 2A.

Dopamine receptor 2

Dopamine receptor 2 (DRD2) is expressed throughout the brain but is found at high levels in the basal ganglia [110]. Recent evidence from structural, functional, clinical, and genetic studies indicates that the role of *DRD2* in mediating the development of OCD merits study. Chronic administration of inositol to rats has been found to result in a significant decrease in DRD2 density [111], which is interesting because inositol has been found to be effective in the treatment of OCD [112]. These findings suggest that a state of hyper-responsiveness of DRD2 may contribute to the pathology of the disorder [111]. Additional support for the role of DRD2 in OCD has been obtained from a recent functional study in which lower left caudate DRD2-binding ratios were observed in patients who had OCD than in controls. The binding ratios in the left caudate were also found to be lower than those in the right caudate in the same patients [113].

A case-control study conducted in a Mexican sample demonstrated an association between the homozygous *A2* genotype of the *Taq*IA polymorphism and patients who had OCD and comorbid tic disorder [66]. Fifty-eight percent of the patients presenting with comorbid tic disorder possessed the *A2/A2* genotype, whilst only 27% of the OCD patients without tic disorder carried the genotype (Table 2B). The investigators, however, did not observe any significant association of the polymorphism when comparing the genotype and allele distribution of the polymorphism in the unstratified sample of patients who had OCD and controls. In a population-based case-control study by Billet and colleagues [108], no statistical significance was observed between either the *DRD2 Taq*IA polymorphism or a serine to cysteine missense mutation occurring in the seventh exon and OCD. These results are summarized in Table 2B.

Dopamine receptor 3

Pharmacologic evidence supports the role of dopamine receptor 3 (DRD3) in anxiety: dopaminergic antagonists acting at the receptor have been found to exhibit anxiolytic properties, and the receptor has been found to possess affinities for typical neuroleptics similar to those of DRD2 [114,115], although it also has been found to exhibit a high affinity for atypical neuroleptics [116]. Moreover, it has been suggested that expression and function of DRD3 are reduced during stress and depression and that chronic treatment with noradrenergic and SRIs increases DRD3 mRNA, thereby reversing the initial effect of stress [117].

One of the most widely studied single-nucleotide polymorphisms in *DRD3* is characterized by an *A*-to-*G* transition occurring in the N-terminal extracellular domain in the first exon. The transition is nonsynonymous, representing a *gly*-to-*ser* amino acid substitution at codon position 9 (*ser9gly*). Although the polymorphism results in a modified protein sequence, the functional consequences have yet to be elucidated. The earliest study conducted to determine whether any association exists between the *ser9gly* variant and OCD, OCD with or without tics, or a family history of OCD and tics was by Catalano and colleagues [118] (see Table 2B). No statistically significant differences were observed in genotype or allele frequencies between the OCD and controls, or between the various OCD sample subsets. The authors note that this investigation should be viewed as preliminary, because the power of the study to detect a small effect was comparatively low (0.30), in view of the small sample size. Neither Nicolini and colleagues [66] nor Billet and colleagues [108] observed any association between the *ser9gly* variant and OCD; the results of these studies are summarized in Table 2B.

The dopamine transporter gene

The dopamine transporter (DAT or SLC6A3) plays a pivotal role in the removal of dopamine from the synapse in the midbrain. The reuptake and diffusion of dopamine by DAT alters the magnitude, duration, and spatial domain of transmitter-induced receptor activation, thereby modifying dopaminergic neurotransmission [119,120]. DAT may constitute an important component in the etiology of OCD, because DAT-knockdown mice have been shown to exhibit excessive sequential stereotypy of behavioral patterns, characteristic of disorders of the basal ganglia such as OCD and Tourette's syndrome [97].

A polymorphic VNTR is found in the genomic sequence encoding the 3' untranslated region of DAT [121–123]. The number of repeats in the VNTR may vary from 3 to 11 [121,124,125]. The function of the polymorphism is presently unclear: investigations have yielded contradictory results [126–128]. The association between the *DAT* 40-bp VNTR and increased susceptibility to OCD has been investigated in four separate studies, all of which yielded negative results (see Table 2B) [44,67,68,108].

Monoamine oxidase A

Monoamine oxidase (MAO) A is a mitochondrial outer membrane enzyme that plays an important role in the degradation of several biogenic amines, including 5-HT and dopamine [129]. The enzyme occurs in two forms, MAO-A and MAO-B, which can be distinguished by molecular weight, substrate affinities, and immunologic properties. MAO-A is present in catecholaminergic neurons in the brain and plays an important role in the metabolic degradation of norepinephrine, epinephrine, and 5-HT [130]. Two polymorphisms, both in linkage disequilibrium and both related to levels of enzymatic activity [131], have been investigated for a possible role in OCD.

Table 2B
Published population and family-based genetic association studies in obsessive-compulsive disorder: dopaminergic candidate genes

Gene/ Variant	Population	Study design	Phenotype investigated	Sample number Affected Case	Families	Control	Results (p-value and allele implicated)	Reference
DRD2								
Taq1A	Mexican	CC	OCD				NS	
			OCD + tics (n = 12) versus control	67		54	P = .014 (CC -genotype implicated as risk factor)	[66]
ser311cys	North American white	CC	OCD	110		110	NS	[108]
DRD3			OCD	97		97	NS	
	Italian	CC	OCD + tics versus OCD − tics	OCD + tics = 19			NS	[118]
ser9gly			FH OCD versus no FH OCD	FH OCD = 9			NS	
	Mexican	CC	OCD	67		54	NS	[66]
	North American white	CC	OCD	103		103	NS	[108]

Gene/polymorphism	Population		Phenotype				Reference
DAT 3' UTR 40bp VNTR	North American white	CC	OCD	103	103	NS	[108]
	Jewish (Ashkenazi [A] and non-A)	CC	OCD	75 (39 A)	172 (112 A)	NS	[44]
	Afrikaners	CC	OCD	71	129	NS	[67]
	South African whites, stratified into Afrikaner	CC	Early-onset[a] OCD versus late-onset OCD	Early-onset = 95 (45 Afrikaner) late-onset = 85 (35 Afrikaner)		NS	[68]

Abbreviations: bp, base pair; *DAT*, dopamine transporter; *DRD2*, dopamine receptor 2; *DRD3*, dopamine receptor 3; CC, case-control; FB, family-based; FH, family history; NS, non-significant ($P > .05$); OCD, obsessive-compulsive disorder; UTR, untranslated region; VNTR, variable number of tandem repeats polymorphism.

[a] Early-onset OCD, age ≤ 15 years.

Table 2C
Published population and family-based genetic association studies in obsessive-compulsive disorder: dopaminergic candidate genes

Gene	Population	Study design	Phenotype investigated	Sample number Affected Case	Families	Control	Results (p-value and allele implicated)	Reference
MAO-A								
		FB	OCD		110		Males: $P = .0186$ for *G*-allele as risk factor	
exon8 *T/G*	North American		OCD + MDD versus OCD − MDD (males only)		25		$P = .0004$ (*G*-allele as risk factor)	[132]
			OCD	122	51 (19 females)	124	CC: Females $P = .024$; FB: Females $P = .022$ (*T*-allele as risk factor)	[133]
Exon14 *T1046C*	Mexican	CC / FB	OCD + MDD versus OCD − MDD	OCD + MDD = 37			Significant in females; data not provided	
	Afrikaner	CC	OCD	71		129	NS	[67]

COMT val158met

Population					Result	Ref.
North American white	CC	OCD	73	148	$P = 2 \times 10^{-4}$ (LL[a] genotype and L-allele as risk factor in males)	[138]
North American white	FB	OCD		110 (54 male)	Males (for L-allele as risk factor); $P = .0079$	[132]
Not specified	FB	OCD		67	Homozygosity for H[b] or L allele as risk factors; $P = .006$[c]	[140]
Afrikaner	CC	OCD	54	54	$P = .0017$ (HL genotype as risk factor)	[141]
Probands collected from Israel, France and United States	FB	OCD		56	$P = .048$ (L-allele as risk factor in females) NS in males	[139]
Japanese	CC	OCD	17	35	NS	[143]
Turkish	CC	OCD	59	114	NS	[142]
Meta-analysis[d]		OCD	144	337	NS	[144]
Brazilian	CC	OCD	79	202	NS	[48]

Abbreviations: CC, case-control; *COMT*, catechol-O-methyltransferase; FB, family-based; *MAO-A*, monoamine oxidase A; MDD, major depressive disorder; OCD, obsessive-compulsive disorder.

[a] L refers to the *COMT val158met* low-activity allele (*met158*, or *A*).

[b] H refers to the *COMT val158met* high activity allele (*val158*, or *G*).

[c] Noninformative matings excluded.

[d] Studies included in meta-analysis [143] included investigations by references 131, 137–140, 142.

Table 3
Published genetic association studies in OCD: *GRIN2B*, *GRIK 2* and *-3*, *GABBR1*, *BDNF* and *MOG* genes

Gene	Population	Study design	Phenotype investigated	Affected Unrelated	Affected Families	Controls	Results (p-value and allele implicated)	Reference
GRIN2B								
5072T/G *5988T/C* *5806A/C*	Canadian	FB	OCD		130		*5072 T*-allele associated with OCD under recessive model (*P* = .014) *5072G-5988T* haplotype associated with OCD under recessive model (*P* = .002)	[145]
			total Y–BOCS score		98		Trend for increased transmission of *5072T*-allele under recessive model	
GRIK2 and *GRIK3* *GRIK2:* rs2227281, rs2227283, rs2235076 (*M867I*) *GRIK3:* rs6691840	European	CC and FB	OCD	156	156	141	FB: *I867*-allele undertransmitted (*P* = .03)	[146]
GABBR1 *A-7265G* *C10497G* *ser491ser* *phe659phe* *A33795G* *T1977G*	Canadian	FB	OCD		159		*–7625A P* = .006 *phe659phe A P* = .032	[147]

BDNF						
SNP1: rs988748 (*C/G*)	N.American	FB	OCD: Early-onset[a] versus late-onset	164 Early-onset = 120	SNP1: *C*-allele *P* = .003 SNP2: *T*-allele *P* = .020 SNP3: *G*-allele *P* = .001 SNP4: *C*-allele *P* = .0025 (*CA*) microsatellite allele 3 overtransmitted in EO	[148]
SNP2: rs2049046 (*A/T*)						
SNP3: rs6265 (*G/A*)						
SNP4: 3′UTR *C/G*						
(*CA*) microsatellite in intron 5						
MOG						
C1334T			OCD	160	*P* = .022 (*MOG4* 2-repeat allele) *MOG4* 2-repeat-*MOG2* 13 repeat haplotype: *P* = .011	[149]
C10991T						
MOG2 dinucleotide repeat	Canadian	FB				
MOG4 tetranucleotide repeat			Total Y–BOCS score	160	*P* = .020 (*MOG4* 2-repeat allele)	

Abbreviations: *BDNF*, brain-derived neurotrophic factor; *GABBR*, gamma-aminobutyric acid type B receptor 1; *GRIK2*, kainate glutamate receptor 2; *GRIK3*, kainate glutamate receptor 3; *GRIN2B*, glutamate receptor subtype 2B *MOG*, myelin oligodendrocyte; OCD, obsessive-compulsive disorder; SNP, single-nucleotide polymorphism; Y–BOCS, Yale Brown Obsessive-Compulsive scale.

[a] Early-onset OCD: age < 18 years.

In a family-based association study, Karayiorgou and colleagues [132] investigated a single nucleotide polymorphism occurring in exon 8 and found that the *G*-allele (correlating with lower enzymatic activity) was associated with OCD in males. Further investigation revealed that this allele was transmitted more frequently in male patients who had OCD presenting with comorbid major depressive disorder than in those without comorbid major depressive disorder. The second variant involves a *T*-to-*C* substitution in exon 14, with the *T*-allele corresponding to lower enzymatic activity [131]. This allele was found to be significantly more frequent among female patients who had OCD in both the family-based and population-based association studies conducted by Camarena and colleagues [133]. These results were not replicated in a subsequent population-based association study in the Afrikaner population, however [67]. Therefore, although the studies by Camarena and colleagues [133] and Karayiourgou and colleagues [131] indicate the possibility of a sexually dimorphic effect of *MAO-A* gene in OCD, the results are difficult to interpret, because different variants were analyzed in each study, and the gender found to be associated with the low-activity allele was different in each case. These results, coupled with the nonsignificant findings by Hemmings and colleagues [67], show the need for investigation in a larger sample that would impart more power to the analysis.

Catechol-O-methyltransferase

Catechol-O-methyltransferase (COMT) is an Mg^{2+}-dependent enzyme that is involved in the inactivation of catecholamines (norepinephrine, epinephrine, and dopamine) [134]. A widely studied polymorphism in *COMT*, a single nucleotide polymorphism involving a valine-to-methionine substitution at codon 158 (*val158met*), has been found to be co-dominantly associated with either the thermolabile (low activity, represented by the *met158* [*A*] allele) or thermostable (high activity; represented by the *val158* [*G*] allele) form of the enzyme [135–137].

COMT is an attractive candidate for OCD genetic studies (Table 2C). Numerous association studies, both family- and population-based, have investigated the possible role of the *val158met* polymorphism in the development of OCD. Initial reports were exciting: Karayiorgou and colleagues [138] observed a significant association between the *met158* (low-activity) allele and *met158/met158* genotype and OCD in a sample of North American males, although no association was observed for the female sample in the same study. Karayiorgou and colleagues [132] replicated these findings in a family-based sample, providing further indications of the role of *COMT* in the disorder. In an attempt to replicate the findings by Karayiourgou and colleagues [132,138], Alsobrook and colleagues [139] observed an association between the *met158/met158* genotype and OCD in females but not in males. Furthermore, although Schindler and colleagues [140] observed an association between homozygosity (either *met158/met158* or *val158/val158* genotypes) at the *val158met* locus and OCD, their findings were not gender-specific. In contrast, the authors' group, Niehaus and colleagues [141], investigated the relationship between the *val158met* polymorphism and OCD in an Afrikaner population and detected a non–gender-based positive association between the heterozygous (*val158/met158*) genotype and susceptibility to OCD.

On the other hand, no association between the polymorphism and OCD was detected in studies by Erdal and colleagues [142], Ohara and colleagues [143], or Meira-Lima and colleagues [48] or in a meta-analysis that included three case-control studies [138,141,143], three family-based studies [132,139,140], and one unpublished study (Veenstra-Vanderweele; see Azzam and colleagues [144]). These results are summarized in Table 2C.

Other plausible candidates

Although monoamine systems may well play a role in mediating OCD, a growing body of research is looking beyond the monoamine systems for alternative biologic underpinnings of the disorder, investigating other potential factors that may be implicated in the disorder, such as multiple downstream cellular pathways or neural circuits and GABAergic, glutaminergic, and peptidergic transmission. Indeed, recent investigations have indicated the possible role that variants in genes encoding glutamate (NMDA) subunit receptor (*GRIN2B*) [145], glutamate ionotropic kainite receptors 1 (*GRIK1*) and 3 (*GRIK3*) [146], GABA Type B receptor 1 (*GABBR1*) [147], brain-derived neurotrophic factor (*BDNF*) [148], and myelin oligodendrocyte glycoprotein (*MOG*) [149] may play in mediating the development of OCD (Table 3).

Summary

During the last 2 decades, a large number of association studies have been dedicated to disentangling the genetic components that may be involved in the etiology of OCD. The preliminary and frequently inconsistent nature of the data represented in the majority of OCD psychiatric genetic-association studies may seem discouraging. Failure to replicate, and thus to confirm, previously identified susceptibility loci could result from a number of reasons, including the potential for population admixture, the clinical heterogeneity of OCD, small sample sizes (and subsequent lack of power), publication bias, epistasis, or failure to account for multiple testing. Various methods of accounting for these confounders do exist and should be implemented in any genetic-association study that is to be regarded as robust and replicable. Discrepancy between results, however, might be ascribed to the underlying genetic differences between the populations in the respective studies (ie, the investigated variant may be in linkage disequilibrium with the causal variant in one population but not in another). Such discrepancies are difficult to reconcile in single-locus association studies; haplotype analyses (in which a number of variants, usually single-nucleotide polymorphisms occurring on the same gene, are analyzed as a unit) may be able to resolve these uncertainties. Investigating epistatic interactions between variants in other genes that might be involved in the same physiologic pathways would be an alternative means of deciphering the reason for discrepant genetic association results.

A valid means of increasing the power (by reducing background noise) would be to stratify the patient sample according to clinically defined subtypes, such as obsession and compulsion subtypes, age at onset of the disorder, and severity of the disorder. Although many of the OCD genetics studies have incorporated investigations of these subtypes [65,66,68,77,84–86,89,107,118,132,133,145,148,149], the number of subjects decreases after stratification, thereby limiting the power of the studies. It may therefore be useful to employ other quantitative approaches in the design of the investigation: the possibility should be considered that OCD symptoms can be broken down into multiple dimensions that are continuous with the normal population [150]. This division would represent an important route to disentangling the complex inheritance of OCD. The results obtained from genetic investigations should be incorporated with clinical and epidemiologic parameters to elucidate correctly the cause of OCD.

Future studies should also be extended to incorporate the screening of more polymorphisms, because high-resolution mapping within specific chromosomes will improve knowledge regarding the impact of genetic diversity within the genes or linked chromosomal regions in OCD. The advantages of a gene-based over a single-nucleotide polymorphism–based approach are becoming ever more apparent [151]. Therefore, a more complete assessment of candidate genes, possibly using haplotype blocks that span larger regions, is proposed. In addition, increasing the amount of information on human genome sequences and polymorphisms will make it possible to characterize the amount of sequence variation expressed in the brain and to delineate the potential effects that these variations may have on the development of OCD. Knowledge of new functional variants will emerge as researchers gain an understanding of the potential for genetic variants in the coding and regulatory regions to impact gene expression.

References

[1] Hettema JM, Neale MC, Kendler KS. A review and meta-analysis of the genetic epidemiology of anxiety disorders. Am J Psychiatry 2001;158(10):1568–78.
[2] Bellodi L, Sciuto G, Diaferia G, et al. Psychiatric disorders in the families of patients with obsessive-compulsive disorder. Psychiatry Res 1992;42(2):111–20.
[3] Nestadt G, Samuels J, Riddle M, et al. A family study of obsessive-compulsive disorder. Arch Gen Psychiatry 2000;57(4):358–63.

[4] Hanna GL, Fischer DJ, Chadha KR, et al. Familial and sporadic subtypes of early-onset obsessive-compulsive disorder. Biol Psychiatry 2005;57(8):895–900.

[5] Pauls DL, Alsobrook JP, Goodman W, et al. A family study of obsessive-compulsive disorder. Am J Psychiatry 1995;152(1):76–84.

[6] Pitman RK, Green RC, Jenike MA, et al. Clinical comparison of Tourette's disorder and obsessive-compulsive disorder. Am J Psychiatry 1987;144(9):1166–71.

[7] Grad LR, Pelcovitz D, Olson M, et al. Obsessive-compulsive symptomatology in children with Tourette's syndrome. J Am Acad Child Adolesc Psychiatry 1987;26(1):69–73.

[8] Inouye E. Similar and dissimilar manifestations of obsessive-compulsive neurosis in monozygotic twins. Am J Psychiatry 1965;121:1171.

[9] Rasmussen SA, Tsuang MT. Clinical characteristics and family history in DSM-III obsessive-compulsive disorder. Am J Psychiatry 1986;143(3):317–22.

[10] Carey G, Gotesman II. Twin and family studies of anxiety, phobic and obsessive disorders. In: Klien DF, Rabkin J, editors. Anxiety: new research and changing concepts. New York: Raven Press; 1981. p. 117–36.

[11] Skre I, Onstad S, Torgersen S, et al. A twin study of DSM-III-R anxiety disorders. Acta Psychiatr Scand 1993;88(2):85–92.

[12] Kim SW, Dysken MW, Kline MD. Monozygotic twins with obsessive-compulsive disorder. Br J Psychiatry 1990;156:435–8.

[13] McGuffin P, Mawson D. Obsessive-compulsive neurosis: two identical twin pairs. Br J Psychiatry 1980;137:285–7.

[14] Clifford CA, Murray RM, Fulker DW. Genetic and environmental influences on obsessional traits and symptoms. Psychol Med 1984;14(4):791–800.

[15] Jonnal AH, Gardner CO, Prescott CA, et al. Obsessive and compulsive symptoms in a general population sample of female twins. Am J Med Genet 2000;96(6):791–6.

[16] Nicolini H, Hanna G, Baxter L, et al. Segregation analyses of obsessive-compulsive and associated disorders: preliminary results. Ursus Medicus 1991;1:25–8.

[17] Cavallini MC, Pasquale L, Bellodi L, et al. Complex segregation analysis for obsessive compulsive disorder and related disorders. Am J Med Genet 1999;88(1):38–43.

[18] Alsobrook IJP II, Leckman JF, Goodman WK, et al. Segregation analysis of obsessive-compulsive disorder using symptom-based factor scores. Am J Med Genet 1999;88(6):669–75.

[19] Nestadt G, Lan T, Samuels J, et al. Complex segregation analysis provides compelling evidence for a major gene underlying obsessive-compulsive disorder and for heterogeneity by sex. Am J Hum Genet 2000;67(6):1611–6.

[20] Hanna GL, Veenstra-VanderWeele J, Cox NJ, et al. Genome-wide linkage analysis of families with obsessive-compulsive disorder ascertained through pediatric probands. Am J Med Genet 2002;114(5):541–52.

[21] Willour VL, Yao SY, Samuels J, et al. Replication study supports evidence for linkage to 9p24 in obsessive-compulsive disorder. Am J Hum Genet 2004;75(3):508–13.

[22] Veenstra-VanderWeele J, Kim SJ, Gonen D, et al. Genomic organization of the SLC1A1/EAAC1 gene and mutation screening in early-onset obsessive-compulsive disorder. Mol Psychiatry 2001;6(2):160–7.

[23] Alexander GE, DeLong MR, Strick PL. Parallel organization of functionally segregated circuits linking basal ganglia and cortex. Annu Rev Neurosci 1986;9:357–81.

[24] Rauch SL, Jenike MA, Alpert NM, et al. Regional cerebral blood flow measured during symptom provocation in obsessive-compulsive disorder using oxygen 15-labeled carbon dioxide and positron emission tomography. Arch Gen Psychiatry 1994;51(1):62–70.

[25] Rauch SL, Savage CR, Alpert NM, et al. Probing striatal function in obsessive-compulsive disorder: a PET study of implicit sequence learning. J Neuropsychiatry Clin Neurosci 1997;9(4):568–73.

[26] Rauch SL. Neuroimaging and neurocircuitry models pertaining to the neurosurgical treatment of psychiatric disorders. Neurosurg Clin N Am 2003;14(2):213–23.

[27] Robinson D, Wu H, Munne RA, et al. Reduced caudate nucleus volume in obsessive-compulsive disorder. Arch Gen Psychiatry 1995;52(5):393–8.

[28] Saxena S, Brody AL, Schwartz JM, et al. Neuroimaging and frontal-subcortical circuitry in obsessive-compulsive disorder. Br J Psychiatry Suppl 1998;35:26–37.

[29] Rosenberg DR, Keshavan MS, O'Hearn KM, et al. Frontostriatal measurement in treatment-naive children with obsessive-compulsive disorder. Arch Gen Psychiatry 1997; 54(9):824–30.

[30] Rosenberg DR, MacMaster FP, Keshavan MS, et al. Decrease in caudate glutamatergic concentrations in pediatric obsessive-compulsive disorder patients taking paroxetine. J Am Acad Child Adolesc Psychiatry 2000;39(9):1096–103.

[31] Lacerda AL, Dalgalarrondo P, Caetano D, et al. Elevated thalamic and prefrontal regional cerebral blood flow in obsessive-compulsive disorder: a SPECT study. Psychiatry Res 2003; 123(2):125–34.

[32] Pujol J, Soriano-Mas C, Alonso P, et al. Mapping structural brain alterations in obsessive-compulsive disorder. Arch Gen Psychiatry 2004;61(7):720–30.

[33] Szeszko PR, MacMillan S, McMeniman M, et al. Brain structural abnormalities in psychotropic drug-naive pediatric patients with obsessive-compulsive disorder. Am J Psychiatry 2004;161(6):1049–56.

[34] Baxter LR Jr, Phelps ME, Mazziotta JC, et al. Local cerebral glucose metabolic rates in obsessive-compulsive disorder. A comparison with rates in unipolar depression and in normal controls. Arch Gen Psychiatry 1987;44(3):211–8.

[35] Baxter LR Jr, Schwartz JM, Mazziotta JC, et al. Cerebral glucose metabolic rates in nondepressed patients with obsessive-compulsive disorder. Am J Psychiatry 1988;145(12): 1560–3.

[36] Baxter LR Jr, Saxena S, Brody AL, et al. Brain mediation of obsessive-compulsive disorder symptoms: evidence from functional brain imaging studies in the human and nonhuman primate. Semin Clin Neuropsychiatry 1996;1(1):32–47.

[37] Volavka J, Neziroglu F, Yaryura-Tobias JA. Clomipramine and imipramine in obsessive-compulsive disorder. Psychiatry Res 1985;14(1):85–93.

[38] Thoren P, Asberg M, Bertilsson L, et al. Clomipramine treatment of obsessive-compulsive disorder. II. Biochemical aspects. Arch Gen Psychiatry 1980;37(11):1289–94.

[39] Ananth J, Pecknold JC, van den SN, Engelsmann F. Double-blind comparative study of clomipramine and amitriptyline in obsessive neurosis. Prog Neuropsychopharmacol 1981;5(3):257–62.

[40] Lesch KP, Bengel D, Heils A, et al. Association of anxiety-related traits with a polymorphism in the serotonin transporter gene regulatory region. Science 1996;274(5292):1527–31.

[41] Heils A, Teufel A, Petri S, et al. Allelic variation of human serotonin transporter gene expression. J Neurochem 1996;66(6):2621–4.

[42] McDougle CJ, Epperson CN, Price LH, et al. Evidence for linkage disequilibrium between serotonin transporter protein gene (SLC6A4) and obsessive compulsive disorder. Mol Psychiatry 1998;3(3):270–3.

[43] Bengel D, Greenberg BD, Cora-Locatelli G, et al. Association of the serotonin transporter promoter regulatory region polymorphism and obsessive-compulsive disorder. Mol Psychiatry 1999;4(5):463–6.

[44] Frisch A, Michaelovsky E, Rockah R, et al. Association between obsessive-compulsive disorder and polymorphisms of genes encoding components of the serotonergic and dopaminergic pathways. Eur Neuropsychopharmacol 2000;10(3):205–9.

[45] Camarena B, Rinetti G, Cruz C, et al. Association study of the serotonin transporter gene polymorphism in obsessive-compulsive disorder. Int J Neuropsychopharmacol 2001;4(3): 269–72.

[46] Cavallini MC, Di Bella D, Siliprandi F, et al. Exploratory factor analysis of obsessive-compulsive patients and association with 5-HTTLPR polymorphism. Am J Med Genet 2002; 114(3):347–53.

[47] Walitza S, Wewetzer C, Gerlach M, et al. Transmission disequilibrium studies in children and adolescents with obsessive-compulsive disorders pertaining to polymorphisms of genes of the serotonergic pathway. J Neural Transm 2004;111(7):817–25.

[48] Meira-Lima I, Shavitt RG, Miguita K, et al. Association analysis of the catechol-o-methyltransferase (COMT), serotonin transporter (5-HTT) and serotonin 2A receptor (5HT2A) gene polymorphisms with obsessive-compulsive disorder. Genes Brain Behav 2004;3(2):75–9.

[49] Chabane N, Millet B, Delorme R, et al. Lack of evidence for association between serotonin transporter gene (5-HTTLPR) and obsessive-compulsive disorder by case control and family association study in humans. Neurosci Lett 2004;363(2):154–6.

[50] Kinnear CJ, Niehaus DJ, Moolman-Smook JC, et al. Obsessive-compulsive disorder and the promoter region polymorphism (5-HTTLPR) in the serotonin transporter gene (SLC6A4): a negative association study in the Afrikaner population. Int J Neuropsychopharmacol 2000;3(4):327–31.

[51] Moreno FA, Delgado PL. Hallucinogen-induced relief of obsessions and compulsions. Am J Psychiatry 1997;154(7):1037–8.

[52] Leonard HL, Rapoport JL. Relief of obsessive-compulsive symptoms by LSD and psilocin. Am J Psychiatry 1987;144(9):1239–40.

[53] Hanes KR. Serotonin, psilocybin, and body dysmorphic disorder: a case report. J Clin Psychopharmacol 1996;16(2):188–9.

[54] Baker RW, Chengappa KN, Baird JW, et al. Emergence of obsessive compulsive symptoms during treatment with clozapine. J Clin Psychiatry 1992;53(12):439–42.

[55] Poyurovsky M, Hermesh H, Weizman A. Fluvoxamine treatment in clozapine-induced obsessive-compulsive symptoms in schizophrenic patients. Clin Neuropharmacol 1996; 19(4):305–13.

[56] Patil VJ. Development of transient obsessive-compulsive symptoms during treatment with clozapine. Am J Psychiatry 1992;149(2):272.

[57] Polesskaya OO, Sokolov BP. Differential expression of the "C" and "T" alleles of the 5–HT2A receptor gene in the temporal cortex of normal individuals and schizophrenics. J Neurosci Res 2002;67(6):812–22.

[58] Khait VD, Huang YY, Zalsman G, et al. Association of serotonin 5-HT2A receptor binding and the T102C polymorphism in depressed and healthy Caucasian subjects. Neuropsychopharmacology 2005;30(1):166–72.

[59] Bray NJ, Buckland PR, Hall H, et al. The serotonin-2A receptor gene locus does not contain common polymorphism affecting mRNA levels in adult brain. Mol Psychiatry 2004; 9(1):109–14.

[60] Parsons MJ, D'Souza UM, Arranz MJ, et al. The -1438A/G polymorphism in the 5-hydroxytryptamine type 2A receptor gene affects promoter activity. Biol Psychiatry 2004; 56(6):406–10.

[61] Spurlock G, Heils A, Holmans P, et al. A family based association study of T102C polymorphism in 5HT2A and schizophrenia plus identification of new polymorphisms in the promoter. Mol Psychiatry 1998;3(1):42–9.

[62] Enoch MA, Kaye WH, Rotondo A, et al. 5–HT2A promoter polymorphism -1438G/A, anorexia nervosa, and obsessive-compulsive disorder. Lancet 1998;351:1785–6.

[63] Enoch MA, Greenberg BD, Murphy DL, et al. Sexually dismorphic relationship of a 5-HT2A promoter polymorphism with obsessive-compulsive disorder. Biol Psychiatry 2001;49:385–8.

[64] Walitza S, Wewetzer C, Warnke A, et al. 5-HT2A promoter polymorphism -1438G/A in children and adolescents with obsessive-compulsive disorders. Mol Psychiatry 2002; 7(10):1054–7.

[65] Tot S, Erdal ME, Yazici K, et al. T102C and -1438 G/A polymorphisms of the 5-HT2A receptor gene in Turkish patients with obsessive-compulsive disorder. Eur Psychiatry 2003; 18(5):249–54.

[66] Nicolini H, Cruz C, Camarena B, et al. DRD2, DRD3 and 5HT2A receptor genes polymorphisms in obsessive-compulsive disorder. Mol Psychiatry 1996;1(6):461–5.

[67] Hemmings SM, Kinnear CJ, Niehaus DJ, et al. Investigating the role of dopaminergic and serotonergic candidate genes in obsessive-compulsive disorder. Eur Neuropsychopharmacol 2003;13(2):93–8.

[68] Hemmings SM, Kinnear CJ, Lochner C, et al. Early- versus late-onset obsessive-compulsive disorder: investigating genetic and clinical correlates. Psychiatry Res 2004;128(2):175–82.

[69] Chou-Green JM, Holscher TD, Dallman MF, et al. Compulsive behavior in the 5-HT2C receptor knockout mouse. Physiol Behav 2003;78(4–5):641–9.

[70] Tsaltas E, Kontis D, Chrysikakou S, et al. Reinforced spatial alternation as an animal model of obsessive-compulsive disorder (OCD): investigation of 5-HT2C and 5-T1D receptor involvement in OCD pathophysiology. Biol Psychiatry 2005;57(10):1176–85.

[71] Prisco S, Esposito E. Differential effects of acute and chronic fluoxetine administration on the spontaneous activity of dopaminergic neurones in the ventral tegmental area. Br J Pharmacol 1995;116(2):1923–31.

[72] Di Maria V, Pierucci M, Esposito E. Selective stimulation of serotonin 2c receptors blocks the enhancement of striatal and accumbal dopamine release induced by nicotine administration. J Neurochem 2004;89(2):418–29.

[73] Lappalainen J, Zhang L, Dean M, et al. Identification, expression, and pharmacology of a Cys23-Ser23 substitution in the human 5-HT2c receptor gene (HTR2C). Genomics 1995;27(2):274–9.

[74] Lappalainen J, Long JC, Virkkunen M, et al. HTR2C Cys23Ser polymorphism in relation to CSF monoamine metabolite concentrations and DSM-III-R psychiatric diagnoses. Biol Psychiatry 1999;46(6):821–6.

[75] Jonsson EG, Bah J, Melke J, et al. Monoamine related functional gene variants and relationships to monoamine metabolite concentrations in CSF of healthy volunteers. BMC Psychiatry 2004;4(1):4.

[76] Okada M, Northup JK, Ozaki N, et al. Modification of human 5-HT(2C) receptor function by Cys23Ser, an abundant, naturally occurring amino-acid substitution. Mol Psychiatry 2004;9(1):55–64.

[77] Cavallini MC, Di Bella D, Pasquale L, et al. 5HT2C CYS23/SER23 polymorphism is not associated with obsessive-compulsive disorder. Psychiatry Res 1998;77(2):97–104.

[78] el Mansari M, Bouchard C, Blier P. Alteration of serotonin release in the Guinea Pig orbito-frontal cortex by selective serotonin reuptake inhibitors. Relevance to treatment of obsessive-compulsive disorder. Neuropsychopharmacology 1995;13(2):117–27.

[79] Zohar J, Kindler S. Serotonergic probes in obsessive compulsive disorder. Int Clin Psychopharmacol 1992;7(Suppl 1):39–40.

[80] Koran LM, Pallanti S, Quercioli L. Sumatriptan, 5-HT(1D) receptors and obsessive-compulsive disorder. Eur Neuropsychopharmacol 2001;11(2):169–72.

[81] Stern L, Zohar J, Cohen R, et al. Treatment of severe, drug resistant obsessive compulsive disorder with the 5HT1D agonist sumatriptan. Eur Neuropsychopharmacol 1998;8(4):325–8.

[82] Gross-Isseroff R, Cohen R, Sasson Y, et al. Serotonergic dissection of obsessive compulsive symptoms: a challenge study with m-chlorophenylpiperazine and sumatriptan. Neuropsychobiology 2004;50(3):200–5.

[83] Mundo E, Richter MA, Sam F, et al. Is the 5-HT(1Dbeta) receptor gene implicated in the pathogenesis of obsessive-compulsive disorder? Am J Psychiatry 2000;157(7):1160–1.

[84] Mundo E, Richter MA, Zai G, et al. 5HT1Dbeta receptor gene implicated in the pathogenesis of obsessive-compulsive disorder: further evidence from a family-based association study. Mol Psychiatry 2002;7(7):805–9.

[85] Di Bella D, Cavallini MC, Bellodi L. No association between obsessive-compulsive disorder and the 5-HT(1Dbeta) receptor gene. Am J Psychiatry 2002;159(10):1783–5.

[86] Camarena B, Aguilar A, Loyzaga C, et al. A family-based association study of the 5-HT-1Dbeta receptor gene in obsessive-compulsive disorder. Int J Neuropsychopharmacol 2004;7(1):49–53.

[87] Walther DJ, Bader M. A unique central tryptophan hydroxylase isoform. Biochem Pharmacol 2003;66(9):1673–80.

[88] Walther DJ, Peter JU, Bashammakh S, et al. Synthesis of serotonin by a second tryptophan hydroxylase isoform. Science 2003;299(5603):76.

[89] Mossner R, Walitza S, Geller F, et al. Transmission disequilibrium of polymorphic variants in the tryptophan hydroxylase-2 gene in children and adolescents with obsessive-compulsive disorder. Int J Neuropsychopharmacol 2005;9:1–6.

[90] Goodman WK, McDougle CJ, Price LH, et al. Beyond the serotonin hypothesis: a role for dopamine in some forms of obsessive compulsive disorder? J Clin Psychiatry 1990;51(Suppl):36–43.

[91] Creese I, Iversen SD. The role of forebrain dopamine systems in amphetamine induced stereotyped behavior in the rat. Psychopharmacologia 1974;39(4):345–57.

[92] Wallach MB. Drug-induced stereotyped behavior: similarities and differences. Psychopharmacol Bull 1974;10(3):12–3.

[93] Nordstrom EJ, Burton FH. A transgenic model of comorbid Tourette's syndrome and obsessive-compulsive disorder circuitry. Mol Psychiatry 2002;7(6):617–25, 524.

[94] Campbell KM, de Lecea L, Severynse DM, et al. OCD-Like behaviors caused by a neuro-potentiating transgene targeted to cortical and limbic D1 + neurons. J Neurosci 1999;19(12):5044–53.

[95] McGrath MJ, Campbell KM, Veldman MB, et al. Anxiety in a transgenic mouse model of cortical-limbic neuro-potentiated compulsive behavior. Behav Pharmacol 1999;10(5):435–43.

[96] McGrath MJ, Campbell KM, Parks CR, et al. Glutamatergic drugs exacerbate symptomatic behavior in a transgenic model of comorbid Tourette's syndrome and obsessive-compulsive disorder. Brain Res 2000;877(1):23–30.

[97] Berridge KC, Aldridge JW, Houchard KR, et al. Sequential super-stereotypy of an instinctive fixed action pattern in hyper-dopaminergic mutant mice: a model of obsessive compulsive disorder and Tourette's. BMC Biol 2005;3(1):4.

[98] Brambilla F, Bellodi L, Perna G, et al. Dopamine function in obsessive-compulsive disorder: growth hormone response to apomorphine stimulation. Biol Psychiatry 1997;42(10):889–97.

[99] Brambilla F, Perna G, Bussi R, et al. Dopamine function in obsessive compulsive disorder: cortisol response to acute apomorphine stimulation. Psychoneuroendocrinology 2000;25(3):301–10.

[100] McDougle CJ, Goodman WK, Leckman JF, et al. Haloperidol addition in fluvoxamine-refractory obsessive-compulsive disorder. A double-blind, placebo-controlled study in patients with and without tics. Arch Gen Psychiatry 1994;51(4):302–8.

[101] McDougle CJ, Epperson CN, Pelton GH, et al. A double-blind, placebo-controlled study of risperidone addition in serotonin reuptake inhibitor-refractory obsessive-compulsive disorder. Arch Gen Psychiatry 2000;57(8):794–801.

[102] Stein DJ, Bouwer C, Hawkridge S, et al. Risperidone augmentation of serotonin reuptake inhibitors in obsessive-compulsive and related disorders. J Clin Psychiatry 1997;58(3):119–22.

[103] Rubinstein M, Phillips TJ, Bunzow JR, et al. Mice lacking dopamine D4 receptors are supersensitive to ethanol, cocaine, and methamphetamine. Cell 1997;90(6):991–1001.

[104] Asghari V, Sanyal S, Buchwaldt S, et al. Modulation of intracellular cyclic AMP levels by different human dopamine D4 receptor variants. J Neurochem 1995;65(3):1157–65.

[105] Van Tol HH, Bunzow JR, Guan HC, et al. Cloning of the gene for a human dopamine D4 receptor with high affinity for the antipsychotic clozapine. Nature 1991;350(6319):610–4.

[106] Wang E, Ding YC, Flodman P, et al. The genetic architecture of selection at the human dopamine receptor D4 (DRD4) gene locus. Am J Hum Genet 2004;74(5):931–44.

[107] Cruz C, Camarena B, King N, et al. Increased prevalence of the seven-repeat variant of the dopamine D4 receptor gene in patients with obsessive-compulsive disorder with tics. Neurosci Lett 1997;231(1):1–4.

[108] Billet EA, Richter MA, Sam F, et al. Investigation of dopamine system genes in obsessive-compulsive disorder. Psychiatr Genet 1998;8:163–9.

[109] Millet B, Chabane N, Delorme R, et al. Association between the dopamine receptor D4 (DRD4) gene and obsessive-compulsive disorder. Am J Med Genet B Neuropsychiatr 2003;116:55–9.

[110] Missale C, Nash SR, Robinson SW, et al. Dopamine receptors: from structure to function. Physiol Rev 1998;78(1):189–225.

[111] Harvey BH, Scheepers A, Brand L, et al. Chronic inositol increases striatal D(2) receptors but does not modify dexamphetamine-induced motor behavior. Relevance to obsessive-compulsive disorder. Pharmacol Biochem Behav 2001;68(2):245–53.

[112] Fux M, Benjamin J, Belmaker RH. Inositol versus placebo augmentation of serotonin reuptake inhibitors in the treatment of obsessive-compulsive disorder: a double-blind crossover study. Int J Neuropsychopharmcol 1999;2(3):193–5.

[113] Denys D, van der WN, Janssen J, et al. Low level of dopaminergic D2 receptor binding in obsessive-compulsive disorder. Biol Psychiatry 2004;55(10):1041–5.

[114] Sokoloff P, Giros B, Martres MP, et al. Molecular cloning and characterization of a novel dopamine receptor (D3) as a target for neuroleptics. Nature 1990;347(6289):146–51.

[115] Sokoloff P, Giros B, Martres MP, et al. Localization and function of the D3 dopamine receptor. Arzneimittelforschung 1992;42(2A):224–30.

[116] Guo N, Klitenick MA, Tham CS, et al. Receptor mechanisms mediating clozapine-induced c-fos expression in the forebrain. Neuroscience 1995;65(3):747–56.

[117] Lammers CH, Diaz J, Schwartz JC, et al. Selective increase of dopamine D3 receptor gene expression as a common effect of chronic antidepressant treatments. Mol Psychiatry 2000; 5(4):378–88.

[118] Catalano M, Sciuto G, Di Bella D, et al. Lack of association between obsessive-compulsive disorder and the dopamine D3 receptor gene: some preliminary considerations. Am J Med Genet 1994;54(3):253–5.

[119] Giros B, Jaber M, Jones SR, et al. Hyperlocomotion and indifference to cocaine and amphetamine in mice lacking the dopamine transporter. Nature 1996;379(6566):606–12.

[120] Frazer A, Gerhardt GA, Daws LC. New views of biogenic amine transporter function: implications for neuropsychopharmacology. Int J Neuropsychopharmcol 1999;2(4):305–20.

[121] Vandenbergh DJ, Persico AM, Hawkins AL, et al. Human dopamine transporter gene (DAT1) maps to chromosome 5p15.3 and displays a VNTR. Genomics 1992;14(4):1104–6.

[122] Vandenbergh DJ, Thompson MD, Cook EH, et al. Human dopamine transporter gene: coding region conservation among normal, Tourette's disorder, alcohol dependence and attention-deficit hyperactivity disorder populations. Mol Psychiatry 2000;5(3):283–92.

[123] Sano A, Kondoh K, Kakimoto Y, et al. A 40-nucleotide repeat polymorphism in the human dopamine transporter gene. Hum Genet 1993;91(4):405–6.

[124] Persico AM, Wang ZW, Black DW, et al. Exclusion of close linkage of the dopamine transporter gene with schizophrenia spectrum disorders. Am J Psychiatry 1995;152(1):134–6.

[125] Doucette-Stamm LA, Blakely DJ, Tian J, et al. Population genetic study of the human dopamine transporter gene (DAT1). Genet Epidemiol 1995;12(3):303–8.

[126] Heinz A, Goldman D, Jones DW, et al. Genotype influences in vivo dopamine transporter availability in human striatum. Neuropsychopharmacology 2000;22(2):133–9.

[127] Jacobsen LK, Staley JK, Zoghbi SS, et al. Prediction of dopamine transporter binding availability by genotype: a preliminary report. Am J Psychiatry 2000;157(10):1700–3.

[128] Martinez D, Gelernter J, Abi-Dargham A, et al. The variable number of tandem repeats polymorphism of the dopamine transporter gene is not associated with significant change in dopamine transporter phenotype in humans. Neuropsychopharmacology 2001;24(5):553–60.

[129] Weyler W, Hsu YP, Breakefield XO. Biochemistry and genetics of monoamine oxidase. Pharmacol Ther 1990;47(3):391–417.

[130] Thorpe LW, Westlund KN, Kochersperger LM, et al. Immunocytochemical localization of monoamine oxidases A and B in human peripheral tissues and brain. J Histochem Cytochem 1987;35(1):23–32.

[131] Hotamisligil GS, Breakefield XO. Human monoamine oxidase A gene determines levels of enzyme activity. Am J Hum Genet 1991;49(2):383–92.

[132] Karayiorgou M, Sobin C, Blundell ML, et al. Family-based association studies support a sexually dimorphic effect of COMT and MAOA on genetic susceptibility to obsessive-compulsive disorder. Biol Psychiatry 1999;45(9):1178–89.

[133] Camarena B, Rinetti G, Cruz C, et al. Additional evidence that genetic variation of MAO-A gene supports a gender subtype in obsessive-compulsive disorder. Am J Med Genet 2001;105(3):279–82.

[134] Axelrod J, Tomchik R. Enzymatic O-methylation of epinephrine and other catechols. J Biol Chem 1958;233(3):702–5.

[135] Grossman MH, Szumlanski C, Littrell JB, et al. Electrophoretic analysis of low and high activity forms of catechol-O-methyltransferase in human erythrocytes. Life Sci 1992;50(7):473–80.

[136] Lachman HM, Papolos DF, Saito T, et al. Human catechol-O-methyltransferase pharmacogenetics: description of a functional polymorphism and its potential application to neuropsychiatric disorders. Pharmacogenetics 1996;6(3):243–50.

[137] Lotta T, Vidgren J, Tilgmann C, et al. Kinetics of human soluble and membrane-bound catechol O-methyltransferase: a revised mechanism and description of the thermolabile variant of the enzyme. Biochemistry 1995;34(13):4202–10.

[138] Karayiorgou M, Altemus M, Galke BL, et al. Genotype determining low catechol-O-methyltransferase activity as a risk factor for obsessive-compulsive disorder. Proc Natl Acad Sci U S A 1997;94(9):4572–5.

[139] Alsobrook JP, Zohar AH, Leboyer M, et al. Association between the COMT locus and obsessive-compulsive disorder in females but not males. Am J Med Genet 2002;114(1):116–20.

[140] Schindler KM, Richter MA, Kennedy JL, et al. Association between homozygosity at the COMT gene locus and obsessive compulsive disorder. Am J Med Genet 2000;96(6):721–4.

[141] Niehaus DJ, Kinnear CJ, Corfield VA, et al. Association between a catechol-o-methyltransferase polymorphism and obsessive-compulsive disorder in the Afrikaner population. J Affect Disord 2001;65(1):61–5.

[142] Erdal ME, Tot S, Yazici K, et al. Lack of association of catechol-O-methyltransferase gene polymorphism in obsessive-compulsive disorder. Depress Anxiety 2003;18(1):41–5.

[143] Ohara K, Nagai M, Suzuki Y, et al. No association between anxiety disorders and catechol-O-methyltransferase polymorphism. Psychiatry Res 1998;80(2):145–8.

[144] Azzam A, Mathews CA. Meta-analysis of the association between the catecholamine-O-methyl-transferase gene and obsessive-compulsive disorder. Am J Med Genet B Neuropsychiatr Genet 2003;123(1):64–9.

[145] Arnold PD, Rosenberg DR, Mundo E, et al. Association of a glutamate (NMDA) subunit receptor gene (GRIN2B) with obsessive-compulsive disorder: a preliminary study. Psychopharmacology (Berl) 2004;174(4):530–8.

[146] Delorme R, Krebs MO, Chabane N, et al. Frequency and transmission of glutamate receptors GRIK2 and GRIK3 polymorphisms in patients with obsessive compulsive disorder. Neuroreport 2004;15(4):699–702.

[147] Zai G, Arnold P, Burroughs E, Barr CL, et al. Evidence for the gamma-amino-butyric acid type B receptor 1 (GABBR1) gene as a susceptibility factor in obsessive-compulsive disorder. Am J Med Genet B Neuropsychiatr Genet 2005;134(1):25–9.

[148] Hall D, Dhilla A, Charalambous A, et al. Sequence variants of the brain-derived neurotrophic factor (BDNF) gene are strongly associated with obsessive-compulsive disorder. Am J Hum Genet 2003;73(2):370–6.

[149] Zai G, Bezchlibnyk YB, Richter MA, et al. Myelin oligodendrocyte glycoprotein (MOG) gene is associated with obsessive-compulsive disorder. Am J Med Genet 2004;129B:64–8.

[150] Leckman JF, Zhang H, Alsobrook JP, et al. Symptom dimensions in obsessive-compulsive disorder: toward quantitative phenotypes. Am J Med Genet 2001;105(1):28–30.

[151] Neale BM, Sham PC. The future of association studies: gene-based analysis and replication. Am J Hum Genet 2004;75(3):353–62.

Immunology of Obsessive-Compulsive Disorder

Tanya K. Murphy, MD*, Muhammad W. Sajid, MD,
Wayne K. Goodman, MD

*Department of Psychiatry, University of Florida School of Medicine,
Gainesville, FL 32610, USA*

With theories of causation ranging from Freud's theory of obsessional neurosis being secondary to substitution of a sexual impulse with obsessive thoughts and compulsive behaviors to a common childhood germ triggering severe obsessive-compulsive disorder (OCD), the pathophysiology of OCD remains one of the most exciting fields of research today. This article focuses on the neuroimmunology of OCD spectrum disorders, on what is known now and what questions remain to be answered by future research.

Basics of autoimmunity

Genetic influences and environmental triggers determine if and when the progression from benign autoimmunity to pathogenic autoimmunity occurs. Three levels of evidence for defining the existence of autoimmunity have been suggested: direct, indirect, and circumstantial [1]. Direct evidence requires transmissibility of the characteristic lesions of the disease from human to human or from human to animal. Indirect evidence requires recreation of the human disease in an animal model. Circumstantial evidence is evidence that suggests the presence of autoimmunity. Box 1 elucidates the currently accepted circumstantial evidence of autoimmune disease. For disorders like OCD, circumstantial evidence is the most compelling, albeit provisional, evidence for an autoimmune causation.

This work was supported by grants #K23 MH01739 and R01 MH063914 from the National Institutes of Mental Health.

* Corresponding author. Department of Psychiatry, University of Florida, P.O. Box 100256, Gainesville, FL 32610.

E-mail address: tmurphy@psychiatry.ufl.edu (T. Murphy).

Box 1. Circumstantial evidence of autoimmune disease

- Presence of infiltrating mononuclear cells in the affected organ or tissue
- Deposition of antigen-antibody complexes in the affected organ or tissue
- Presence in the same patient of other known autoimmune diseases*
- Preferential usage of certain major histocompatibility complex class II alleles
- Improvement of symptoms with the use of immunosuppressive drugs*
- High serum levels of IgG autoantibodies*
- Positive family history for the same disease or for other diseases known to be autoimmune*

---

* Some support exists

An autoimmune form of obsessive-compulsive disorder?

During investigations into neuropsychiatric aspects of rheumatic fever (RF), subjects who had SC were found to present frequently with classic OCD symptoms [2,3]. Although the initial focus was on the OCD symptoms observed in patients who had SC, tic disorders, emotional lability, separation anxiety, inattention, and hyperactivity were also reported frequently in these patients [2]. Around the same time, an increased incidence of tic disorders was noted to have coincided with a group A streptococcus (GAS) outbreak in a developmental pediatric practice [4]. Reasoning that if RF and SC are secondary to GAS infections, then the higher incidence of OCD and tics also could be GAS related, the National Institutes of Mental Health group coined the term "pediatric autoimmune neuropsychiatric disorders associated with streptococcus" (PANDAS) [5]. Box 2 shows the current criteria necessary for a PANDAS diagnosis. More than a decade later, the phenomenon of PANDAS continues to be met with both skepticism and interest concerning the possibility that a common pathogen might set into motion a pediatric psychiatric disorder that can evolve into chronic disabling OCD in adulthood.

The phenotype for pediatric autoimmune neuropsychiatric disorders associated with streptococcus

In 1998, 50 children were described who had an acute and dramatic onset/exacerbations of OCD/or tics. These children had symptom changes that

---

Box 2. Current diagnostic criteria for PANDAS

- The presence of obsessive compulsive disorder or a tic disorder
- Pediatric onset of symptoms (age 3 years to puberty)
- Episodic or sawtooth course of symptom severity
- An association with group A streptococcal infection (a positive throat culture for streptococcus or history of scarlet fever)
- Evidence of concurrent neurological abnormalities (motoric hyperactivity or adventitious movements, such as choreiform movements)

---

followed GAS infection, GAS exposure, or non-cultured pharyngitis [5]. These children frequently were observed to have symptoms of separation anxiety, nightmares, personality change, oppositional behaviors, and deterioration in math skills and handwriting in addition to a diagnosis of OCD or tics [5]. In addition to tics, abnormalities such as hyperactivity or choreiform movements were noted on the neurologic examination during periods of symptom exacerbation. Symptom presentation is also influenced by gender, with boys more likely to present with tics and girls more likely to present with chorea-like movements. Gender dimorphism is evident in PANDAS, tics, OCD, and SC with regards to age of onset, with male predominance more likely before the age of 10 years [5–7].

Pathogenesis of group A streptococcus

Multiple characteristics of GAS, from proteins shared with humans to changing genetics, make it an interesting suspect in the saga of infection-triggered psychiatric disorders. GAS is a bacterial pathogen whose strains are responsible for both suppurative infections, such as pharyngitis, scarlet fever, toxic shock syndrome, necrotizing fasciitis, septicemia and impetigo, and nonsuppurative sequelae, such as rheumatic fever, glomerulonephritis, and reactive arthritis. Recent concern about GAS has focused on strains identified as the "flesh-eating" bacteria that destroy infected soft tissues or limbs [8]. The general public is more familiar with GAS as the most common bacterial cause of sore throat ("strep throat") which routinely affects school-aged children 5 to 15 years of age. As a pathogen, GAS has developed complex virulence mechanisms to avoid host defenses including capsule formation and antiphagocytic factors. In the last decade, the incidence and severity of GAS infections has increased significantly, and a greater degree of allelic diversity has been recognized. GAS produces a number of toxic factors, including opacity factor (which is hemolytic), streptolysin O and streptolysin S (both hemolytic and cytotoxic), hyaluronidase (which hydrolyzes hyaluronic acid), NADase (which enables tissue invasion), streptokinase (which is involved in nephritis), and M-like proteins (which bind to immunoglobulins and possibly interfere with complement). To date, more than 80 serotypes of GAS have been described; 150 alleles of the M protein, 89 alleles of speB, and 269 alleles of the Sic protein are known to exist. Some of the suspected virulence factors were not present in earlier strains of GAS, possibly because random re-assortment of the GAS genome over time increased the chance of new virulence factors developing [9]. Clinical evidence that GAS may be changing is reflected in changes in the clinical manifestations of illnesses caused by GAS. In the outbreaks of RF in the mid-1980s, a higher representation of certain serotypes and mucoid strains of GAS was noted, and a large proportion of individuals had only a mild or no history of prior pharyngitis. All indications are that GAS fluctuated in virulence and clinical manifestations in the last several decades.

Genetics

Genetics plays an important role in an individual's vulnerability to infection-triggered neuropsychiatric disorders. Because SC is a model for understanding PANDAS, the genetics of SC may give insights into understanding hereditary susceptibility to PANDAS. Family-based studies support a genetic predisposition to RF. Epidemiologic studies showing the ability of the same streptococcal strain to cause infection of varying severity in different individuals further suggest that host factors play an important role in determining the severity and outcome of GAS infections [10]. Only recently have researchers linked a receptor involved in innate immunity (Toll like receptor-2 polymorphism) [11] and tumor necrosis factor-alpha (TNFα) [12] to susceptibility to RF. Such polymorphisms may increase an individual's response to GAS infections. In fact, patients who have a propensity to produce high levels of proinflammatory cytokines in response to GAS products are noted to exhibit severe clinical manifestations [13]. Although there is clear evidence supporting a hereditary predisposition to developing OCD and tics [14,15], more investigation into the genetic and environmental interactions involved in the vulnerability to these illnesses is needed. Most of the studies investigating genetic loci have focused on neurotransmitter receptors and transporters, not on immune-based genes. One study has found a significant relationship between OCD and a polymorphism of myelin oligodendrocyte glycoprotein by Family Based Association Test [16]. Myelin oligodendrocyte glycoprotein is a protein implicated in the pathology of multiple sclerosis. Other than age, risk factors for developing a PANDAS phenotype of OCD are not known. To date, only one report has looked specifically at the family histories of patients who have PANDAS [17]. In this study, Lougee and colleagues [17] evaluated the first-degree relatives of 54

PANDAS probands for tics, OCD, subclinical OCD, and other disorders listed in Axis I of the *Diagnostic and Statistical Manual of Mental Disorders,* fourth edition. The rates of OCD and tic disorders in first-degree relatives of patients who had PANDAS mirrored those previously reported in probands that had childhood-onset OCD and TS. Other psychiatric disorders that are commonly comorbid with OCD and TS, including attention-deficit hyperactivity disorder (ADHD), major depressive disorder, and phobias, also were observed in a number of the family members of patients who had PANDAS. A child's risk of developing PANDAS is related to his or her genetic predisposition and to pathogen and environmental factors and should prove to be an intriguing area of exploration.

Evidence for association of group A streptococcus and neuropsychiatric disorders

Support for the association of GAS infections with OCD or tics continues to accumulate, with observations that have attributed onset or exacerbation of OCD or tics to recent streptococcal or respiratory infection or to categorically elevated GAS titers [5,18–25]. For instance, a pediatric group examined all children who presented with a sudden onset of a neuropsychiatric problem (such as OCD, a tic disorder, or late-age–onset ADHD) for GAS and found 12 such children over a 3-year period, all of whom had OC symptoms. They reported that these children also had a high prevalence of urinary frequency, and two children had high anti-deoxyribonuclease B (DNaseB) titers. They found that the neuropsychiatric symptoms remitted rapidly with antibiotic therapy [21]. Other examples also suggest an infectious trigger for the onset of neuropsychiatric symptoms. In a retrospective survey of 80 children (5–17 years of age) diagnosed as having a tic disorder, 53% of patients described acute and severe onset or worsening of their tic symptoms. Of those, 21% reported that abrupt changes occurred within 6 weeks following a streptococcal infection [23]. A study found elevated anti-streptolysin O titer in a significant percentage of 150 children at initial evaluation of tic disorders: 38% had an anti-streptolysin O titer above 500 IU/mL, compared with 2% of healthy controls (n = 150) [26].

Titer elevations found in cross-sectional analyses of children who have OCD and tics do not prove recent streptococcal infection, however. Unless serial titers are performed on a child before, during, and after OCD/tic onset, titer characteristics remain undefined because elevated titers are a common finding in this age group [27]. Some children who have tics and OCD, similar to reports in RF [28], may have persistent immune activation to GAS leading to titer elevations lasting 6 months to a year without clear evidence of preceding streptococcal infection. This chronic immune response may heighten sensitivity to central nervous system (CNS) perturbations. For example, Murphy and colleagues [25] found that patients who had a dramatically fluctuating neuropsychiatric symptom course had more evidence of persistent elevations in one or more streptococcus titers than those who had a course inconsistent with PANDAS [25]. This finding may result from the relative proximity of the streptococcal infection at the time of study enrollment, with repeated streptococcal exposures leading to more severe and turbulent symptoms. A corollary of this finding is the report of increased percentages of B cells in patients who have tic disorders that seem to be secondary to recent infection or immune activation [29]. The increased percentage of B cells may be secondary to alterations in other lymphocyte subclasses or result from an increase in antibody machinery related to antibody-mediated autoimmunity or to a nonspecific reaction to a recent streptococcal infection. Other types of infections, as well as stress, are believed to trigger OCD/tic symptoms [30,31], with a chronically activated immune system predisposing the triggering of the symptoms.

Frequent GAS infections may be one of the main reasons for chronic titer elevations and have been found to predispose children to neuropsychiatric sequelae [24] (T.K. Murphy, unpublished data). Many patients seen by the authors in research and clinic settings report onset of neuropsychiatric symptoms after a bout of repeated streptococcal infections that occur over the course of a few months (T.K. Murphy, unpublished data). Much more compelling support is an epidemiologic study that found that the odds of developing a tic disorder were significantly increased with prior history of multiple GAS infections [24]. Similarly, a case study of 12 patients found that the number of prior GAS infections correlated with a more severe course and a greater incidence of relapse [21]. A school study examining motoric signs and behavior while obtaining monthly GAS cultures from 693 school children found that those who had repeated GAS infections during the 8-month study had more frequent neuropsychiatric findings (T.K Murphy, unpublished data). Most of the recurrences are relapses (ie, infection by the same streptococcal type rather than new infections of a different type). Possible causes could include poor compliance or inadequate duration of antibiotic therapy, poor antibiotic penetration into tonsillar tissue, inactivation of antibiotic caused by beta-lactamase–producing bacteria, lack of protective oral flora, or immunologic defects. The reasons for GAS recurrence probably are complex; if and why recurrence increases neuropsychiatric risk is undetermined.

Correlating timing and certainty of a GAS infection with neuropsychiatric onset is often difficult. The main confounding issues with the timing are differentiating true inciting GAS infections, whether clinical or subclinical, from GA-carrier states. In the outbreaks of RF in the mid-1980s, a higher representation of certain serotypes and mucoid strains of GAS was noted [32], and a large proportion of individuals (75% in one study) had only a mild or no history of prior pharyngitis [33]. It is conceivable, therefore, that some cases of new-onset OCD or tics will have an undetected association with GAS, because prior infections with the same serotype of GAS are less likely to elicit symptoms of a clinical pharyngitis [34]. Others argue that overall immunity to GAS has changed over time to decrease the severity of clinical presentation but not to susceptibility to infection [35].

GAS association is assumed, for the most part, when elevated levels of GAS antibody are observed, because a long time lag often exists between the suspected infection and the onset of symptoms. Other RF symptoms, such as carditis, certainly add support for GAS etiology. The clinical significance of elevated streptococcal antibodies in a child presenting with a dramatic onset of OCD has been met with skepticism, however [36]. To make an unmistakable diagnosis of a new-onset GAS infection, a positive 24-hour culture of a subtype that was not previously cultured in that child, along with an acute and convalescent streptococcal titers showing a rise of 0.2 log or higher in a child who did not receive antibiotics is recommended [37]. This level of rigor is uncommon in clinical practice, because serotype determinations and serial titers are not standard practice or practical for documenting acute GAS in the office of the child's primary care provider. In fact, 79% of physicians indicated they would prescribe antibiotics for pharyngitis without obtaining a laboratory culture [38]. Moreover, GAS carriage rates are typically low [39–41], so that 90% of positive GAS rapid streptococcus tests or cultures should reflect acute infection.

Although it is a weaker argument, seasonal variations in the onset of autoimmune illness often correlate with seasonal variations of infectious illness [42]. For example, the incidence of RF peaks from January to March, shortly after peak rates of GAS infection, with lower rates of acute RF reported in the summer months [43]. Tic symptoms are increased in fall and winter months [25,44], also correlating with peak rates of streptococcal pharyngitis. Increased rates of upper respiratory infection and school-based stress probably are contributing factors, however.

Anti-brain antibodies

The presence of anti-brain antibodies in patients who have OCD would provide circumstantial evidence for CNS autoimmunity. The mechanism by which systemic autoantibodies might traverse the blood–brain barrier (BBB) and gain access to the CNS is not known, but a variety of mechanisms have been proposed. Inflammatory toxins may lead to a breakdown of the BBB. Cytokines can cross the BBB through the circumventricular organs and, when infused peripherally, are known to activate inflammatory cells on the CNS side of the BBB. Peripheral B cells that are cross-reactive to a CNS epitope also have been shown to induce intrathecal production of antibody [45]. Therefore, the induction of intrathecal antibodies by peripheral B cells, activation of CNS inflammatory cells by peripheral cytokines, and the traversing of the BBB by peripheral B cells and antibodies are all viable explanations by which autoantibodies produced in response to a peripheral antigen are able to react with neural structures.

One mechanism of antibody interaction with self-proteins is through molecular mimicry. Molecular mimicry is the phenomenon in which a microbial protein resembles a host protein. An injury or loss of the normally impermeable BBB may lead to the host proteins becoming recognizable by the immune system. The CNS manifestations characteristic of SC are thought to be related to production of antibodies to streptococcal antigens associated with the M protein of streptococcus that cross-react with epitopes on neuronal tissue [46]. Remarkable homology among various epitopes of the streptococcal M protein and tissue molecules (such as tropomyosin) suggests a humoral-mediated mechanism of autoimmunity in the pathogenesis of RF. The finding of increased antibodies to caudate in patients who have TS [19] parallels findings of increased anti-basal ganglia antibodies (ABGA) in patients who have SC [47]. Some studies in OCD or TS show few differences of antibody binding when compared with control groups [4,48,49], even when varied techniques and epitopes are used [50]; these results suggest lack of test sensitivity or possibly controls with benign autoimmunity. Other groups, however, consistently have found evidence of ABGA in post-streptococcal neuropsychiatric disorders [51,52]. In a study specific to OCD, Western immunoblotting revealed significant ABGA binding (as seen in SC) in 42% of the OCD group compared with 2% to 10% of neurologic and streptococcal control groups, respectively ($P < .001$ in all comparisons) [51].

An examination of the potential of these antibodies to elicit relevant neuropsychiatric behaviors in animals has led to contradictory findings [53,54], although recent studies suggest these antibodies may be involved in neuronal signaling [55]. Ultimately, improvement and standardization of reagents, techniques, and subject selection [56] should help resolve some of the differences among different research centers. Potential mechanisms by which autoantibodies cause clinical manifestations in CNS diseases such as SC and PANDAS include direct stimulation or blockade of receptors in the basal ganglia or immune complexes promoting inflammation of these brain regions. Studies in patients who have SC have found that increased antineuronal antibody binding to basal ganglia tissue correlates well with symptom severity [47], with research supporting antibody-mediated neuronal cell signaling in the pathogenesis of SC [55].

Monoclonal antibodies in patients who had SC that were targeted to N-acetyl-beta-D-glucosamine, the dominant epitope of GAS, showed specificity to mammalian lysoganglioside, a CNS ganglioside that influences neuronal signal transduction. Sera from these patients contained antibodies that targeted human neuronal cells and specifically induced calcium/calmodulin–dependent protein (CaM) kinase II activity, whereas sera from convalescing patients or from patients who had other streptococcal-related diseases lacked activation of this enzyme. Activation of CaM kinase II has been shown to cause increased release of dopamine in brain tissue, a mechanism by which clinical symptoms might ensue [57]. Sera from patients who have

SC also have been found to modify intracellular calcium levels in PC12 cells by a complement-independent mechanism. Ca2+ levels in sera of patients who have SC correlated directly with the ELISA optical density values for ABAGs [58]. The binding of autoantibodies to these neuronal cell surface antigens may promote signal transduction, leading to the release of excitatory neurotransmitters. The potential mechanism by which symptoms occur in SC may also explain the pathogenesis of PANDAS.

Other obsessive-compulsive disorder–immune relationships

Although patients who have SC seem to be at greatest risk for developing OCD, those who have RF without chorea also have an increased risk for developing OCD over expected prevalence [59]. The symptoms observed among the patients who have SC (aggressive thoughts and fears of contamination) were similar to those previously noted among samples of pediatric patients who had primary OCD but differed from those reported by patients who had tic disorder. This symptom overlap might suggest a shared neuropathology between childhood-onset OCD and SC that differs from that of tic disorders [60]. Tic symptoms have been reported to occur in patients who have SC, however. Studies support an increased risk for OCD and ADHD in those with acute and persistent SC [3,61] as well as an increase in OCD in non-SC RF [59]. Pre-existing ADHD may be a risk factor for developing SC [59], but in theory ADHD could be an earlier sequela to GAS encountered in the preschool years. The risk of developing OCD seems to occur only during acute episodes of RF. One study compared the adult prevalence of OCS in patients who had a history of RF to those who had diabetes mellitus and found no increased prevalence of OCS in either group [62].

The high rate of OCD symptoms in SC has prompted further exploration of a potential autoimmune basis for OCD in a subset of patients. Comorbid OCD in patients who have other autoimmune diseases, such as systemic lupus erythematosus, thyroid dysfunction [63], and multiple sclerosis [64,65], has been reported. Slattery and colleagues [66] demonstrated a significantly higher prevalence of OCD in a cohort of 50 patients who had systemic lupus erythematosus [66]. OCD was 10 to 15 times more common in this study group than in community-based studies of OCD. Likewise, Miguel and colleagues [65] reported a higher prevalence of OCD in patients who had multiple sclerosis [65]. Conversely, a chart-review study [67] concluded that adult patients who had OCD seemed to have an increased rate of immune-related diseases beyond that seen in other psychiatric disorders. Future research concerning the association of OCD with other autoimmune disorders seems warranted.

Measurement of peripheral cytokine profiles, lymphocyte subsets, and antibodies to viruses and self-proteins have been the primary focus of efforts to study alterations in immune indices in adults who have OCD [68–71], following in the steps of studies that support the role of cell-mediated mechanisms in the pathogenesis of RF [72,73]. Some studies found evidence of an altered or imbalanced immune function in adult patients who had OCD [69,74], but others failed to find humoral evidence of autoimmunity [68,71] or cytokine alterations [68,75,76]. These studies highlight the need for further exploration of the role immune processes play in the development and maintenance of OCD or tic symptoms. Sample sizes in previous studies often have been small, and the degree to which hypothalamo-pituitary-axis alterations (caused by stress versus autoimmunity) have affected results has yet to be resolved.

In a study of adults who have OCD, Denys and colleagues [77] found a significant decrease in the production of TNF-α and natural killer (NK) activity in patients who had OCD compared with controls. Patients who had first-degree relatives who had OCD had significantly lower NK activity than patients whose relatives did not exhibit OCD. Also, those who had childhood-onset OCD had significantly lower numbers of NK cells than patients who had adult-onset illness. Alterations in cytokine measures also have been found in TS. Leckman and colleagues [78], in a study of 46 patients who had TS or childhood-onset OCD compared with 31 age-matched controls, found interleukin-12 and TNF-α elevated at baseline in patients and a further increase of both markers during symptom exacerbation. In a longitudinal study, a higher level of D8/17-reactive cells and neopterin was found in children who had tic disorders or OCD than in control subjects at baseline; however, no significant change was seen when comparing baseline and exacerbation visits [79]. Table 1 presents an overview of immune parameters found in OCD and related disorders.

Peripheral markers of autoimmunity

Peripheral markers of CNS disease could result from CNS injury or inflammation with resultant release of protein and escape of the marker through a breached BBB or from overproduction of a protein in the CNS or peripherally. Identification of an immune marker in OCD/TS could help determine the patient subtype best suited for immune therapies. The search for markers of CNS injury in neurologic illnesses has led to findings of increased levels of the CNS proteins S-100 and enolase in both cerebral spinal fluid and serum [92]. Peripheral levels of S-100 were elevated in patients who had TS relative to age-matched controls, supporting the hypothesis that CNS inflammation is involved in this disorder [93]. Pediatric patients (7–17 years of age) who had TS or OCD (n = 47) and healthy control subjects (n = 19) were monitored prospectively for newly acquired GAS infections and for nonspecific markers of acute inflammatory responses [79]. Neopterin, a pyrazinopyrimidine compound that serves as a marker of cellular immune system activation, was higher in the patients than in controls (22% versus 0%), but no difference was observed in C-reactive protein.

Table 1
Overview of immune parameters in patients who have OCD-spectrum disorders

Immune parameter	Reference #	Author	Findings
ABGA	4,19	Kiessling et al (1993,1994)	↑ tic, OCD
	49	Murphy et al (1997)	↑ OCD, tic
	48,80	Singer et al 1998, (2004)	± tic; ± PANDAS
	81	Wendlandt et al (2001)	↑ tic
	82	Morshed et al (2001)	↑ tic
	52	Pavone et al (2004)	↑ PANDAS
	51	Dale et al (2005)	↑ OCD
Type 1 cytokines	74	Mittleman et al (1997)	↑ OCD
IL-12, TNF-α	78	Leckman et al (2005)	↑ tic
D8/17	83	Swedo et al (1997)	↑ PANDAS
	84	Niehaus et al (1999)	↑ OCD
	49,85	Murphy et al (1997, 2001)	↑ OCD, tic
	86	Hoekstra et al (2001)	↑ tic
	87	Eisen et al (2001)	± OCD
	88	Sokel et al (2002)	↑ AN
	89	Inoff-Germain et al (2003)	± OCD, tic
Streptococcus association			
Titers	49	Murphy et al (1997)	± OCD, tic
	20	Muller et al (2000)	↑ tic
	90	Peterson et al (2000)	± tic/OCD, ↑ADHD
	82	Morshed et al (2001)	↑ tic
	25	Murphy et al (2004)	↑ OCD
Infections	5	Swedo et al (1998)	↑ OCD, tic
	18	Giulino et al (2002)	↑ OCD
	21	Murphy et al (2002)	↑ OCD
	91	Perrin et al (2004)	± OCD, tic
	79	Luo et al (2004)	± tic, OCD
	24	Mell et al (2005)	↑ OCD, tic

Abbreviations: ABGA, anti-basal ganglia antibodies; ADHD, attention deficit hyperactivity disorder; AN, anorexia nervosa; IL-12, interleukin 12; OCD, obsessive compulsive disorder; PANDAS, pediatric autoimmune neuropsychiatric disorders associated with streptococcus TNF-α, tumor necrosis factor-alpha; ↑, positive association or increased over control population; ±, minimal or nonsignificant finding.

One of the most exciting but ultimately disappointing prospects for finding a marker for immune-mediated OCD/tics began as an extension of studies of a putative peripheral marker of susceptibility to RF. Monoclonal antibodies (mAbs) to D8/17, an alloantigen found on B lymphocytes, was originally isolated from a patient who had rheumatic carditis and since has been found to react with epitopes expressed on expanded populations of B lymphocytes in a majority of patients who have documented RF [94]. Because the diagnosis of SC is often a diagnosis of exclusion, increased expression of D8/17 has been proposed to help differentiate SC from other forms of chorea. Subsequently, the possibility of an immune-mediated pathogenesis of OCD/TS has generated interest in the potential of mAb D8/17 in identifying patients at risk for streptococcal-precipitated neuropsychiatric disorders [49,83]. In two flow cytometric studies, increased binding was observed in neuropsychiatric patients compared with controls, but a subpopulation of D8/17+ B cells was not found [86,95]. The potential for D8/17 to serve as marker of immune function at points of neuropsychiatric exacerbation would suggest that it might be a state marker instead of trait marker as suggested in the RF literature. Although patients who had OCD/TS demonstrated significantly higher levels of D8/17-reactive cells than control subjects, there was no consistent pattern of change in D8/17 levels when exacerbation time points were compared with baseline or follow-up time points [79]. To date, because of concerns about methodology and reagents [29,85,95], an assay for the alloantigen D8/17 has not been correlated reliably with suspected PANDAS cases, leaving the diagnostic potential of this antibody and its relationship to the pathophysiology of psychiatric disorders doubtful [80,96]. Weisz and colleagues [29] failed to demonstrate an elevated percentage of D8/17+ B cells in patients who had either acute RF or TS. They did find a significant increase in CD19+ B cells in patients who had RF or TS compared with normal controls, and the increase correlated with streptococcus titers. The authors' group found that CD19 levels were inversely related to the level of D8/17 binding (T.K. Murphy, unpublished data) but had no correlation with elevated streptococcus titers [49]. They concluded that the D8/17 antibody is a nonspecific immunoglobulin that binds to increased cell surface markers during periods of immune activation and that the level of this binding is highly sensitive to the dilution of the mAb (T.K.Murphy, unpublished data). In mixed support of the notion that D8/17 may reflect immune activation, Luo and colleagues [79] found that D8/17 percentages showed more fluctuations in patients who had tics but did not correlate with symptom exacerbations or titer elevations [79]. The D8/17 story hints at the possibility of immune alterations in patients who have tics or OCD, but results have been too tenuous to allow interpretation of D8/17's significance.

Neurologic and cardiac concerns in the pediatric autoimmune neuropsychiatric disorders associated with streptococcus phenotype

The classic CNS autoimmune complication of GAS is RF and its neuropsychiatric expression, SC [97]. In PANDAS, studies have indicated that an overall worsening of neurologic performance occurs with or after the appearance of OCD/tic symptoms [25]. Choreiform movements that represented an overall worsening of neurologic performance occurred about 3 months following a tic exacerbation [25]. Such a lag is consistent with the finding that OCD symptoms precede the appearance of any motoric manifestation by days or weeks in patients who have RF [59]. Similarly, in a study of 673 children (pre-kindergarten through sixth grade), behavior changes were observed with or 1 month subsequent to GAS ($P = .03$) (T.K. Murphy, unpublished data). Delayed associations at 2 to 3 months were also found more often in the younger age group ($P = .002$). The presence of neurologic soft signs, such as choreiform movements and pronator sign/drift, are a frequently observed comorbidity among childhood-onset OCD, tics, and ADHD. The significance of neurologic soft signs in relationship to GAS infections has never been examined prospectively. Certainly, GAS has the propensity to produce CNS deficits as evidenced by SC. More recently, neurologic sequelae, including myoclonus, poststreptococcal basal ganglia encephalopathy, and restless legs syndrome, have been reported to be associated with GAS [51].

In addition to choreiform movements, other subtle signs of neurologic impairment have been reported to be associated with PANDAS. Parents occasionally comment on deterioration in handwriting (bigger, sloppier letters) or a decrease in motor skills (a good baseball player becomes a mediocre player). Parents are more likely to be concerned with new-onset or severe worsening of OCD or tic symptoms, increased moodiness, or increased ADHD behaviors such as inability to focus, increased hyperactivity, or greater distractibility. In a comparison of fine-motor functioning of 19 children who had PANDAS and 19 age- and gender-matched controls, the motor performance was significantly slower during exacerbations of streptococcal-triggered OCD or tics, and these motor skills improved when neuropsychiatric symptoms were in remission (D. Becker, personal communication, 2000). There are enough differences between SC and PANDAS that this subtype of OCD/TS may a distinct pathophysiology, however [98]. GAS is known to elicit a wide array of phenotypes that have varying degrees of overlap with RF. For example, post-streptococcal reactive arthritis (PSRA) has similarities to the arthritis seen in RF, but the criteria for RF are not met because there are few reports of carditis and no CNS involvement. Pathophysiologically, PSRA may differ from RF in that PSRA has been associated with non–group A streptococcus, the serotypes of GAS differ from those associated with RF, and serologies are dissimilar [99]. The absence of frank chorea and absence of carditis differentiate PANDAS from SC. It is estimated that rheumatic carditis is found in 30% to 64% of all patients child originally presenting with who have SC, but no data suggest that a child presenting with OCD or tics is at increased risk of developing rheumatic carditis [100]. The delineation of neurologic symptoms severe enough to meet criteria for SC but not severe enough for PANDAS is not always easy.

Diagnosis and treatment issues

The difficulty in distinguishing PANDAS from other phenotypes of OCD or tics, and occasionally from SC, makes it difficult to establish practical treatment protocols. Areas of contention (eg, the GAS association, course definition, and the neurologic demarcation of SC from PANDAS) contribute to this difficulty. It remains to be shown that onset, severity, or course of tic/OC symptom episodes can reliably separate PANDAS from other etiologic forms of tics/OCD, even though this nosology offers the best framework for studying the GAS association. Moreover, factors that determine whether the symptoms of PANDAS remit after an acute episode or progress to a more chronic illness are not yet known. Nonetheless, the symptoms and characteristic course of PANDAS are often typical of OCD and tics early in the illness. During the history-gathering process, careful attention should be given to reports of repeated, frequent infections, evidence of GAS in a young child (eg, unexplained abdominal pain accompanied by fever), scarlet fever, brief episodes of tics, OCD, or compulsive urination that remitted, and especially sudden-onset of OCD or tics accompanying an infectious illness. In patients who have abnormal neurologic examination evidenced by muscle weakness, abnormal reflexes (slow return of patellar reflex), or chorea, further work-up is indicated. In patients who have new-onset OCD or tics or recent symptom exacerbation, a throat culture is a relatively benign procedure that will help rule out the possibility that symptoms are triggered by a subclinical GAS infection. Streptococcal titers obtained at symptom onset should be repeated to check for a rise in titers 4 to 6 weeks later. In patients who experienced onset of OCD more than 4 weeks before examination, streptococcal titers add support but do not provide definitive proof of a streptococcal trigger.

Streptococcus pharyngitis in preschool children presents with less evidence of tonsillar exudates and cervical adenopathy and more evidence of gastroenteritis than seen in school-aged children. Although development of RF is rare in children under the age of 5 years, the impact of early GAS infections on future immune response to GAS and neuropsychiatric vulnerability is unknown. Having a tonsillectomy at an early age may be associated with increased risk of OCD/TS [25]. Many children undergo tonsillectomy and adenoidectomy secondary to sleep apnea from adenoid hypertrophy or recurrent pharyngeal GAS infections. Although symptomatic GAS infections have been shown to decrease after tonsillectomy [101], the role of non–carrier state subclinical infections has not been documented. Recent research has shown that children who have hypertrophy of adenoids and tonsils exhibit both local and general changes in immunologic parameters [102]. Both humoral (IgA, IgG, (gM) and cellular (CD3, CD4, CD8) parameters significantly decreased postoperatively, but at the 6-month postoperative examination these parameters had normalized. The impact of tonsillectomy and adenoidectomy on the development of autoimmune sequelae has not been studied.

Although the PANDAS hypothesis remains unsettled, the current treatment for patients meeting the PANDAS criteria continues to be the standard-of-care practices for patients who have OCD or TS. Although increasing evidence supports a link between GAS and neuropsychiatric disorders, the incidence of pediatric streptococcal infections is extremely high, not all streptococcal infections are detected, and only a minority of children develops a neuropsychiatric illness. Standard-of-care practices notwithstanding, many practitioners prescribe antibiotics to patients who have OCD or tics, not always with PANDAS phenotype (T.K. Murphy, unpublished data), despite substandard support of this practice. Although prophylactic antibiotic therapy in patients who have SC seems to prevent neuropsychiatric exacerbations [103], other investigators report that about a third will have a recurrence [104]. Studies in which patients who had SC received monthly prophylactic injections of benzathine penicillin G showed that not all SC recurrences seem to be triggered by GAS [105] and that recurrences may occur after infections too mild or too brief to be detected easily [106]. These studies suggest that some improvement in course occurs after prophylactic antibiotics, but the number enrolled was small, none of the reports was blinded, and (because most patients who have SC are advised to take prophylactic antibiotics until their late teens) no data exist comparing the overall neuropsychiatric severity of those receiving treatment and those who were not treated [7,103].

Protocols for diagnosis and treatment of PANDAS are provisional, given that a definitive association between GAS and OCD or tics has yet to be established. Studies have been criticized for design and small sample size [36]. No conclusive evidence that the antibiotics reduced clinical exacerbations was found in a clinical trial involving the use of prophylactic oral penicillin in treating apparent episodes of PANDAS [107]. The sample size was small, however, and the lack of efficacy may have been caused by questionable compliance. Additionally, the initial 8-month crossover design of penicillin and placebo (4 months on each compound) was found to be suboptimal because of the short duration of observation during each phase and the possibility of carry-over effects. Given these potential confounds, the National Institutes of Metal Health study was changed to a 12-month parallel design comparing penicillin and azithromycin. Eleven subjects were maintained on penicillin, and 12 were maintained on azithromycin during the 12-month study [108]. Subjects assigned randomly to either drug had a reduced number of streptococcal infections and a reduced number of neuropsychiatric exacerbations during the study year. There were no reports of side effects or of any adverse effects from the medications. The authors suggest that both antibiotics may be safe and effective in preventing GAS infection and in decreasing the number of neuropsychiatric exacerbations in these children without any significant differences between groups. This study was limited by the comparison of retrospective data for the baseline year with prospective data of the treatment year using an active comparator. This study does, however, support the feasibility of comparing the efficacy of an antibiotic with a placebo in a similar study design.

Finding literature to support the use of one antibiotic over the other for a prophylaxis trial is extremely difficult for a variety of reasons. For

PANDAS, the study size was small, and studies in RF are limited by failure of prophylactic antibiotics to prevent recurrences of RF and SC and lack of a placebo arm because of ethical issues. Although penicillin remains the standard antibiotic for GAS and RF, its efficacy is questioned throughout the literature [109,110]. For example a Cochrane analysis reported that intramuscular penicillin seemed to be more effective than oral penicillin in preventing recurrence of RF and streptococcal throat infections, but the evidence was based on poor-quality trials [111]. Compliance is another concern because of the need to take the medication every 12 hours for long-term prophylaxis.

Penicillin may serve an additional, non-antimicrobial role in the treatment of some disorders, although such a role has not yet been supported by clinical studies. A recent screening of Food and Drug Administration–approved medications discovered that beta-lactam antibiotics such as ceftriaxone and penicillin promoted the expression of the glutamate transporter GLT1 and demonstrated a neuroprotective role in vivo and in vitro when used in models of ischemic injury and motor neuron degeneration, both based in part on glutamate toxicity. These findings indicate that positive promoters of glutamate expression may have a fundamental neuroprotective role in neurologic disorders such as amyotrophic lateral sclerosis [112].

Macrolides have been used frequently in the past for treating many upper respiratory infections, including GAS pharyngitis, with adequate efficacy ($> 90\%$). Azithromycin has a longer duration of action, allowing a shorter course of treatment. Because of its tolerability and shortened treatment regimen, compliance is easier to maintain. The main drawback to using azithromycin has been reported macrolide-resistant GAS [113] and an increased risk of selection for endemic resistant pathogens over a longer course of treatment [114]. The longest study of azithromycin prophylaxis was by Snider and colleagues [108]. Although the medication seemed to be well tolerated in this small sample, cultures were not examined for resistance. Although the finding was not statistically significant, azithromycin seemed to be less effective than penicillin in reducing neuropsychiatric exacerbations (11 versus 6; $P =$ not significant).

The results of a trial of plasmapheresis or intravenous immunoglobulin (IVIG) in the treatment of children who had PANDAS add additional support for an immune-mediated pathology of OCD and tics [115]. Study participants showed marked improvements in OCD severity, anxiety, and overall functioning, and tic symptoms improved significantly in those receiving plasma exchange. These improvements were noted in the first week with plasma exchange and after 3 weeks of IVIG therapy and were maintained at 1-year follow-up in 82% of the children (subjects received prophylactic antibiotics after immune therapy was completed). Approximately half of the children were able to decrease or discontinue their neuropsychotropic medications. The use of plasma exchange or IVIG acutely for an exacerbation of neuropsychiatric symptoms in patients who have PANDAS requires further research before being considered the standard of care, however.

These treatment benefits seem to be specific to children who clearly meet the criteria for PANDAS, because plasma exchange in four children who had severe chronic OCD did not result in significant improvements [116]. For these patients, it is possible that an immune-mediated process resulted in irreversible neurologic insults that are less responsive to immune therapies. This group, however, might represent children who have non–immune-mediated causes of their illness. Also, the response of neuropsychiatric symptoms to immune therapies is not specific to streptococcal-triggered symptoms. Allen and colleagues [30] reported on two children who had evidence of viral-triggered symptoms that improved after immune therapies. These results should be interpreted with caution, because the typical duration of untreated infection-triggered OCD may be shorter than that of classic OCD.

Two presentations of pediatric autoimmune neuropsychiatric disorders associated with streptococcus

Case 1

Tom, a 9-year-old white boy presented with both parents at the office of a local psychiatrist with the complaint of new-onset nightmares causing him to awaken each morning at 4:00 AM followed by an inability to sleep because of fears of robbers, killers, sex offenders, terrorists, and that the ceiling and roof would fall in because the sheet rock was unable to support the weight. Three weeks before symptom onset, his mother and sibling had developed a sore throat that resolved spontaneously. A few days later, Tom was noted to have a persistent low-grade fever and a sore throat. An appointment was made with his pediatrician but was canceled when his symptoms also spontaneously resolved. Tom also disclosed a compulsive need to touch his pencil five times before he could pick it up. A straight-A student last year, he has "struggled" during the last few weeks according to his parents' report. His parents also report notable irritability, inattentiveness, impaired ability to concentrate and follow instructions, and an increased level of activity that began about the same time as his sleep difficulties. Approximately 6 weeks later his parents noted unusual movements and posturing of hands that occurred even during sleep but stopped during purposeful hand movements. The frequency and severity of the movements varied over the course of the following several weeks. The parents also noted a marked deterioration in handwriting. A brief review of early-childhood records revealed early onset and frequent reoccurrence of otitis media, sinus infections, and mild, but persistent asthma, all before the age of 1 year, and a hospitalization at 13 months for viral pneumonia. He had recurring episodes of strep throat at 3 years and scarlet fever at age 3.5 years. Pregnancy, delivery, and developmental milestones were all normal. When assessed for entry into a research protocol 3 months later, Tom was diagnosed as having OCD, transient tic disorder with choreiform type tics, and ADHD/combined type. His stressed neurologic examination showed difficulty maintaining supinated extensor position with choreiform movements and overflow on stressed gait. His anti-streptolysin O titer was not elevated, but his DNAseB titer had increased during the 3 months since symptom onset.

Comment

Tom is an example of OCD onset without strong evidence of GAS infection because of the possibility of spontaneous recovery without treatment. He also shows chorea-like tics, making the distinction from SC less certain.

Case 2

Ted, an intelligent 8-year-old white boy with an unremarkable medical history, woke up one morning with urinary frequency and urgency. He also began voicing fears that he would "injure someone"—specifically his mother and father. Extremely anxious, he also began asking repeatedly for reassurance about everything he did (eg, he would say, "I moved that fork. Is that OK?"). He also began exhibiting hyperactivity and fear of separation from his parents. Three weeks after presentation of symptoms, his parents took him to a psychiatrist who advised them to have his pediatrician test for streptococcus infection. The resulting throat culture was positive, and a 10-day course of amoxicillin was initiated. Three days after the antibiotic was started, his OCD symptoms resolved. About 2 months later, Ted was seen for entry into the authors' research protocol. His culture was negative, but rising titers were observed between onset and examination, suggesting that the positive findings of the first culture were not caused by a carrier state. Neurologic examination was relevant for neurologic soft signs including mild choreiform movements. He was diagnosed as having OCD, mild transient tics, separation anxiety, and dysgraphia.

Comment

Ted is a good example of sudden-onset severe OCD with many of the core features described in the literature for PANDAS but presented with subclinical pharyngitis.

Controversy concerning pediatric autoimmune neuropsychiatric disorders associated with streptococcus

Adhering to the criteria proposed for PANDAS, these children have dramatic and undeniable presentations [117]. The clinical entity of PANDAS still encounters some skepticism, however [36]. PANDAS criteria have been criticized as being narrow and arbitrary, ignoring the possible clinical spectrum of the disorder. Criteria 1 (presence of OCD/tics) may eventually include additional neuropsychiatric manifestations such as anorexia nervosa [88] and ADHD [83]. The proposed pediatric age range for the onset of PANDAS and a waxing-and-waning clinical course can be problematic in distinguishing these children from those who simply have TS or OCD. Making a conclusive case for GAS association, given the uncertainties of carrier states, missed infections, and chronic titer elevations, adds to the diagnostic quagmire. Nevertheless, PANDAS provides an intriguing phenotypical and theoretical basis for investigating genetic, environmental, and immune-based relationships in OCD spectrum disorders.

Summary

Childhood OCD often develops into a chronic illness that lasts decades. Proof that some type of immunotherapy (such as antibiotic prophylaxis) could significantly reduce recurrence or exacerbation of symptoms of OC or tics would suggest a supportive role for immune triggers in the onset or worsening of these conditions and provide additional tools for improving outcome. The validity of PANDAS will continue to be questioned, however, because demonstrating a clear causation will be difficult on a background of a common childhood illness. Along with the previously mentioned immunotherapy study, validation of the PANDAS phenotype (broadly interpreted) would be advanced from new and continued research in the following areas: (1) prospective studies to identify infectious triggers in the onset and exacerbations of OCD spectrum disorders, (2) biological measures for immune and genetic susceptibility, and (3) large scale epidemiological studies demonstrating the relationship between infection and OCD spectrum disorders. The assimilation of these study results should allow for elucidation of the immune system's role in the onset and maintenance of OCD.

Acknowledgments

Paula J. Edge provided personal and technical assistance in the writing and editing of this article.

References

[1] Rose NR, Bona C. Defining criteria for autoimmune diseases (Witebsky's postulates revisited). Immunol Today 1993;14(9):426–30.
[2] Swedo SE. Sydenham's chorea. A model for childhood autoimmune neuropsychiatric disorders. JAMA 1994;272(22):1788–91.
[3] Asbahr FR, Negrao AB, Gentil V, et al. Obsessive-compulsive and related symptoms in children and adolescents with rheumatic fever with and without chorea: a prospective 6-month study. Am J Psychiatry 1998;155(8):1122–4.
[4] Kiessling LS, Marcotte AC, Culpepper L. Antineuronal antibodies in movement disorders. Pediatrics 1993;92(1):39–43.

[5] Swedo SE, Leonard HL, Garvey M, et al. Pediatric autoimmune neuropsychiatric disorders associated with streptococcal infections: clinical description of the first 50 cases. Am J Psychiatry 1998;155(2):264–71.

[6] Leonard HL, Swedo SE, Rapoport JL, et al. Tourette syndrome and obsessive-compulsive disorder. Adv Neurol 1992;58:83–93.

[7] Carapetis JR, Currie BJ. Rheumatic chorea in northern Australia: a clinical and epidemiological study. Arch Dis Child 1999;80(4):353–8.

[8] Cunningham MW. Pathogenesis of group A streptococcal infections. Clin Microbiol Rev 2000;13(3):470–511.

[9] Proft T, Webb PD, Handley V, et al. Two novel superantigens found in both group A and group C streptococcus. Infect Immun 2003;71(3):1361–9.

[10] Haukness HA, Tanz RR, Thomson RB Jr, et al. The heterogeneity of endemic community pediatric group a streptococcal pharyngeal isolates and their relationship to invasive isolates. J Infect Dis 2002;185(7):915–20.

[11] Berdeli A, Celik HA, Ozyurek R, et al. TLR-2 gene Arg753Gln polymorphism is strongly associated with acute rheumatic fever in children. J Mol Med 2005;83(7):535–41.

[12] Sallakci N, Akcurin G, Koksoy S, et al. TNF-alpha G-308A polymorphism is associated with rheumatic fever and correlates with increased TNF-alpha production. J Autoimmun 2005;25(2):150–4.

[13] Norrby-Teglund A, Chatellier S, Low DE, et al. Host variation in cytokine responses to superantigens determine the severity of invasive group A streptococcal infection. Eur J Immunol 2000;30(11):3247–55.

[14] Hanna GL. Clinical and family-genetic studies of childhood obsessive-compulsive disorder. In: Goodman WK, Rudorfer MV, Maser JD, editors. Obsessive-compulsive disorder: contemporary issues in treatment. Mahwah (NJ): Lawrence Erlbaum Associates; 2000. p. 87–103.

[15] Pauls DL, Leckman JF. The inheritance of Gilles de la Tourette's syndrome and associated behaviors. Evidence for autosomal dominant transmission. N Engl J Med 1986;315(16):993–7.

[16] Zai G, Bezchlibnyk YB, Richter MA, et al. Myelin oligodendrocyte glycoprotein (MOG) gene is associated with obsessive-compulsive disorder. Am J Med Genet B Neuropsychiatr Genet. 2004;129(1):64–8.

[17] Lougee L, Perlmutter SJ, Nicolson R, et al. Psychiatric disorders in first-degree relatives of children with pediatric autoimmune neuropsychiatric disorders associated with streptococcal infections (PANDAS). J Am Acad Child Adolesc Psychiatry 2000;39(9):1120–6.

[18] Giulino L, Gammon P, Sullivan K, et al. Is parental report of upper respiratory infection at the onset of obsessive-compulsive disorder suggestive of pediatric autoimmune neuropsychiatric disorder associated with streptococcal infection? J Child Adolesc Psychopharmacol 2002;12(2):157–64.

[19] Kiessling LS, Marcotte AC, Culpepper L. Antineuronal antibodies: tics and obsessive-compulsive symptoms. J Dev Behav Pediatr 1994;15(6):421–5.

[20] Muller N, Riedel M, Forderreuther S, et al. Tourette's syndrome and *Mycoplasma pneumoniae* infection. Am J Psychiatry 2000;157(3):481–2.

[21] Murphy ML, Pichichero ME. Prospective identification and treatment of children with pediatric autoimmune neuropsychiatric disorder associated with group A streptococcal infection (PANDAS). Arch Pediatr Adolesc Med 2002;156(4):356–61.

[22] Perlmutter SJ, Garvey MA, Castellanos X, et al. A case of pediatric autoimmune neuropsychiatric disorders associated with streptococcal infections. Am J Psychiatry 1998;155(11):1592–8.

[23] Singer HS, Giuliano JD, Zimmerman AM, et al. Infection: a stimulus for tic disorders. Pediatr Neurol 2000;22(5):380–3.

[24] Mell LK, Davis RL, Owens D. Association between streptococcal infection and obsessive-compulsive disorder, Tourette's syndrome, and tic disorder. Pediatrics 2005;116(1):56–60.

[25] Murphy TK, Sajid M, Soto O, et al. Detecting pediatric autoimmune neuropsychiatric disorders associated with streptococcus in children with obsessive-compulsive disorder and tics. Biol Psychiatry 2004;55(1):61–8.

[26] Cardona F, Orefici G. Group A streptococcal infections and tic disorders in an Italian pediatric population. J Pediatr 2001;138(1):71–5.

[27] Kaplan EL, Rothermel CD, Johnson DR. Anti-streptolysin O and anti-deoxyribonuclease B titers: normal values for children ages 2 to 12 in the United States. Pediatrics 1998; 101(1):86–8.

[28] Quinn RW, Liao SJ. A comparative study of antihyaluronidase, antistreptolysin "O", antistreptokinase and streptococcal agglutination titers in patients with rheumatic fever, acute hemolytic streptococcal infections, rheumatoid arthritis and non-rheumatoid forms of arthritis. J Clin Invest 1950;29(9):1156–66.

[29] Weisz JL, McMahon WM, Moore JC, et al. D8/17 and CD19 expression on lymphocytes of patients with acute rheumatic fever and Tourette's disorder. Clin Diagn Lab Immunol 2004;11(2):330–6.

[30] Allen AJ, Leonard HL, Swedo SE. Case study: a new infection-triggered, autoimmune subtype of pediatric OCD and Tourette's syndrome. J Am Acad Child Adolesc Psychiatry 1995;34(3):307–11.

[31] Fallon BA, Nields JA. Lyme disease: a neuropsychiatric illness. Am J Psychiatry 1994; 151(11):1571–83.

[32] Schwartz B, Facklam RR, Breiman RF. Changing epidemiology of group A streptococcal infection in the USA. Lancet 1990;336(8724):1167–71.

[33] Congeni BL. The resurgence of acute rheumatic fever in the United States. Pediatr Ann 1992;21(12):816–20.

[34] Lee LH, Ayoub E, Pichichero ME. Fewer symptoms occur in same-serotype recurrent streptococcal tonsillopharyngitis. Arch Otolaryngol Head Neck Surg 2000;126(11):1359–62.

[35] Quinn RW. Epidemiology of group A streptococcal infections—their changing frequency and severity. Yale J Biol Med 1982;55(3–4):265–70.

[36] Kurlan R, Kaplan EL. The pediatric autoimmune neuropsychiatric disorders associated with streptococcal infection (PANDAS) etiology for tics and obsessive-compulsive symptoms: hypothesis or entity? Practical considerations for the clinician. Pediatrics 2004;113(4):883–6.

[37] Shet A, Kaplan EL. Clinical use and interpretation of group A streptococcal antibody tests: a practical approach for the pediatrician or primary care physician. Pediatr Infect Dis J 2002;21(5):420–6 [quiz: 427–30].

[38] Paluck E, Katzenstein D, Frankish CJ, et al. Prescribing practices and attitudes toward giving children antibiotics. Can Fam Physician 2001;47:521–7.

[39] Ginsburg CM, McCracken GH, Crow SD, et al. Seroepidemiology of the group-A streptococcal carriage state in a private pediatric practice. Am J Dis Child 1985;139(6):614–7.

[40] Hoffmann S. The throat carrier rate of group A and other beta hemolytic streptococci among patients in general practice. Acta Pathol Microbiol Immunol Scand 1985;93(5): 347–51.

[41] Pichichero ME, Marsocci SM, Murphy ML, et al. Incidence of streptococcal carriers in private pediatric practice. Arch Pediatr Adolesc Med 1999;153(6):624–8.

[42] Dowell SF. Seasonal variation in host susceptibility and cycles of certain infectious diseases. Emerg Infect Dis 2001;7(3):369–74.

[43] Tolaymat A, Goudarzi T, Soler GP, et al. Acute rheumatic fever in north Florida. South Med J 1984;77(7):819–23.

[44] Snider LA, Seligman LD, Ketchen BR, et al. Tics and problem behaviors in schoolchildren: prevalence, characterization, and associations. Pediatrics 2002;110:331–6.

[45] Knopf PM, Harling-Berg CJ, Cserr HF, et al. Antigen-dependent intrathecal antibody synthesis in the normal rat brain: tissue entry and local retention of antigen-specific B cells. J Immunol 1998;161(2):692–701.

[46] Bronze MS, Dale JB. Epitopes of streptococcal M proteins that evoke antibodies that cross-react with human brain. J Immunol 1993;151(5):2820–8.

[47] Kotby AA, El Badawy N, El Sokkary S, et al. Antineuronal antibodies in rheumatic chorea. Clin Diagn Lab Immunol 1998;5(6):836–9.

[48] Singer HS, Giuliano JD, Hansen BH, et al. Antibodies against human putamen in children with Tourette syndrome. Neurology 1998;50(6):1618–24.

[49] Murphy TK, Goodman WK, Fudge MW, et al. B lymphocyte antigen D8/17: a peripheral marker for childhood-onset obsessive-compulsive disorder and Tourette's syndrome? Am J Psychiatry 1997;154(3):402–7.

[50] Singer HS, Hong JJ, Rippel CA, et al. The need for caution in considering the diagnostic utility of antibasal ganglia antibodies in movement disorders. Arch Dis Child 2004;89(7):595–7.

[51] Dale RC, Heyman I, Giovannoni G, et al. Incidence of anti-brain antibodies in children with obsessive-compulsive disorder. Br J Psychiatry 2005;187:314–9.

[52] Pavone P, Bianchini R, Parano E, et al. Anti-brain antibodies in PANDAS versus uncomplicated streptococcal infection. Pediatr Neurol 2004;30(2):107–10.

[53] Hallett JJ, Harling-Berg CJ, Knopf PM, et al. Anti-striatal antibodies in Tourette syndrome cause neuronal dysfunction. J Neuroimmunol 2000;111(1–2):195–202.

[54] Loiselle CR, Lee O, Moran TH, et al. Striatal microinfusion of Tourette syndrome and PANDAS sera: failure to induce behavioral changes. Mov Disord 2004;19(4):390–6.

[55] Kirvan CA, Swedo SE, Heuser JS, et al. Mimicry and autoantibody-mediated neuronal cell signaling in Sydenham chorea. Nat Med 2003;9(7):914–20.

[56] Rippel CA, Hong JJ, Yoon DY, et al. Methodologic factors affect the measurement of anti-basal ganglia antibodies. Ann Clin Lab Sci 2005;35(2):121–30.

[57] Kantor L, Hewlett GH, Gnegy ME. Enhanced amphetamine- and K + -mediated dopamine release in rat striatum after repeated amphetamine: differential requirements for Ca2 + - and calmodulin-dependent phosphorylation and synaptic vesicles. J Neurosci 1999;19(10):3801–8.

[58] Teixeira AL Jr, Guimaraes MM, Romano-Silva MA, et al. Serum from Sydenham's chorea patients modifies intracellular calcium levels in PC12 cells by a complement-independent mechanism. Mov Disord 2005;20(7):843–5.

[59] Mercadante MT, Busatto GF, Lombroso PJ, et al. The psychiatric symptoms of rheumatic fever. Am J Psychiatry 2000;157(12):2036–8.

[60] Asbahr FR, Garvey MA, Snider LA, et al. Obsessive-compulsive symptoms among patients with Sydenham chorea. Biol Psychiatry 2005;57(9):1073–6.

[61] Maia AS, Barbosa ER, Menezes PR, et al. Relationship between obsessive-compulsive disorders and diseases affecting primarily the basal ganglia. Rev Hosp Clin Fac Med Sao Paulo 1999;54(6):213–21.

[62] Asbahr FR, Ramos RT, Costa AN, et al. Obsessive-compulsive symptoms in adults with history of rheumatic fever, Sydenham's chorea and type I diabetes mellitus: preliminary results. Acta Psychiatr Scand 2005;111(2):159–61.

[63] Placidi GP, Boldrini M, Patronelli A, et al. Prevalence of psychiatric disorders in thyroid diseased patients. Neuropsychobiology 1998;38(4):222–5.

[64] George MS, Kellner CH, Fossey MD. Obsessive-compulsive symptoms in a patient with multiple sclerosis. J Nerv Ment Dis 1989;177(5):304–5.

[65] Miguel EC, Stein MC, Rauch SL, et al. Obsessive-compulsive disorder in patients with multiple sclerosis. J Neuropsychiatry Clin Neurosci 1995;7(4):507–10.

[66] Slattery MJ, Dubbert BK, Allen AJ, et al. Prevalence of obsessive-compulsive disorder in patients with systemic lupus erythematosus. J Clin Psychiatry 2004;65(3):301–6.

[67] Dinn WM, Harris CL, McGonigal KM, et al. Obsessive-compulsive disorder and immunocompetence. Int J Psychiatry Med 2001;31(3):311–20.

[68] Carpenter LL, Heninger GR, McDougle CJ, et al. Cerebrospinal fluid interleukin-6 in obsessive-compulsive disorder and trichotillomania. Psychiatry Res 2002;112(3):257–62.

[69] Marazziti D, Presta S, Pfanner C, et al. Immunological alterations in adult obsessive-compulsive disorder. Biol Psychiatry 1999;46(6):810–4.

[70] Ravindran AV, Griffiths J, Merali Z, et al. Circulating lymphocyte subsets in obsessive compulsive disorder, major depression and normal controls. J Affect Disord 1999; 52(1–3):1–10.

[71] Black JL, Lamke GT, Walikonis JE. Serologic survey of adult patients with obsessive-compulsive disorder for neuron-specific and other autoantibodies. Psychiatry Res 1998;81(3): 371–80.

[72] Hutto JH, Ayoub EM. Cytotoxicity of lymphocytes from patients with rheumatic carditis in vitro. In: Read SE, Zabriskie JB, editors. Streptococcal diseases and the immune response. New York: Academic Press; 1987. p. 733–8.

[73] Tomai M, Kotb M, Majumdar G, et al. Superantigenicity of streptococcal M protein. J Exp Med 1990;172(1):359–62.

[74] Mittleman BB, Castellanos FX, Jacobsen LK, et al. Cerebrospinal fluid cytokines in pediatric neuropsychiatric disease. J Immunol 1997;159(6):2994–9.

[75] Maes M, Meltzer HY, Bosmans E. Psychoimmune investigation in obsessive-compulsive disorder: assays of plasma transferrin, IL-2 and IL-6 receptor, and IL-1 beta and IL-6 concentrations. Neuropsychobiology 1994;30(2–3):57–60.

[76] Monteleone P, Catapano F, Fabrazzo M, et al. Decreased blood levels of tumor necrosis factor-alpha in patients with obsessive-compulsive disorder. Neuropsychobiology 1998; 37(4):182–5.

[77] Denys D, Fluitman S, Kavelaars A, et al. Decreased TNF-alpha and NK activity in obsessive-compulsive disorder. Psychoneuroendocrinology 2004;29(7):945–52.

[78] Leckman JF, Katsovich L, Kawikova I, et al. Increased serum levels of interleukin-12 and tumor necrosis factor-alpha in Tourette's syndrome. Biol Psychiatry 2005;57(6): 667–73.

[79] Luo F, Leckman JF, Katsovich L, et al. Prospective longitudinal study of children with tic disorders and/or obsessive-compulsive disorder: relationship of symptom exacerbations to newly acquired streptococcal infections. Pediatrics 2004;113(6):e578–85.

[80] Singer HS, Loiselle CR, Lee O, et al. Anti-basal ganglia antibodies in PANDAS. Mov Disord 2004;19(4):406–15.

[81] Wendlandt JT, Grus FH, Hansen BH, et al. Striatal antibodies in children with Tourette's syndrome: multivariate discriminant analysis of IgG repertoires. J Neuroimmunol 2001; 119(1):106–13.

[82] Morshed SA, Parveen S, Leckman JF, et al. Antibodies against neural, nuclear, cytoskeletal, and streptococcal epitopes in children and adults with Tourette's syndrome, Sydenham's chorea, and autoimmune disorders. Biol Psychiatry 2001;50(8):566–77.

[83] Swedo SE, Leonard HL, Mittleman BB, et al. Identification of children with pediatric autoimmune neuropsychiatric disorders associated with streptococcal infections by a marker associated with rheumatic fever. Am J Psychiatry 1997;154(1):110–2.

[84] Niehaus DJ, Knowles JA, van Kradenberg J, et al. D8/17 in obsessive-compulsive disorder and trichotillomania. S Afr Med J 1999;89(7):755–6.

[85] Murphy TK, Benson N, Zaytoun A, et al. Progress toward analysis of D8/17 binding to B cells in children with obsessive compulsive disorder and/or chronic tic disorder. J Neuroimmunol 2001;120(1–2):146–51.

[86] Hoekstra PJ, Bijzet J, Limburg PC, et al. Elevated D8/17 expression on B lymphocytes, a marker of rheumatic fever, measured with flow cytometry in tic disorder patients. Am J Psychiatry 2001;158(4):605–10.

[87] Eisen JL, Leonard HL, Swedo SE, et al. The use of antibody D8/17 to identify B cells in adults with obsessive-compulsive disorder. Psychiatry Res 2001;104(3):221–5.

[88] Sokol MS, Ward PE, Tamiya H, et al. D8/17 expression on B lymphocytes in anorexia nervosa. Am J Psychiatry 2002;159(8):1430–2.

[89] Inoff-Germain G, Rodriguez RS, Torres-Alcantara S, et al. An immunological marker (D8/17) associated with rheumatic fever as a predictor of childhood psychiatric disorders in a community sample. J Child Psychol Psychiatry 2003;44(5):782–90.

[90] Peterson BS, Leckman JF, Tucker D, et al. Preliminary findings of antistreptococcal antibody titers and basal ganglia volumes in tic, obsessive-compulsive, and attention deficit/hyperactivity disorders. Arch Gen Psychiatry 2000;57(4):364–72.

[91] Perrin EM, Murphy ML, Casey JR, et al. Does group A beta-hemolytic streptococcal infection increase risk for behavioral and neuropsychiatric symptoms in children? Arch Pediatr Adolesc Med 2004;158(9):848–56.

[92] Lamers KJ, van Engelen BG, Gabreels FJ, et al. Cerebrospinal neuron-specific enolase, S-100 and myelin basic protein in neurological disorders. Acta Neurol Scand 1995;92(3):247–51.

[93] van Passel R, Schlooz WA, Lamers KJ, et al. S100B protein, glia and Gilles de la Tourette syndrome. Eur J Paediatr Neurol 2001;5(1):15–9.

[94] Zabriskie JB. Rheumatic fever: a model for the pathological consequences of microbial-host mimicry. Clin Exp Rheumatol 1986;4(1):65–73.

[95] Murphy T, Goodman W. Genetics of childhood disorders: XXXIV. Autoimmune disorders, part 7: D8/17 reactivity as an immunological marker of susceptibility to neuropsychiatric disorders. J Am Acad Child Adolesc Psychiatry 2002;41(1):98–100.

[96] Hamilton CS, Garvey MA, Swedo SE. Sensitivity of the D8/17 assay. Am J Psychiatry 2003;160(6):1193–4 [author reply: 1194].

[97] Dale RC. Post-streptococcal autoimmune disorders of the central nervous system. Dev Med Child Neurol 2005;47(11):785–91.

[98] Murphy TK, Goodman WK, Ayoub EM, et al. On defining Sydenham's chorea: where do we draw the line? Biol Psychiatry 2000;47(10):851–7.

[99] Jansen TL, Janssen M, Traksel R, et al. A clinical and serological comparison of group A versus non-group A streptococcal reactive arthritis and throat culture negative cases of post-streptococcal reactive arthritis. Ann Rheum Dis 1999;58(7):410–4.

[100] Snider LA, Sachdev V, MaCkaronis JE, et al. Echocardiographic findings in the PANDAS subgroup. Pediatrics 2004;114(6):e748–51.

[101] Paradise JL, Bluestone CD, Colborn DK, et al. Tonsillectomy and adenotonsillectomy for recurrent throat infection in moderately affected children. Pediatrics 2002;110(1 Pt 1):7–15.

[102] Zielnik-Jurkiewicz B, Jurkiewicz D. Implication of immunological abnormalities after adenotonsillotomy. Int J Pediatr Otorhinolaryngol 2002;64(2):127–32.

[103] Gebremariam A. Sydenham's chorea: risk factors and the role of prophylactic benzathine penicillin G in preventing recurrence. Ann Trop Paediatr 1999;19(2):161–5.

[104] Terreri MT, Roja SC, Len CA, et al. Sydenham's chorea—clinical and evolutive characteristics. Sao Paulo Med J 2002;120(1):16–9.

[105] Korn-Lubetzki I, Brand A, Steiner I. Recurrence of Sydenham chorea: implications for pathogenesis. Arch Neurol 2004;61(8):1261–4.

[106] Berrios X, Quesney F, Morales A, et al. Are all recurrences of "pure" Sydenham chorea true recurrences of acute rheumatic fever? J Pediatr 1985;107(6):867–72.

[107] Garvey MA, Perlmutter SJ, Allen AJ, et al. A pilot study of penicillin prophylaxis for neuropsychiatric exacerbations triggered by streptococcal infections. Biol Psychiatry 1999;45(12):1564–71.

[108] Snider LA, Lougee L, Slattery M, et al. Antibiotic prophylaxis with azithromycin or penicillin for childhood-onset neuropsychiatric disorders. Biol Psychiatry 2005;57(7):788–92.

[109] Brook I, Gober AE. Antimicrobial resistance in the nasopharyngeal flora of children with acute otitis media and otitis media recurring after amoxicillin therapy. J Med Microbiol 2005;54(Pt 1):83–5.

[110] Kaplan EL. Pathogenesis of acute rheumatic fever and rheumatic heart disease: evasive after half a century of clinical, epidemiological, and laboratory investigation. Heart 2005; 91:3–4.

[111] Manyemba J, Mayosi BM. Penicillin for secondary prevention of rheumatic fever. Cochrane Database Syst Rev 2002;(3):CD002227.

[112] Rothstein JD, Patel S, Regan MR, et al. Beta-lactam antibiotics offer neuroprotection by increasing glutamate transporter expression. Nature 2005;433(7021):73–7.

[113] Richter SS, Heilmann KP, Beekmann SE, et al. Macrolide-resistant *Streptococcus pyogenes* in the United States, 2002–2003. Clin Infect Dis 2005;41(5):599–608.

[114] Guchev IA, Gray GC, Klochkov OI. Two regimens of azithromycin prophylaxis against community-acquired respiratory and skin/soft-tissue infections among military trainees. Clin Infect Dis 2004;38(8):1095–101.

[115] Perlmutter SJ, Leitman SF, Garvey MA, et al. Therapeutic plasma exchange and intravenous immunoglobulin for obsessive-compulsive disorder and tic disorders in childhood. Lancet 1999;354(9185):1153–8.

[116] Nicolson R, Swedo SE, Lenane M, et al. An open trial of plasma exchange in childhood-onset obsessive- compulsive disorder without poststreptococcal exacerbations. J Am Acad Child Adolesc Psychiatry 2000;39(10):1313–5.

[117] Swedo SE, Leonard HL, Rapoport JL. The pediatric autoimmune neuropsychiatric disorders associated with streptococcal infection (PANDAS) subgroup: separating fact from fiction. Pediatrics 2004;113(4):907–11.

PSYCHIATRIC
CLINICS
OF NORTH AMERICA

ELSEVIER
SAUNDERS

Psychiatr Clin N Am 29 (2006) 471–486

Tourette's Syndrome

Roseli Gedanke Shavitt, MD, PhD*,
Ana Gabriela Hounie, MD, PhD,
Maria Conceição Rosário Campos, MD, PhD,
Eurípedes C. Miguel, MD, PhD

*Department of Psychiatry, University of São Paulo Medical School,
Rua Dr. Ovidio Pires de Campos, Sao Paulo 05430-010, Brazil*

The essential features of Tourette's syndrome (TS) are chronic motor and vocal tics. According to the *Diagnostic and Statistical Manual of Mental Disorders*, edition 4, symptoms should start before age 18 years and persist for at least 1 year; symptom-free intervals should last no longer than 3 months [1].

TS is a category within the spectrum of tic disorders that affects about 1% of school-aged children, whereas the estimated prevalence rates for all tic disorders (TS, chronic motor or vocal tic disorder, and transient tic disorder) range from 4% to 18% [2]. TS is four times more frequent in males than in females [2].

A waxing-and-waning course is typical of TS, and the natural history of TS is characterized by improvement over time [3]. The average age of onset of symptoms is 7 years but typically ranges from 3 to 8 years. Tic severity is usually greater around ages 7 to 12 years, with a steady decline until age 20 years [3]. To date, no clinical measures have been identified that can predict which patients' tic symptoms will persist into adulthood.

The frequent association of TS with obsessive-compulsive symptoms (OCS) and obsessive-compulsive disorder (OCD) is widely recognized [2,4]. Evidence suggests that TS and OCD are disorders that might be considered part of one spectrum because of similar clinical characteristics, familial/ genetic background, and neurobiologic hypotheses [5–7]. The clinical

This work was supported by grants from Fundação de Amparo à Pesquisa do Estado de São Paulo (FAPESP) - #99/08560- and Conselho Nacional de Desenvolvimento Científico e Tecnológico (CNPQ), Brazil - #521369/96-7.
    * Corresponding author.
    E-mail address: roseli@protoc.com.br (R.G. Shavitt).

association between tics and OCS was noted in the original description by
Itard, in 1825, of the Marquise de Dampierre, a noblewoman who presented
motor and vocal tics and obsessive thoughts [8]. In 1885, Gilles de la Tourette
published the first report on patients who presented a combination of multiple motor tics and involuntary vocalizations, with the occasional appearance
of eruptive cursing that he designated "coprolalia" [8]. Current evidence regarding comorbidity and family and molecular genetic, neuroimaging, and
treatment studies suggest that TS, OCD, and chronic tic disorder arise
from a common neurobiologic pathway [6]. The relationship of TS and
this postulated spectrum of disorders is reviewed in the following sections.

Clinical features of tics

A tic is a sudden, repetitive movement, gesture, or utterance that typically
mimics some fragment of normal behavior. Tics have brief duration and often occur in periodic bouts, with a frequency that may vary from few times
a week to uncountable bursts occurring more than 100 times per minute [3].
Tics vary in intensity and forcefulness, typically diminish during sleep or activities that need concentration, and can be intensified by anxiety, stress, fatigue, and excitement [9]. Tics can be suppressed by voluntary effort, but this
suppression frequently leads to a heightened emotional state, which is commonly described by patients as an energy that builds up until the tics are performed. Although tics can be totally involuntary, they often are preceded by
subjective experiences—general feelings, premonitory urges, or bodily sensations—that occur immediately before or during the tics and can be as dis-
turbing as the tics themselves [3,10].
      TS typically starts with simple motor tics of the eyes, face, or head and
may progress to tics involving the shoulders, trunk, and extremities [9].
Examples of simple motor tics include eye blinking, head jerks, or shoulder
shrugs. Complex motor tics manifest as purposeful-appearing behaviors,
such as facial expressions or gestures, and might involve dystonic movements. Symptoms may be relatively mild (eg, slapping or tapping) or, less
frequently, may be more severe (eg, punching one side of the face, biting
a wrist, or gouging eyes to the point of blindness or bone fractures) [9].
      Phonic or vocal tics are sounds, noises, or utterances made by the airflow
through the nose or mouth. On average, phonic tics begin many years after
the onset of motor tics and usually are simple in character [3]. They can
range from simple throat clearing, grunting, and squeaking to more complex
vocalizations, including dramatic and abrupt changes in the rhythm, rate,
and volume of speech, echolalia, palilalia, and, less frequently, coprolalia
(obscene speech) [11].
      Varying degrees of disability may result from TS symptoms, depending
on the presence of additional disorders, the level of support from the relatives, and the patient's individual abilities. Social isolation, difficulty in making friends, and family conflicts are frequent complications [9].

Complex tics may involve ritualized behaviors that resemble compulsions. The difference between some complex tics and compulsions can be subtle. For instance, according to current nosology, a ticlike compulsion such as touching someone with one hand after touching with the other can be conceptualized as a complex motor tic or as a compulsion without an obsession. Likewise, an eye blink performed to relieve the fear that something tragic will happen to a close relative may be erroneously classified as a tic, when it should be considered a compulsion. Taking into account all the evidence suggesting a common pathophysiology between TS and OCD, the authors have suggested the term "intentional repetitive behavior" (ie, the patient mentally determines the need to perform the behavior) to describe a continuum of these complex clinical phenomena (for more detail, see [12]). The intentional repetitive behaviors may be preceded or accompanied by certain subjective experiences, also called "sensory phenomena," described as general feelings, urges, bodily sensations, or "just-right" perceptions. As discussed later, these sensory phenomena may differentiate subgroups of OCD patients who have or do not have comorbid TS [10].

Comorbidity in Tourette's syndrome

The most frequent comorbidities in patients who have TS are attention-deficit hyperactivity disorder (ADHD), OCS, and OCD [2,4,13]. High rates of mood and anxiety disorders have also been reported in TS samples [4,13]. In comparing TS alone, OCD alone, and TS plus OCD, Coffey and colleagues [13] found that the pattern of comorbidity for the TS plus OCD group was closer to that of TS alone than to that of OCD alone, suggesting that TS plus OCD is a more severe phenotype than TS or OCD and etiologically may be more closely linked to TS than to OCD (Table 1).

This article addresses TS with comorbid OCD. ADHD, thricotillomania, body dysmorphic disorder, and other associated conditions are discussed in other articles in this issue.

Tourette's syndrome with comorbid obsessive-compulsive disorder

Many studies have emphasized that the clinical characteristics of OCD in patients who have TS differ from those found in patients who have OCD alone and have described the clinical features that characterize the tic-related OCD phenotype. The differences between tic-related and non–tic-related OCD are shown in Table 1.

Patients who have OCD with and without tics also differ in the subjective experiences that precede or accompany their repetitive behaviors. Such subjective experiences may be described as cognitions (ie, thoughts, ideas, or images), autonomic anxiety (ie, somatic feelings of anxiety), and sensory phenomena (for a detailed description, see [10]). To assess these variables, the authors' group developed a structured interview in which patients are

Table 1
Clinical features that are more frequent in patients who have tic-related OCD than in patients who have non–tic-related OCD

Phenotypic features	Study
Presence of sensory phenomena	Miguel et al, 1995 [12]; 1997 [14]; 2000 [10]
Intrusive, violent, and sexual images or thoughts, hoarding, and counting rituals	Rasmussen & Tsuang, 1986 [15]; Pitman, 1987 [16]; George et al, 1993 [17]; Holzer et al, 1994 [18]; Eapen et al, 1997 [19]; Miguel et al, 1997 [14]; Petter et al, 1998 [20]; Swerdlow et al, 1999 [21]
"Ticlike" compulsions (need to touch, tap, or rub items, or blinking and staring to relieve the distress caused by obsessions)	George et al, 1993 [17]; Holzer et al, 1994 [18]; Leckman et al, 1994 [22]; Miguel et al, 1997 [14]; Eapen et al, 1997 [19]; Petter et al, 1998 [20]; Rosario-Campos et al, 2001 [23]
Symmetry/hoarding symptoms	Baer, 1994 [24]; Mataix-Cols et al, 1999 [25]
Aggressive, sexual and religious obsessions and related compulsions and symmetry/ordering symptoms	George et al, 1993 [17]; Leckman et al, 1997 [26]
Higher number and variety of OCS	Miguel et al, 1997 [14]
Higher comorbidity with trichotillomania, body dysmorphic disorder, bipolar disorder, attention deficit/hyperactive disorder, social phobia, substance abuse	Coffey et al, 1998 [13]

Abbreviations: OCD, obsessive-compulsive disorder; OCS, obsessive-compulsive symptoms.
Adapted from Hounie AG, Rosario-Campos MC, Diniz JB, et al. Obsessive-compulsive disorder in Tourette syndrome. Adv Neurol 2006;99:22–38.

asked to identify the phenomena that precede or accompany their repetitive behaviors [12]. When compared with patients who have TS alone, patients who have OCD alone report a higher frequency of cognitive and autonomic anxiety phenomena and a lower frequency of sensory phenomena preceding repetitive behaviors. Patients who have OCD plus TS report a higher frequency of sensory phenomena than patients who have OCD alone, similar that in patients who have TS alone [10,14].

Another study by the authors' group has measured the impact of TS and chronic motor tics in the clinical profile of OCD by comparing three groups [27]. Group 1 comprised patients who had OCD without tics (ie, OCD); patients in group 2 had OCD plus chronic motor/vocal tics (CMVT; ie, OCD plus CMVT); and patients in group 3 had OCD plus TS. In patients who had OCD the frequency of intrusive sounds, repeating behaviors, counting compulsions, and ticlike compulsions was lower than in the other two groups. Patients who had OCD plus CMVT had intermediate scores for somatic obsessions, bodily sensations, just-right perceptions, presence of sensory phenomena, number of psychiatric comorbidities, age at interview, and age at OCS onset. On the other hand, patients who had OCD plus CMVT had significantly higher scores than patients who had OCD or patients who had OCD plus TS on religious obsessions and depressive mood disorders. These findings suggest that the OCD phenotype may vary according to the presence of chronic tics or TS [27].

Tourette's syndrome, obsessive-compulsive disorder, and the search for quantitative phenotypes

It is often difficult to define mutually exclusive OCD or TS subtypes, and the categorical approach does not allow researchers to deal with the consistent overlap in patients who belong simultaneously to different subgroups. Therefore, there have been attempts to deal with the phenotypic heterogeneity in OCD and TS in a dimensional approach.

For instance, Alsobrook and Pauls [28], using an agglomerative hierarchical cluster analysis and factor analysis, have identified four TS symptom dimensions: (1) aggressive phenomena (eg, kicking, temper fits, argumentativeness), (2) purely motor and phonic tic symptoms, (3) compulsive phenomena (eg, touching of others or objects, repetitive speech, throat clearing), and (4) tapping and absence of grunting. Of interest, the third factor has been associated with a greater risk for ADHD, but not for OCD, in the probands, and a greater risk for ADHD and OCD in the relatives [28].

In OCD, there have been at least 12 factor-analytic studies published, involving more than 2000 patients [29]. These studies have consistently identified three to five symptom-factors or dimensions, accounting for nearly 70% of the variance [24,26]. Some studies have associated tic-related OCD with high scores on the dimension "aggression/sexual/religious obsessions and related compulsions" and the dimension "symmetry and ordering obsessions and compulsions" [24,26]. Leckman and colleagues [30] found that these same dimensions correlated significantly in sibling pairs concordant for TS and also noted that mother–child correlations were significant for these two factors. The "aggression," the "symmetry," and the "hoarding" dimensions were more frequently found in patients who had tic-related OCD than in patients who had non–tic-related OCD. These studies suggest that some OCD symptom dimensions correlate with comorbid tic disorders and also might be associated with higher familial loading.

Pathogenesis

Genetics

Genetic epidemiologic studies
Family and twin studies have demonstrated that genetic factors participate in the vertical transmission of TS and associated conditions [31,32]. Results from segregation analysis studies suggest that the pattern of transmission within TS families is consistent with autosomal transmission [5,30].

Family studies provide the most compelling evidence for the association between TS and OCD. First-degree relatives of TS probands have higher frequencies of OCS, OCD, and TS than seen in relatives of controls, regardless of whether the proband has a concomitant diagnosis of TS [5,33]. Similarly, first-degree relatives of OCD probands have higher frequencies of

OCD and tic disorders than seen in relatives of controls [6,34,35]. Studies with OCD probands indicated that the earlier the age at onset of OCS in the proband, the higher the genetic loading in the family for both OCD and tics [6,34].

Rosario-Campos and colleagues [36] evaluated the effects of an early on-set of OCS in 106 childhood probands and the recurrence risks of OCD and tics in 325 first-degree relatives. These rates were compared with 44 control probands and 140 first-degree family members. The study results were consistent with earlier reports of early-onset OCD cases, indicating that the familial aggregation of OCD is largely concentrated among families with early-onset OCD probands. The risk of morbidity among case relatives was the highest reported so far (odds ratio, 25.2) [36].

Molecular studies

A study of a large French Canadian family identified evidence for linkage at chromosome region 11q23 [37]. This study used markers previously identified in linkage studies of population isolates in South Africa [38]. Alternatively, in a sibling-pair study undertaken by the Tourette Syndrome International Consortium for Genetics, the areas on chromosome 4q and 8p were suggestive of linkage [39]. A genome scan using the affected-pedigree method on a series of multigenerational families revealed loci on chromosomes 5, 10, and 13 as markers of possible linkage in at least one of the families [40].

Two studies of patients who had TS plus OCD have shown interesting results. One did a genome scan of the hoarding phenotype and reported significant allele sharing for markers at 4q34-35, 5q35, and 17q25 [41]. The other completed univariate and complex segregation analyses using quantitative OCS dimension scores [31]. Segregation analyses were consistent with dominant major gene effects for both dimension 1 (aggression obsessions and related compulsions) and dimension 2 (symmetry obsessions and related compulsions), whereas the findings for dimension 3 (contamination/cleaning) and dimension 4 (hoarding symptoms) were consistent with recessive inheritance [31].

The candidate genes that have been examined in association studies with patients who have TS and controls include various dopamine receptors (DRD1, DRD2, DRD4, and DRD5), the dopamine transporter, various noradrenergic genes (ADRA2a, ADRA2C, and DBH) and some serotonergic genes (5-HTT) [3]. The current view is that these alleles could have a cumulative effect rather than be a major source of vulnerability to TS [3].

Findings regarding cytogenetic abnormalities in patients who have TS include a de novo duplication of the long arm of chromosome 7 [42], a balanced translocation between chromosomes 6 and 8 with a translocation breakpoint on chromosome 8q [43], an 18q21.1-q22.2 inversion [44], and alterations in chromosomes 2 and 7 affecting the gene for a membrane protein at nodes of Ranvier [45]. More recently, Abelson and colleagues [46] were able to identify Slit and Trk-like 1 (*SLITRK1*) as a candidate gene on chromosome 13q31.1. These authors also reported a frameshift mutation and two independent occurrences of the identical variant in the binding site for microRNA hsa-miR-189 among 174 unrelated probands. These variants were absent from 3600 control chromosomes, and *SLITRK1* mRNA and *hsa-miR-189* showed an overlapping expression pattern in brain regions previously implicated in TS [46].

To conclude, even though the genes involved in TS expression and their respective patterns of transmission have not been identified so far, there are some promising results, and future research will probably add some heuristic data.

Immunologic aspects: the role of streptococcal infection and rheumatic fever

The designation "pediatric autoimmune neuropsychiatric disorders associated with streptococcal infection" (PANDAS) has been proposed to describe prepubertal children in whom OCD or TS symptoms begin abruptly or exacerbate after infection with a group A beta hemolytic streptococcus (GABHS) [47]. Further studies have described a higher prevalence of OCD or TS in rheumatic fever, even without Sydenham's chorea, both in active [48,49] and nonactive phases [50,51]. Supporting this proposal is evidence from one study that reported improvement in OCD and TS symptoms in cases of PANDAS after plasmapheresis [52]. Familial aggregation of OCD/TS has been described in cases of rheumatic fever (Hounie AG, Pauls DL, Rosário-Campos MC, et al. Obsessive-compulsive spectrum disorder and rheumatic fever: a family study; unpublished manuscript) as well as in PANDAS [53]. Relatives of patients who have PANDAS/OCD have shown the same rate of OCD as relatives of children who have OCD, which may suggest that classic early-onset OCD shares underlying mechanisms with OCD triggered by streptococcal infections. Higher rates of rheumatic fever were also described in parents and grandparents of patients who had PANDAS than in parents and grandparents of controls [47].

The hypothesized mechanism underlying the relationship between streptococcal infection, rheumatic fever, and the OCD spectrum is the molecular mimicry between bacteria and host. This assumption has been widely supported by several studies showing higher levels of autoantibodies in patients who had OCD [49]. Moreover, Muller and colleagues [54] reported higher titers of antibodies against M proteins (the major virulence factor of GABHS) in 25 adult patients who had TS than in 25 healthy controls. An animal-model study suggested that autoantibodies from a patient who had Sydenham's chorea might activate neurons binding transmembrane lysoganglioside, suggesting the possibility of a pathway through which antibodies could act within the neuronal circuitries involved in this disorder

[55]. A trial of neuropsychiatric symptom prophylaxis with oral penicillin in children who had PANDAS was unsuccessful, however [56], and two prospective longitudinal studies failed to demonstrate a clear relation between new GABHS infections and the development or exacerbation of tic symptoms [57,58]. Therefore the PANDAS concept remains controversial.

Perinatal events

Risk factors for the development of TS include pre- and perinatal adverse events. Delivery complications, especially forceps deliveries, and fetal exposure to high levels of coffee, cigarettes, or alcohol were associated with male gender and OCD in a sample of TS probands [59]. In a later study, males were more likely to have experienced birth complications in a cohort of 148 TS patients, suggesting that perinatal brain injury may be implicated in the etiology of TS in some boys [4]. Future studies of potential epigenetic risk factors should clarify their contribution to the manifestation of TS.

Neuroimaging

Volumetric MRI studies have shown larger dorsolateral prefrontal regions in children but significantly smaller volumes in adults who have TS [60]. Aberrant laterality in TS was suggested by the reduced or reversed basal ganglia asymmetry, mainly in male subjects who had TS [61]. In a group of patients who had TS, the cross-sectional area of the corpus callosum was reduced when compared with normal controls [61]. On the other hand, children who had TS showed larger volumes in four subregions of the corpus callosum, mainly in the rostral body, formed by axons connecting premotor and supplementary motor areas of both hemispheres [62]. A recent prospective, longitudinal study in 43 children measured before age 14 years investigated the association of basal ganglia volumes with the severity of tics and OCS at the time of childhood MRI and at follow-up after an average of 7.5 years [63]. The volumes of caudate nucleus correlated significantly and inversely with the severity of tics and OCS in early adulthood but did not correlate with the severity of symptoms at the time of the MRI scan, suggesting that morphologic disturbances of the caudate nucleus within cortico-striatal-thalamocortical circuits are central to the persistence of both tics and OCS into adulthood [63].

Functional neuroimaging studies have found that voluntary tic suppression involves deactivation of the putamen and globus pallidus, coupled with partial activation of prefrontal cortex and caudate nucleus. The smaller the difference between right caudate activation and other subcortical areas deactivation, the more severe are the symptoms [64]. Apparently, patients who have TS exhibit decreased activity in the caudate and thalamus, together with increased activity of the lateral and medial premotor cortex, supplementary motor areas, anterior cingulate gyrus, dorsolateral-rostral prefrontal cortex, inferior parietal cortex, putamen, caudate, primary motor cortex,

Broca's area, superior temporal gyrus, insula, and claustrum [65]. Vocal tics, including coprolalia, seem to activate pre-rolandic and post-rolandic language regions, insula, caudate, thalamus, and cerebellum, whereas motor tics seem to be associated with activity in sensorimotor cortex [65].

Positron-emission tomography and single-photon emission CT data from subjects who have TS suggest an increased density of presynaptic dopamine transporters and postsynaptic dopamine D2 receptors, as well as a greater dopamine release in the putamen when compared with healthy controls [66]. These data suggest a relevant role of dopamine in TS, and are consistent with the efficacy of dopamine antagonists for the treatment of TS. Nevertheless, the glutamatergic, serotonergic, cholinergic, noradrenergic, and opioid systems may also be implicated, once they are present in the cortico-striatal-thalamocortical circuits and interact with the dopaminergic system [66].

In conclusion, there is evidence that the manifestation of both TS and OCD involves abnormalities in cortico-striatal-thalamocortical pathways. Compared with OCD, TS seems associated with activation of cortical areas other than the orbitofrontal cortex, especially sensorimotor areas.

Treatment of Tourette's syndrome

Patients who have mild symptoms can be managed with nonpharmacologic approaches, such as proper education, counseling, and behavioral techniques. The temporal pattern of tics can help the doctor decide whether to begin anti-tic drug treatment or simply provide monitoring and support [3]. For more severe cases, medication can be considered. A successful treatment does not necessarily mean the complete suppression of tics but rather a substantial reduction in their frequency and intensity, so that the patient is not significantly disturbed by them. Patient associations have been essential in propagating information about TS and putting affected families in touch with one another [3]. Several patient associations have been founded around the world after the pioneer model of the Tourette Syndrome Association in the United States, including the Brazilian Association of TS, Tics and OCD (ASTOC/www.astoc.org.br).

The best-studied behavioral intervention for TS is habit reversal, which consists of various techniques focused at increasing the awareness of tics and developing a competing response to replace the target tic when the patient is first aware that tics are about to occur [67]. Additional research on habit reversal is needed to identify factors associated with symptom maintenance. For instance, Wilhelm and colleagues [67] suggested that relapse prevention and booster sessions could help patients maintain the benefits acheived.

Pharmacotherapy

Several medications have been studied in TS, but only a few have been evaluated in placebo-controlled studies. The use of the $\alpha 2$-adrenergic drugs clonidine and guanfacine is supported by controlled studies [68,69]. Typical antipsychotics, once the treatment of choice because of their greater effectiveness [70], are now second-line agents because of side effects such as extrapyramidal symptoms and tardive dyskinesia. A few initial controlled studies with atypical antipsychotics have been published. Trials of different anticonvulsant drugs, such as levetiracetam [71], topiramate, and gabapentin [66], are under way.

Clonidine (daily dose range, 0.10–0.30 mg in divided doses) [68] and guanfacine (daily dose range, 0.5–3.0 mg in divided doses) [69] should be tried for patients who have milder symptoms, starting with low doses and with gradual increases if needed. Their main adverse effect is sedation. Baclofen [66] or clonazepam [72] could be alternatives.

Typical and atypical neuroleptics have been used to treat TS because they block postsynaptic dopamine D2 receptors. Among the available agents are the typical neuroleptics pimozide and haloperidol [70], the substituted benzamides sulpiride [73] and tiapride [74], and the atypical neuroleptics risperidone [75], ziprasidone [76], olanzapine [77], and quetiapine [78]. Good results have been reported with aripiprazole, a stabilizer of the dopamine/serotonin system [79,80]. Of note, a double-blind, placebo-controlled comparison of fluvoxamine versus sulpiride, followed by single-blind combined therapy in subjects who had TS plus OCD, showed that sulpiride monotherapy significantly reduced tics but not OCS. Fluvoxamine, either alone or combined with sulpiride, did not ameliorate tics but reduced OCS [73]. These findings suggest that combined treatment may be best for patients who have TS plus OCD.

Adverse effects common to neuroleptics include sedation, dysphoria, weight gain, and acute dystonic reactions. Ziprasidone may cause less weight gain but has a greater risk of prolonging the QT interval, as does pimozide [3].

Other medications that have data supporting their effect in reducing tics are tetrabenazine [81], pergolide [82], ropinirole [83], nicotine gum or patches in combination with neuroleptics [84], and botulinum toxin [85]. There is preliminary evidence supporting the use of delta-9-tetrahydrocannabinol, donepezil, and ondansetron [66].

For more severe and refractory cases, direct interventions in neural pathways may be of help, although larger controlled studies are still needed. Initial reports on surgical interventions for patients who had TS appeared in the 1960s [86], but serious side effects were associated with the various approaches. More recently, bilateral capsulotomy has been associated with at least 50% improvement in both motor and vocal tics in 12 patients who had TS, with no severe side effects [87]. Deep brain stimulation has been successfully employed in three patients who had TS, with few minor side effects [88]. In addition, in a severe case of TS with coprolalia and self-injuries, great improvement was reported after deep brain stimulation in which target regions were the centromedian-parafascicular complex of the thalamus and the internal part of the globus pallidus [89].

*Treatment implications of comorbid Tourette's syndrome
and obsessive-compulsive disorder*

Some authors suggest that the presence of tics may predict a worse response to monotherapy of OCD with selective serotonin reuptake inhibitors (SSRIs) [90,91]. Nevertheless, results of a blind study developed by the authors' group did not confirm the presence of tics as predicting poor response in 41 patients who had OCD and who were treated with clomipramine [92]. One explanation for the improvement in patients who had tic-related OCD could be the noradrenergic properties of clomipramine, which might have had a positive effect on tics (previous studies used SSRIs). Another study by the same group comparing patients who had respondent and refractory OCD, tic disorders were distributed equally in the two groups (Ferrão YA, Shavitt RG, Bedin N, et al. Clinical features associated with treatment refractory obsessive-compulsive disorder; unpublished manuscript). In the available literature, few clinical trials include patients who have OCD and comorbid TS; often, TS is an exclusion criterion in OCD clinical trials. Consequently, the extent to which tics represent a worse predictor of treatment response in OCD is open to further investigation [7].

In view of the findings described here, treatment of OCD with a comorbid tic disorder should start with a first-line option for each disorder. The treatment of OCD is addressed in another article of this issue. It is relevant to this discussion that approximately one third of patients who have OCD do not have a satisfactory response to a first-line therapy. For those cases, evidence supports the use of combined therapy of a serotonin reuptake inhibitor with typical [91] or atypical antipsychotics [93–96]. The presence of a comorbid tic disorder, once believed to be predictive of a good response to such a combination therapy [91], does not seem necessary for the combination to be effective for patients who have OCD [93]. Conversely, tic symptoms of patients who have tic-related OCD whose OCD symptoms do not respond to SSRIs might benefit from the combined therapy with atypical antipsychotics.

Summary

This article has focused on TS, and the relationship between TS and OCD has been addressed from different perspectives. In patients who have OCD, the presence of TS seems to have some impact in the clinical manifestation of OCD symptoms. One of the main features of tic-related OCD is the frequent presence of sensory phenomena preceding the compulsions, in the absence of obsessions. Genetic epidemiologic studies provide consistent evidence for the association between TS and OCD. Although no major loci have been identified so far, family and segregation analysis studies support the assumption that genes play a major role in the etiology of TS and related disorders. Genes interact with environmental factors, which can modulate the expression of TS or OCD and determine the onset of these disorders. Neuroimaging studies suggest that the pathophysiology of TS encompasses projections of primary, secondary, and somatosensory cortex to the putamen, dorsolateral caudate nucleus, and globus pallidus, whereas the pathophysiology of OCD involves more ventral structures, such as orbitofrontal-caudate-thalamic-cortical areas. Current treatment strategies for TS include education, behavioral therapy, pharmacotherapy, and support from patients associations. Alfa-adrenergic agents such as guanfacine and clonidine are first-choice treatments for TS; typical antipsychotics are more effective but are troublesome because of their long-term side-effect profiles. For comorbid TS plus OCD, each condition should be treated with its respective first-line option. Nonetheless, for patients who have tic-related OCD who are unresponsive to monotherapy with serotonin reuptake inhibitors, augmentation of serotonin reuptake inhibitors with atypical antipsychotics may be of benefit. Despite important advances, research is needed to clarify further the biologic and behavioral aspects of TS and its relationship with the frequently associated conditions, with particular attention to their management and prognosis.

Acknowledgments

This work represents an extension of some papers published by the authors' group (Maria Conceição do Rosario-Campos, MD, PhD, Roseli G. Shavitt, MD, PhD Ygor Ferrão, MD, MSc, Antonio Carlos Lopes, MD, Marcos Tomanik Mercadante, MD, PhD, Geraldo Busatto, MD, PhD, Priscila Chacon, BS, Eurípedes Miguel, MD, PhD) in collaboration with several distinguished researchers. James F. Leckman, MD, Scott Rauch, MD, and David L. Pauls, PhD, contributed to this paper.

The authors thank Antonio Carlos Lopes, MD, for reviewing the text on interventions in neural pathways of Tourette's syndrome.

References

[1] American Psychiatric Association. Diagnostic and statistical manual of mental disorders. 4th edition. Washington (DC): American Psychiatric Association; 1994.
[2] Robertson MM. Diagnosing Tourette syndrome: is it a common disorder? J Psychosom Res 2003;55:3–6.
[3] Leckman JF. Tourette's syndrome. Lancet 2002;360:1577–86.
[4] Eapen V, Fox-Hiley P, Banerjee S, et al. Clinical features and associated psychopathology in a Tourette syndrome cohort. Acta Neurol Scand 2004;109:255–60.
[5] Pauls DL, Leckman JF. The inheritance of Gilles de la Tourette's syndrome and associated behaviors: evidence for autosomal dominant transmission. N Engl J Med 1986;315:993–7.
[6] Pauls DL, Alsobrook JP II, Goodman W, et al. A family study of obsessive-compulsive disorder. Am J Psychiatry 1995;152(1):76–84.
[7] Miguel EC, Rosario-Campos MC, Shavitt RG, et al. The tic-related obsessive-compulsive disorder phenotype. Adv Neurol 2001;85:43–55.

[8] Kushner HI. A cursing brain? The histories of Tourette syndrome. Cambridge (MA): Harvard University Press; 1999.

[9] Leckman JF, Peterson BS, Pauls DL, et al. Tic disorders. Psychiatr Clin North Am 1997; 20(4):839–61.

[10] Miguel EC, Rosário-Campos MC, Prado HS, et al. Sensory phenomena in obsessive-compulsive disorder and Tourette's disorder. J Clin Psychiatry 2000;61:150–6.

[11] Hounie A, Petribú K. Síndrome de Tourette—revisão bibliográfica e relato de casos. Rev Bras Psiquiatr 1999;21(1):50–63.

[12] Miguel EC, Coffey BJ, Baer L, et al. Phenomenology of intentional repetitive behaviors in obsessive-compulsive disorder and Tourette's disorder. J Clin Psychiatry 1995;56:420–30.

[13] Coffey BJ, Miguel EC, Biederman J, et al. Tourette's disorder with and without obsessive-compulsive disorder in adults: are they different? J Nerv Ment Dis 1998;186:201–6.

[14] Miguel EC, Baer L, Coffey BJ, et al. Phenomenological differences appearing with repetitive behaviours in obsessive-compulsive disorder and Gilles de la Tourette Syndrome. Br J Psychiatry 1997;170:140–5.

[15] Rasmussen SA, Tsuang MT. Clinical characteristics and family history in DSM-III obsessive-compulsive disorder. Am J Psychiatry 1986;143(3):317–22.

[16] Pitman RK, Green RC, Jenike MA, et al. Clinical comparison of Tourette's disorder and obsessive-compulsive disorder. Am J Psychiatry 1987;144:1166–71.

[17] George MS, Trimble MR, Ring HA, et al. Obsessions in obsessive compulsive disorder with and without Gilles de la Tourette's syndrome. Am J Psychiatry 1993;150:93–7.

[18] Holzer JC, Goodman WK, McDougle CJ, et al. Obsessive-compulsive disorder with and without a chronic tic disorder. A comparison of symptoms in 70 patients. Br J Psychiatry 1994;464:469–73.

[19] Eapen V, Robertson MM, Alsobrook JP II, et al. Obsessive-compulsive symptoms in Gilles de la Tourette's syndrome and obsessive-compulsive disorder: Differences by diagnosis and family history. Am J Med Genet 1997;74:432–8.

[20] Petter T, Richter MA, Sandor P. Clinical features distinguishing patients with Tourette's syndrome and obsessive-compulsive disorder form patients with obsessive-compulsive disorder without tics. J Clin Psychiatry 1998;59:456–9.

[21] Swerdlow RN, Zinner S, Farber HR, et al. Symptoms in obsessive-compulsive disorder and Tourette syndrome: a spectrum? CNS Spectr 1999;4(3):21–33.

[22] Leckman JF, Goodman WK, North WG, et al. Elevated cerebrospinal fluid levels of oxytocin in obsessive-compulsive disorder: comparison with Tourette's syndrome and healthy controls. Arch Gen Psychiatry 1994;51(10):782–92.

[23] Rosario-Campos MC, Leckman JF, Mercadante MT, et al. Adults with early-onset obsessive-compulsive disorder. Am J Psychiatry 2001;158:1899–903.

[24] Baer L. Factor analysis of symptom subtypes of obsessive compulsive disorder and their relation to personality and tic disorders. J Clin Psychiatry 1994;55:18–23.

[25] Mataix-Cols D, Rauch SL, Manzo PA, et al. Use of factor-analyzed symptom dimensions to predict outcome with serotonin reuptake inhibitors and placebo in the treatment of obsessive-compulsive disorder. Am J Psychiatry 1999;156:1409–16.

[26] Leckman JF, Grice DE, Boardman J, et al. Symptoms of obsessive-compulsive disorder. Am J Psychiatry 1997;154(7):911–7.

[27] Diniz JB. Rosário-Campos MC, Hounie AG, et al. Chronic tics and Tourette syndrome in patients with obsessive-compulsive disorder. J Psychiatr Res, in press.

[28] Alsobrook JP, Pauls DL. A factor analysis of tic symptoms in Gilles de la Tourette's syndrome. Am J Psychiatry 2002;159:291–6.

[29] Mataix-Cols D, Rosario-Campos MC, Leckman JF. A multidimensional model of obsessive-compulsive disorder. Am J Psychiatry 2005;162(2):228–38.

[30] Leckman JF, Pauls DL, Zhang H, Rosario-Campos MC, et al. Obsessive-compulsive symptom dimensions in affected sibling pairs diagnosed with Gilles de la Tourette syndrome. Am J Med Genet B Neuropsychiatr Genet 2003;116(1):60–8.

[31] Walkup JT, Leckman JF, Price RA, et al. The relationship between Tourette syndrome and obsessive compulsive disorder: a twin study. Psychopharmacol Bull 1988;24:375–9.

[32] Price RA, Kidd KK, Cohen DJ, et al. A twin study of Tourette syndrome. Arch Gen Psychiatry 1985;42:815–20.

[33] Hebebrand J, Klug B, Fimmers R, et al. Rates for tic disorders and obsessive compulsive symptomatology in families of children and adolescents with Gilles de la Tourette syndrome. J Psychiatr Res 1997;31(5):519–30.

[34] Nestadt G, Samuels J, Riddle M, et al. A family study of obsessive-compulsive disorder. Arch Gen Psychiatry 2000;57:358–63.

[35] Grados M, Riddle MA, Samuels JF, et al. The familial phenotype of obsessive-compulsive disorder in relation to tic disorders: the Hopkins OCD family study. Biol Psychiatry 2001; 50:559–65.

[36] Rosario-Campos MC, Leckman J, Curi M, et al. A family study of early-onset obsessive-compulsive disorder. Am J Med Genet B Neuropsychiatr Genet. 2005;136(1):92–7.

[37] Merette C, Brassard A, Potvin A, et al. Significant linkage for Tourette syndrome in a large French Canadian family. Am J Hum Genet 2000;67:1008–13.

[38] Simonic I, Nyholt DR, Gericke GS, et al. Further evidence for linkage of Gilles de la Tourette syndrome (GTS) susceptibility loci on chromosomes 2p11, 8q12 and 11q23–24 in South African Afrikaners. Am J Med Genet 2001;105:163–7.

[39] The Tourette Syndrome Association International Consortium for Genetics. A complete genome screen in sib-pairs affected with Gilles de la Tourette syndrome. Am J Hum Genet 1999;65:1428–36.

[40] Barr CL, Wigg KG, Pakstis AJ, et al. Genome scan for linkage to Gilles de la Tourette syndrome. Am J Med Genet 1999;88(4):437–45.

[41] Zhang H, Leckman JF, Pauls DL, et al. Tourette Syndrome Association International Consortium for Genetics. Genomewide scan of hoarding in sib pairs in which both sibs have Gilles de la Tourette syndrome. Am J Hum Genet 2002;70(4):896–904.

[42] Kroisel PM, Petek E, Emberger W, et al. Candidate region for Gilles de la Tourette syndrome at 7q31. Am J Med Genet 2001;101:259–61.

[43] Crawford FC, Ait-Ghezala G, Morris M, et al. Translocation breakpoint in two unrelated Tourette syndrome cases, within a region previously linked to the disorder. Hum Genet 2003;113:154–61.

[44] State MW, Greally JM, Cuker A, et al. Epigenetic abnormalities associated with a chromosome 18(q21-q22) inversion and a Gilles de la Tourette syndrome phenotype. Proc Natl Acad Sci U S A 2003;100(8):4684–9.

[45] Verkerk AJ, Matheus CA, Joosse M, et al. CNTNAP2 is disrupted in a family with Gilles de la Tourette syndrome and obsessive compulsive disorder. Genomics 2003;82:1–9.

[46] Abelson JF, Kwan KY, O'Roak BJ, et al. Sequence variants in SLITRK1 are associated with Tourette's syndrome. Science 2005;310(5746):317–20.

[47] Swedo SE. Pediatric autoimmune neuropsychiatric disorders associated with streptococcal infections (PANDAS). Mol Psychiatry 2002;7(Suppl 2):S24–5.

[48] Asbahr FR, Negrão AB, Gentil V, et al. Obsessive-compulsive and related symptoms in children and adolescents with rheumatic fever with and without chorea: a prospective 6-month study. Am J Psychiatry 1998;155(8):1122–4.

[49] Mercadante MT, Filho GB, Lombroso PJ, et al. Rheumatic fever and co-morbid psychiatric disorders. Am J Psychiatry 2000;157(12):2036–8.

[50] Hounie AG, Pauls DL, Mercadante MT, et al. Obsessive-compulsive spectrum disorders in rheumatic fever with and without Sydenham's chorea. J Clin Psychiatry 2004;65(7):994–9.

[51] Alvarenga PG, Hounie AG, Mercadante MT, et al. Obsessive-compulsive symptoms in adults with non-active rheumatic fever. J Neuropsychiat Clin Neurosci, in press.

[52] Perlmutter SJ, Leitman SF, Garvey MA. Therapeutic plasma exchange and intravenous immunoglobulin for obsessive-compulsive disorder and tic disorders in childhood. Lancet 1999;354(9185):1153–8.

[53] Lougee L, Perlmutter SJ, Nicolson R, et al. Psychiatric disorders in first degree relatives of children with PANDAS. J Am Acad Child Adolesc Psychiatry 2000;39(10):1313–5.

[54] Muller N, Kroll B, Schwarz MJ, et al. Increased titers of antibodies against streptococcal M12 and M19 proteins in patients with Tourette's syndrome. Psychiatry Res 2001;101(2): 187–93.

[55] Kirvan CA, Swedo SE, Heuser JS, et al. Mimicry and autoantibody-mediated neuronal cell signaling in Sydenham chorea. Nat Med 2003;9(7):914–20.

[56] Garvey MA, Perlmutter SJ, Allen AJ, et al. A pilot study of penicillin prophylaxis for neuropsychiatric exacerbations triggered by streptococcal infections. Biol Psychiatry 1999; 45(12):1564–71.

[57] Luo F, Leckman JF, Katsovich L, et al. Prospective longitudinal study of children with tic disorders and/or obsessive-compulsive disorder: relationship of symptom exacerbations to newly acquired streptococcal infections. Pediatrics 2004;113:e578–85.

[58] Perrin EM, Murphy ML, Casey JR, et al. Does group A beta-hemolytic streptococcal infection increase risk for behavioral and neuropsychiatric symptoms in children? Arch Pediatr Adolesc Med 2004;158:848–56.

[59] Santangelo SL, Pauls DL, Goldstein J, et al. Tourette's syndrome: what are the influences of gender and comorbid obsessive-compulsive disorder? J Am Acad Child Adolesc Psychiatry 1994;33:795–804.

[60] Peterson BS, Staib L, Scahill L, et al. Regional brain and ventricular volumes in Tourette syndrome. Arch Gen Psychiatry 2001;58(5):427–40.

[61] Peterson BS, Thomas P, Kane MJ, et al. Basal ganglia volumes in patients with Gilles de la Tourette syndrome. Arch Gen Psychiatry 2003;60(4):415–24.

[62] Baumgardner TL, Singer HS, Denckla MB. Corpus callosum morphology in children with Tourette syndrome and attention deficit hyperactivity disorder. Neurology 1996;47(2): 477–82.

[63] Bloch MH, Leckman JF, Zhu H, et al. Caudate volumes in childhood predict symptom severity in adults with Tourette syndrome. Neurology 2005;65(8):1253–8.

[64] Peterson BS, Skudlarski P, Anderson AW, et al. A functional magnetic resonance imaging study of tic suppression in Tourette syndrome. Arch Gen Psychiatry 1998;55(4):326–33.

[65] Stern E, Silbersweig DA, Chee KY, et al. A functional neuroanatomy of tics in Tourette syndrome. Arch Gen Psychiatry 2000;57(8):741–8.

[66] Singer HS. Tourette's syndrome: from behavior to biology. Lancet Neurol 2005;4:149–59.

[67] Wilhelm S, Deckersbach T, Coffey BJ, et al. Habit reversal versus supportive psychotherapy for Tourettés disorder: a randomized controlled trial. Am J Psychiatry 2003;1670:1175–7.

[68] Leckman JF, Hardin MT, Riddle MA, et al. Clonidine treatment of Gilles de la Tourette's syndrome. Arch Gen Psychiatry 1991;48(4):24–8.

[69] Scahill L, Chappell PB, Kim YS, et al. A placebo-controlled study of guanfacine in the treatment of children with tic disorders and attention deficit hyperactivity disorder. Am J Psychiatry 2001;158:1067–74.

[70] Shapiro E, Shapiro AK, Fulop G, et al. Controlled study of haloperidol, pimozide and placebo for the treatment of Gilles de la Tourette's syndrome. Arch Gen Psychiatry 1989;46(8): 722–30.

[71] Awaad Y, Michon AM, Minarik S. Use of levetiracetam to treat tics in children and adolescents with Tourette syndrome. Mov Disord 2005;20(6):714–8.

[72] Gonce M, Barbeau A. Seven cases of Gilles de la Tourette's syndrome: partial relief with clonazepam: a pilot study. Can J Neurol Sci 1977;4:279–83.

[73] George MS, Trimble MR, Robertson MM. Fluvoxamine and sulpiride in comorbid obsessive-compulsive disorder and Gilles de la Tourette syndrome. Hum Psychopharmacol 1993; 8:327–34.

[74] Eggers C, Rothenberger A, Berghaus U. Clinical and neurobiological findings in children suffering from tic disease following treatment with tiapride. Eur Arch Psychiatry Neurol Sci 1988;237:223–9.

[75] Scahill L, Leckman JF, Schultz RT, et al. A placebo-controlled trial of risperidone in Tourette syndrome. Neurology 2003;60(7):1130–5.

[76] Sallee FR, Kurlan R, Goetz CG, et al. Ziprasidone treatment of children and adolescents with Tourette's syndrome: a pilot study. J Am Acad Child Adolesc Psychiatry 2000;39(3): 292–9.

[77] Budman CL, Gayer A, Lesser M, et al. An open-label study of the treatment efficacy of olanzapine for Tourette's disorder. J Clin Psychiatry 2001;62:290–4.

[78] Mukaddes NM, Abali O. Quetiapine treatment of children and adolescents with Tourette's disorder. J Child Adolesc Psychopharmacol 2003;13:295–9.

[79] Hounie A, Mathis MA, Sampaio AS, et al. Aripiprazole and Tourette syndrome. Rev Bras Psiquiatr 2004;26(3):213.

[80] Murphy TK, Bengtson MA, Soto O, et al. Case series on the use of aripiprazole for Tourette syndrome. Int J Neuropsychopharmacol 2005;8(3):489–90.

[81] Jancovic J, Orman J. Tetrabenazine therapy of dystonia, chorea, tics, and other dyskinesias. Neurology 1988;38:391–4.

[82] Gilbert DL, Dure L, Sethuraman G, et al. Tic reduction with pergolide in a randomized controlled trial in children. Neurology 2003;60(4):606–11.

[83] Anca MH, Giladi N, Korczyn AD. Ropinirole in Gilles de la Tourette syndrome. Neurology 2004;62:1626–7.

[84] Silver AA, Shytle RD, Sheehan KH, et al. Multicenter, double-blind, placebo-controlled study of mecamylamine monotherapy for Tourette's disorder. J Am Acad Child Adolesc Psychiatry 2001;40(9):1103–10.

[85] Marras C, Andrews D, Sime E, et al. Botulinum toxin for simple motor tics: a randomized, double-blind, controlled clinical trial. Neurology 2001;56:605–10.

[86] Cooper IS. Dystonia reversal by operation in the basal ganglia. Arch Neurol 1962;7:64–74.

[87] Sun B, Krahl SE, Zhan S, et al. Improved capsulotomy for refractory Tourette's syndrome. Stereotact Funct Neurosurg 2005;83(2–3):55–6.

[88] Vandewalle V, van der Linden C, Groenewegen HJ, et al. Stereotactic treatment of Gilles de la Tourette syndrome by high frequency stimulation of thalamus. Lancet 1999;353 (9154):724.

[89] Houeto JL, Karachi C, Mallet L, et al. Tourette's syndrome and deep brain stimulation. J Neurol Neurosurg Psychiatry 2005;76:992–5.

[90] McDougle CJ, Goodman WK, Leckman JF, et al. The efficacy of fluvoxamine in obsessive-compulsive disorder: effects of comorbid chronic tic disorder. J Clin Psychopharmacol 1993; 13:354–8.

[91] Mc Dougle CJ, Goodman WK, Leckman JF, et al. Haloperidol addition in fluvoxamine-refractory obsessive-compulsive disorder: a double-blind, placebo controlled study in patients with and without tics. Arch Gen Psychiatry 1994;51:302–8.

[92] Shavitt RG, Belotto C, Curi M, et al. Clinical features associated with treatment response in obsessive-compulsive disorder. Compr Psychiatry, in press.

[93] McDougle CJ, Epperson CN, Pelton GH, et al. A double-blind, placebo-controlled study of risperidone addition in serotonin reuptake inhibitor-refractory obsessive-compulsive disorder. Arch Gen Psychiatry 2000;57(8):794–801.

[94] Metin O, Yazici K, Tot S, et al. Amisulpiride augmentation in treatment resistant obsessive-compulsive disorder: an open trial. Hum Psychopharmacol 2003;18(6):463–7.

[95] Bystritsky A, Ackerman DL, Rosen RM, et al. Augmentation of serotonin reuptake inhibitors in refractory obsessive-compulsive disorder using adjunctive olanzapine: a placebo-controlled trial. J Clin Psychiatry 2004;65(4):565–8.

[96] Denys D, de Geus F, van Megen HJ, et al. A double-blind, randomized, placebo-controlled trial of quetiapine addition in patients with obsessive-compulsive disorder refractory to serotonin reuptake inhibitors. J Clin Psychiatry 2004;65(8):1040–8.

ELSEVIER
SAUNDERS

PSYCHIATRIC
CLINICS
OF NORTH AMERICA

Psychiatr Clin N Am 29 (2006) 487–501

Understanding and Treating Trichotillomania: What We Know and What We Don't Know

Douglas W. Woods, PhD[a],*, Christopher Flessner, MS[a],
Martin E. Franklin, PhD[b], Chad T. Wetterneck, MS[a],
Michael R. Walther, BA[b], Emily R. Anderson, MS[c],
Dodanid Cardona, MD[d]

[a]Department of Psychology, 211 Garland Hall, University of Wisconsin – Milwaukee,
Milwaukee, WI 53201, USA
[b]University of Pennsylvania School of Medicine, Philadelphia, PA, USA
[c]University of Nebraska–Lincoln, Lincoln, NE, USA
[d]The Children's Hospital of Philadelphia, Philadelphia, PA, USA

Trichotillomania (TTM) is currently classified as an impulse-control disorder, but there has been considerable debate as to whether it would be classified more appropriately as a disorder on the obsessive-compulsive spectrum [1]. In either case, TTM involves repetitive hair pulling that results in significant hair loss (criterion A in the *Diagnostic and Statistical Manual of Mental Disorders*, fourth edition [DSM-IV]). To receive a diagnosis of TTM, an individual must also meet the following criteria [2]:

1. There is an increasing level of tension immediately before hair pulling or during attempts to avoid pulling
2. There is a sensation of relief, pleasure, or gratification during hair pulling
3. The pulling is not explained better by a general medical condition or other mental disorder
4. Significant distress or impairment in occupational, social, or other areas of functioning is experienced as a result of the pulling

This article was supported in part by a grant from the National Institute of Mental Health (MH61457), and a grant from the Trichotillomania Learning Center, Santa Cruz, CA.
* Corresponding author.
E-mail address: dwoods@uwm.edu (D.W. Woods).

   This article summarizes current research on TTM while focusing on information that may be particularly relevant to practitioners. After discussing
diagnostic considerations and epidemiologic data, it discusses comorbidities
and etiologic findings and then considers potential subtypes. The article then
describes the various assessment tools available to clinicians and reviews the
current status of TTM treatment research. Significant gaps remain in the
knowledge of TTM, and the final section of the article outlines a direction
for future research and highlights some work being done to ameliorate the
situation.

Diagnostic considerations and epidemiology

   Substantial controversy remains as to whether the criteria described in
DSM-IV, text revised (TR), are too restrictive. Specifically, there is concern
that the inclusion of criteria B (tension before pulling) and C (reduction of
tension after pulling) actually excludes a large percentage of individuals who
repetitively pull their hair to the point of hair loss and functional impairment but who do not experience antecedent tension or its subsequent reduction. Preliminary epidemiologic research supports this concern. Estimates
suggest that the prevalence of pulling in the absence of both criteria B
and C is approximately 3.4% of college women, whereas the prevalence
of TTM as defined by the full DSM-IV criteria is 0.6% [3]. Unfortunately,
the extent to which criteria B and C produce any incremental validity in
terms of predicting functional impairment, treatment response, or course
of the disorder has not been addressed as yet. A large study, currently underway and funded by the Trichotillomania Learning Center (TLC), should
begin to clarify this diagnostic issue.
   Regardless of diagnostic label, the locations and methods of pulling show
great individual variation. Hair may be pulled from any body region but is
most commonly pulled, one hair at a time, from the scalp, lashes, and brows
[4]. Pulling typically is done with the fingers, but tools such as tweezers,
brushes, or combs may also be used. Often, those who have TTM engage
in a variety of postpulling behaviors including manipulating the pulled
hair using the mouth, hands, or face or chewing or ingesting the hair [5].
   In adult samples, the average age of onset is approximately 13 years [5],
but when children who engage in chronic hair pulling are sampled, the average age of onset seems to be around 18 months [6]. In younger children,
feelings of tension and relief from tension may not be reported [6–8].
   TTM seems to be more common among females, although it remains unclear whether this sex difference results from a true differences in the occurrence of the disorder, reflects a female treatment-seeking bias, or reflects
a tacit societal acceptability of hair loss in men [9]. The gender distribution
in children is less clear, but it seems that the younger the sample, the more
equal the gender distribution [10].

Functional impact and comorbidity

Early research on small samples of persons who had TTM suggests that the disorder can have numerous negative effects on physical and psychosocial functioning [11–13]. Physically, the most notable consequence is hair loss, but recurrent hair pulling can also produce follicle damage, changes in the structure and appearance of regrown hair, scalp irritation, enamel erosion and gingivitis (from hair mouthing) [9], and repetitive strain injury [14]. Those who ingest the hair are susceptible to trichobezoars, which may lead to anorexia, vomiting, weight loss, and possible death [15].

Psychosocially, TTM also seems to have a great impact [11,16,17]. For example, Stemberger and colleagues [17] found that more than 60% of adults who had TTM avoided swimming and getting haircuts, more than 20% avoided well-lit public places, and more than 30% were uncomfortable with windy weather. Additionally, more than 50% reported low self-esteem, depression, irritability, and feelings of unattractiveness. Although existing studies indicate that TTM may contribute to significant impairment in daily functioning, it is clear that the small samples and the use of psychosocial impact measures that are nonspecific to the disorder significantly limit what is known about the functional impact of TTM.

TTM seems to have a broad psychosocial impact, and it frequently co-occurs with other psychiatric conditions. As many as 55% of individuals who have TTM have comorbid psychiatric diagnoses, most commonly mood and anxiety disorders [12]. In another study, 27% of a sample who had TTM had a mood disorder, 26% had an obsessive-compulsive disorder, 23% had another anxiety disorder, and 55% had a comorbid personality disorder [18]. Similar comorbidity rates were found by Christenson and colleagues [3], who found that 23% of the sample also had major depression, and 18% had panic disorder.

Although hair pulling at a young age may be simply a benign habit [19], psychiatric comorbidity seems to be evident in some younger children who have TTM, with recent research on toddlers showing that 50% of the toddlers in the sample met requirements for a comorbid anxiety disorder, 40% displayed developmental problems, 20% had chronic pediatric concerns, and 100% of the sample had family stressors such as parental separation, homelessness, unemployment, or parent mental illness [6].

Etiologic and maintaining factors

Like the limited research on the utility of diagnostic criteria, functional impact, and psychiatric comorbidity, the research on etiologic and maintaining factors is sparse. In research on both biologic and environmental factors, studies are beset by generally small samples and lack of experimental designs. Therefore the literature reviewed here should be viewed not as definitive but rather as a basis for additional work.

Biologic underpinnings

Although a specific TTM gene has not been identified in humans, a genetic basis for TTM has been suggested [17,20,21]. Similarly, no experimental studies have been conducted linking a specific neurochemical deficit to pulling severity, but outcome studies suggesting favorable responses to selective serotonin reuptake inhibitors and dopamine blockers have led some to suggest that dysregulations of the serotonin and dopamine systems are functionally related to the severity of hair pulling [22,23]. Likewise the apparent efficacy of naltrexone (an opiate blocker) in reducing hair pulling has led to the belief that endogenous opiate activity is involved in TTM, [24] but studies evaluating whether those who have TTM experience decrease in pain sensitivity (a possible prediction of the opioid hypothesis) have not been supportive [25,26]. Limited research in neurostructural and neurofunctional deficits has shown that patients who have TTM have significantly reduced left putamen and left ventriculate volumes compared with healthy controls [27–29] and have increased right and left cerebellar and right superior parietal functioning [30]. Persons who have more severe hair pulling exhibit a greater decrease of activity in the frontal and parietal regions and left caudate [31].

Environmental factors

A number of different events, including specific features of the hair, cognitions, emotional experiences, or particular settings, may trigger an episode of pulling. Physical features of the hair that may evoke pulling include a particular color (eg, gray), shape (eg, curly or split ends), or texture (eg, coarse) [5,9]. Specific cognitions may also trigger pulling for some individuals [5]. Typically, these thoughts are about the hair or its perceived appearance (eg, "My eyebrows should be symmetrical" or "Gray hairs are bad, and I need to remove them"), but pulling severity has also been correlated with negative beliefs about appearance, shame-related cognitions, and fear of being negatively evaluated (Norberg MM, Woods DW, Wetterneck CT. Examination of the mediating role of psychological acceptance in relationships between cognitions and the severity of chronic hairpulling; unpublished manuscript). Although a direct causal relation is often assumed between such cognitions and pulling, recent research suggests that these cognition–pulling relationships may be mediated by a third variable, experiential avoidance, which refers to a person's general tendency to control or escape from unpleasant private experiences such as thoughts or emotions (Norberg MM, Woods DW, Wetterneck CT. Examination of the mediating role of psychological acceptance in relationships between cognitions and the severity of chronic hairpulling; unpublished manuscript) [32,33].

A third common trigger for pulling is the experience of negative affective states such as anxiety and tension [12,34], loneliness, fatigue, guilt, anger, indecision, frustration, and excitement [5,12]. A final class of events that has been found to trigger pulling in persons who have TTM is specific settings, such as studying or reading, sitting at work or in class, watching television, talking on the telephone, driving, or being in the bathroom or bedroom [12,35].

In addition to a variety of pulling triggers, a number of pulling consequences may serve to maintain the behavior through positive or negative reinforcement. Positive reinforcers can include tactile sensations created by rubbing the pulled hair against a person's body, on the face or lips, or between the fingers, the visual stimuli produced by pulling certain types of hair (eg, thick hairs or those with plump roots) [36–38], or satisfying or pleasurable feelings derived from the act of pulling [5]. Negative reinforcers for pulling include the removal of an aversive stimulus or emotional experience contingent on pulling. For example, it has been suggested that hair pulling may be reinforced by distracting an individual from a stressful event, undesired emotions, or boredom [5], and when asked to rate their emotional experiences before, during, and after pulling, people who have TTM report a reduction in anxiety and tension across the pulling episode [12]. In the same study, feelings such as guilt, sadness, and anger were found to have increased across the course of a hair-pulling session, suggesting that pulling may also create a rise in unpleasant feelings which then sets the occasion for additional hair-pulling episodes.

Possible subtypes of pulling

Evidence from the studies on environmental factors involved in TTM maintenance suggests the disorder may have different subtypes. Preliminary findings suggest two types of pulling may exist, and both types may be present in many of those who have the disorder. Focused pulling is viewed as an intentional act used to control aversive private experiences, such as an urge, bodily sensation (eg, itching or burning), or cognition. In contrast, nonfocused or automatic pulling seems to occur outside the person's awareness and often occurs during sedentary activities. Generally, this behavior is considered an "habitual" type of pulling, occurring independent of any well-defined specific emotional or cognitive experience. Estimates of how automatic and focused pulling are distributed in those who have TTM vary greatly. Primarily focused pulling has been estimated to occur in 15% to 34% of pullers, automatic pulling in 5% to 47%, and both types in 19% to 80% [39,40]. Clearly, there is discrepancy in this research, much of which can be attributed to the lack of a common measurement instrument and use of slightly different subtype definitions.

The existence of the focused and nonfocused subtypes is still debatable, but recent research conducted in the authors' laboratory lends support to the distinction. In this research, a 10-item survey designed to measure focused and nonfocused pulling was administered to 43 adults who had TTM. A factor analysis was conducted using a varimax rotation, and separate focused and nonfocused factors emerged. Results showed that the two factors were unrelated ($r = -0.092$; $P > .05$), thus increasing the validity of the focused/nonfocused construct. In addition, the focused factor, but not the nonfocused factor, was significantly and positively correlated with measures of negative affect, including the Beck Depression Inventory ($r = 0.31$; $P < .05$), and the State Trait Anxiety Inventory ($r = .33$; $P < .05$). A recently completed study, the Milwaukee Dimensions of Trichotillomania Survey (M-DOTS) further refined a focused/nonfocused pulling scale, and results generally confirmed earlier findings, lending even more support to the validity of the focused/nonfocused distinction (Flessner CA, Woods DW, Franklin M, et al. The Milwaukee-Dimensions of Trichotillomania Scale (M-DOTS): development, exploratory factor analysis, and psychometric properties; unpublished manuscript).

Assessment of trichotillomania

The review of etiologic/maintaining factors indicates that much information is needed for a more complete understanding of TTM. Unfortunately, one of the larger limitations to such an advance is the paucity of assessment instruments available to researchers and clinicians. This section describes the components of an assessment for TTM and then briefly reviews the existing instruments specifically designed to assess TTM.

A comprehensive assessment of TTM should include multiple components. Care should be taken to diagnose the disorder, its severity, and potential subtypes accurately, and clinicians should assess the physical and functional impact of the disorder and possible comorbid diagnoses. Although a discussion of strategies to assess comorbidities and functional impact is beyond the scope of this article, the assessments developed to assess the severity and possible subtypes of TTM are reviewed briefly.

Assessing severity of trichotillomania

Several assessment strategies, both direct and indirect, have been developed to measure severity of TTM. Direct strategies include measures of pulling frequency, duration, or amount of hair loss using self-monitoring, live or videotaped observation, or product-based techniques. In self-monitoring, the client records either the number of pulling episodes or the actual number of hairs pulled each day [41]. Although there may be a treatment benefit with self-monitoring because of reactivity, the accuracy and reliability of data collected with this procedure are suspect [42]. Live or videotaped observation by a clinician is rarely used because of the time commitment on the part of the practitioner and because most individuals who have TTM (particularly adults) do not pull in front of others [43,44]. Finally, some have used product-based strategies such as collecting or counting hairs, weighing pulled hairs [45], or photographing pulled areas [42], but these methods also have several limitations including (1) an inability to confirm that the product was produced by pulling, (2) failure of the client to collect pulled hair accurately, (3) possible embarrassment or reactivity experienced by client, and (4) difficulty in photographing certain body sites because of practical or personal reasons (eg, pubic region, chest, legs) [43].

Indirect methods involve self- or clinician-rated scales and typically assess TTM in a more global fashion. Three clinician-rated scales have been developed: the Yale-Brown Obsessive Compulsive Scale-Trichotillomania (Y–BOCS-TM) [46], the Psychiatric Institute Trichotillomania Scale (PITS) [47], and the National Institute of Mental Health (NIMH) Trichotillomania Severity and Impairment Scales (NIMH-TSS and -TIS) [22]. In addition, two self-report measures, the Massachusetts General Hospital-Hairpulling Scale (MGH-HS) [48] and the Trichotillomania Scale for Children (TSC) [49], have been developed for adults and children, respectively. In recent examinations of the clinician-rated measures, the PITS and NIMH-TIS demonstrated acceptable inter-rater reliability, but the internal consistency of the PITS, Y–BOCS-TM, and NIMH-TSS fell below minimally acceptable levels [50,51].

Research has also examined the psychometric properties of self-report measures for adults (eg, the MGH-HS) [48] and children (TSC) [49]. O'Sullivan and colleagues [52] showed that the MGH-HS demonstrated good test–retest reliability, convergent and divergent validity, and sensitivity to change in hair pulling. Recent research has confirmed the good test–retest reliability and internal consistency of the MGH-HS but has provided more limited support for convergent validity when using ratings of hair loss, the NIMH-TIS, self-reported number of hairs pulled, or a scale of global severity as concurrent measures (Flessner CA, Wetterneck CT, Woods DW. Assessment of trichotillomania (TTM): revisiting the Massachusetts General Hospital-Hairpulling Scale (MGH-HS); unpublished manuscript) [51]. Although there is a dearth of literature examining adequate measures for the assessment of the severity of TTM in adults, only one study has attempted to extend this line of research to children. Research on the TSC is less extensive, but the measure seems have promise, because it has shown strong internal consistency and test–retest reliability as well as strong convergent validity with existing measures of pulling severity such as the PITS [49].

Assessing subtypes

To date, most clinician-rated and self-report measures have concentrated on assessing the severity of TTM. Much less research has focused on developing assessments to differentiate between the possible subtypes of TTM (ie, focused and nonfocused pulling). To the authors' knowledge, their research group is the first to develop and examine the psychometric properties of a scale designed to identify symptoms thought to be characteristic of these two subtypes.

The M-DOTS originated as a 24-item scale with questions designed to assess both focused pulling (eg, "I pull my hair when I am anxious or upset") and automatic pulling (eg, "I pull my hair when I am concentrating on another activity") (Flessner CA, Woods DW, Franklin M, et al. The Milwaukee-Dimensions of Trichotillomania Scale (M-DOTS): development, exploratory factor analysis, and psychometric properties; unpublished manuscript). The M-DOTS was administered to 1697 individuals who had TTM in a Web-based survey, and an exploratory factor analysis revealed two distinct dimensions of TTM, including a 12-item focused pulling scale and a six-item automatic pulling scale. Subsequent analyses revealed good internal consistency and construct validity for both scales. These findings provide empirical evidence supporting the distinction between focused and automatic pulling and offer a potentially useful tool for measuring the two types.

Psychometrically strong assessment options are lacking. Only a handful of studies have been conducted with the expressed purpose of developing new and evaluating existing methods for the assessment of TTM, and only one study has extended this research to children who have TTM. Continued work is necessary in the development of additional measures of both TTM severity and subtypes [50]. Continued work in this area may prove increasingly beneficial for researchers and clinicians examining the efficacy of existing interventions for both adults and children who have TTM.

Does treatment work?

Research on the pharmacologic and nonpharmacologic treatment of TTM is scarce, and this scarcity is reflected in what care providers know about the disorder and its management. A survey of general practitioners, psychiatrists, and psychologists suggested that such providers were relatively uninformed about TTM [53]. In addition, 72% of providers thought medication was an effective treatment for TTM, whereas only 54% thought cognitive behavioral therapy (CBT) was an effective treatment option. Unfortunately, the available treatment evidence is not consistent with these beliefs.

A review of the literature reveals that although numerous single-subject experimental designs and case-study methods have been used to evaluate a wide array of treatments [54], only nine randomized trials have been conducted thus far with adults. This section reviews each of these trials and then describes the authors' recently completed randomized, controlled trial, which to their knowledge is the only randomized, controlled trial of any treatment for pediatric TTM. In general, knowledge about TTM treatments for adults is limited by small sample sizes, lack of specificity regarding sample characteristics, nonrandom assignment to treatment, dearth of long-term follow-up data, exclusive reliance on patient self-report measures, and lack of information regarding rates of treatment refusal and dropout.

Only six randomized, controlled trials evaluating the efficacy of pharmacotherapy have been conducted to date. Swedo and colleagues [22] conducted a double-blind crossover study with 14 women and found clomipramine superior to desipramine at posttreatment evaluation. Long-term response to clomipramine varied widely, with an overall 40% reduction in symptoms maintained at 4-year follow-up [55]. Another double-blind crossover study by Christenson and colleagues [56] failed to demonstrate the superiority of fluoxetine over placebo. In fact, neither condition improved hair pulling significantly. Streichenwein and Thornby [57] also failed to show any difference between fluoxetine and placebo in reducing hair pulling despite lengthening the treatment phase and increasing the maximum fluoxetine dose to 80 mg. In the first controlled trial directly comparing pharmacologic interventions with psychotherapy, Ninan and colleagues [58] compared clomipramine, CBT, and placebo. CBT produced greater changes in severity of hair pulling and in associated impairment and a higher rate of response than either double-blinded clomipramine and placebo; differences between clomipramine and placebo approached but did not achieve statistical significance. Another randomized, controlled trial found behavior therapy superior to fluoxetine and wait-list but failed to find a significant treatment effect for fluoxetine [59]. Research on the opioid-blocking compound naltrexone showed that the drug was superior to placebo in reducing TTM symptoms [24]. Taken together, results from these controlled studies of pharmacotherapy are equivocal at best. Much more work is needed in the development of pharmacotherapy for TTM in adults, and the absence of a single randomized, controlled trial in pediatric TTM severely limits treatment recommendations that can be made to parents whose children suffer from this disorder.

With respect to nonpharmacologic/CBT interventions, a variety of specific techniques have been applied, including awareness training, self-monitoring, aversion, covert sensitization, negative practice, relaxation training, habit-reversal training, stimulus control, and overcorrection [54]. Although the state of the CBT literature justifies only cautious recommendations, experts generally think that habit reversal, awareness training, and stimulus control are core interventions required for TTM, with other intervention strategies such as cognitive techniques to be used on an as-needed basis [1].

Only four randomized trials have been investigated the efficacy of CBT for TTM, all of which involved adult samples. Woods and colleagues [60] found a combination of acceptance and commitment therapy (ACT) and habit reversal superior to wait-list, although the study design did not allow conclusions to be made about the separate contributions of ACT and habit reversal, respectively. As described previously, Ninan and colleagues [58] found CBT superior to both clomipramine and placebo at posttreatment evaluation. Similarly, in their report of a completed randomized, controlled trial involving behavioral therapy, fluoxetine, and wait-list, van Minnen and colleagues [59] found behavioral therapy superior to fluoxetine or wait-list. Azrin and colleagues [41] found that habit reversal was more effective than negative practice, another behavioral approach. Patients using habit reversal reported a 99% reduction in number of hair-pulling episodes, compared with a 58% reduction in patients using negative practice. Moreover, the habit-reversal group maintained their gains at 22-month follow-up, with patients reporting 87% reduction compared with pretreatment. Although encouraging, this particular study is limited by a number of methodologic problems including exclusive reliance upon patient self-report, substantial attrition (7 of 19 subjects) during the follow-up phase, and the absence of a formal treatment manual that would allow replication.

As noted previously, none of the existing randomized trials has focused exclusively on pediatric TTM. There is some evidence from single-subject experimental designs and multiple uncontrolled case studies that children and adolescents may benefit from CBT [61]. Studies that include larger sample sizes and randomization are sorely needed to evaluate the efficacy of CBT for pediatric TTM.

To address this issue, the authors' research group recently completed a randomized, controlled trial examining a CBT package that included awareness training, stimulus control, and habit-reversal training. Initial findings from that study were encouraging and attest the efficacy and durability of CBT for TTM: CBT was clearly superior to minimal attention control at posttreatment evaluation, and patients assigned randomly to CBT tended to maintain their gains through an 8-week maintenance phase and through the 6-month naturalistic follow-up phase [62].

Generally speaking, the limited literature on treatment of TTM strongly suggests that there is neither a universal or complete response to any treatments for TTM. Likewise, the limited body of literature suggests that treatment gains may be difficult to sustain [63–67]. Given that monotherapy with CBT or pharmacotherapy is likely to produce only partial symptom reduction in the long run, these therapies might yield superior improvement when combined. Unfortunately, the absence of any controlled studies comparing the efficacy of CBT treatments involving habit reversal, pharmacotherapy, and their combination weakens this suggestion considerably.

Future directions

The research presented in this article shows that much empirical work is needed to develop a better understanding of TTM and its treatment. Recognizing this problem and the importance of stimulating new research on TTM, the National Institute of Mental Health co-sponsored a meeting with the TLC in November of 2004 (http://www.nimh.nih.gov/scientific-meetings/trichotillomania.pdf). The purpose of the meeting was to provide a critical evaluation of the state of TTM research and to create an agenda for future work. The Scientific Advisory Board of the TLC discussed these recommendations and formed a plan for addressing critical gaps.

One clear outcome from the NIMH-sponsored meeting was the need for a broad-spectrum investigation of the impact of TTM on the lives of those it affects. To address this issue, the TLC commissioned the Trichotillomania Impact Project for Adults (TIP-A) and children (TIP-C). These studies use parallel methodologies involving anonymous Internet sampling of adults and children (along with parents of the children) who have TTM. In each study, the impact on various funcional domains is assessed, as are various phenomenologic features of the disorder. To date, the TIP-A (with more than 1600 participants) has been completed, and the TIP-C is under way. After the on-line portion of the studies, the TIP will begin broad-scale field trials in which data from extensive face-to-face phenotyping and ascertainment of functional impact will be collected. Currently plans are being made to link this extensive phenotyping with the systematic collection and storage of genetic data as a means of elucidating possible genetic markers of TTM.

A second direction for future research involves determining the prevalence and developmental course of the disorder. A large-scale epidemiologic study should be conducted to determine the point and lifetime prevalence rates of TTM in pediatric and adult samples. If the small-scale prevalence studies conducted so far are accurate, a larger, more credible epidemiologic effort would highlight the need to direct resources toward the scientific study of this problem. Further longitudinal research is also needed to determine the percentage of youngsters who experience this problem. Examination of factors associated with maintenance of pulling behavior over time may help determine which pullers should be targeted for earlier intervention.

A third area for future research is the development of additional psychometrically sound assessment instruments, a process that has already begun in adult TTM and is now under way with younger samples [48,49,52]. Because TTM is often episodic, such instruments must be sensitive to this feature of the condition. Further, the preferred pulling site must be taken into account when rating frequency of pulling and severity of alopecia. Also, as described earlier in the discussion of the M-DOTS, the development of assessments must focus not only on pulling severity but must consider the possible need to assess subtypes of the disorder that may emerge in subsequent research. Once available, the measures will enable the needed epidemiologic and longitudinal studies already described and the experimental psychopathology and treatment development studies discussed later.

It is also imperative to improve the understanding of factors contributing to and controlling TTM. As described previously and discussed more broadly in reference to treatments [68], improved theoretical understanding of the core psychopathology of TTM will beget the development of better treatments. A major problem in TTM involves the insufficient experimental study of its psychopathology, with the resulting gap in the understanding of its etiologic and maintaining factors. Studies linking psychological and biological methods would help close the current gaps in knowledge and perhaps would stimulate a more interdisciplinary approach to the treatment of this condition.

The final area of future research involves treatment development and dissemination. The meager treatment-outcome literature and the equivocal findings from randomized, controlled trials in adults suggest that there is much work to do with adults. The relative absence of pediatric studies compounds the issue in children. Successful treatment development, demonstration of efficacy, dismantling of treatment packages found efficacious, and dissemination are still a long way off. Successful progression through each of these critical stages is hindered by the lack of conceptual clarity about the disorder as well as by the paucity of experimental psychopathology findings, epidemiologic evidence, and data on functional impairment clearly documenting that TTM is worthy of additional attention from researchers and, by extension, from funding agencies. Further, because research in TTM is in its infancy, pooling resources across the laboratories conducting the preliminary work in this area might allow larger sample sizes, more definitive conclusions, and better publications and thereby might begin to answer the many questions that must be addressed to enable significant progress in the conceptualization and ultimately in the treatment of those who suffer from this disorder.

References

[1] Franklin ME, Tolin DF, Diefenbach GJ. Trichotillomania. In: Hollander E, Stein DJ, editors. Clinical manual of impulse control disorders. Washington (DC): American Psychiatric Press, Inc.; 2006. p. 149–73.

[2] American Psychiatric Association. Diagnostic and statistical manual of mental disorders. 4th edition text revision. Washington (DC): American Psychiatric Association; 2000.

[3] Christenson GA, Pyle RL, Mitchell JE. Estimated lifetime prevalence of trichotillomania in college students. J Clin Psych 1991;52:415–7.

[4] Stein DJ, Christenson GA, Hollander E, editors. Trichotillomania. Washington (DC): American Psychiatric Press; 1991.

[5] Mansueto CS, Townsley-Stemberger RM, McCombs-Thomas A, et al. Trichotillomania: a comprehensive behavioral model. Clin Psych Rev 1991;17:567–77.

[6] Wright HH, Holmes GR. Trichotillomania (hair pulling) in toddlers. Psych Rep 2003;92: 228–30.

[7] Hanna GL. Trichotillomania and related disorders in children and adolescents. Child Psychiatry Hum Dev 1997;27:255–68.

[8] King RA, Scahill L, Vitulano LA, et al. Childhood trichotillomania: clinical phenomenology, comorbidity, and family genetics. J Am Acad Child Adolesc Psychiatry 1995;34:1451–9.

[9] Christenson GA, Mansueto CS. Trichotillomania: descriptive characteristics and phenomenology. In: Stein DJ, Christenson GA, Hollander E, editors. Trichotillomania. Washington (DC): American Psychiatric Press, Inc.; 1999. p. 1–42.

[10] Reeve E. Hair pulling in children and adolescents. In: Stein DJ, Christenson GA, Hollander E, editors. Trichotillomania. Washington (DC): American Psychiatric Press, Inc.; 1999. p. 201–24.

[11] Diefenbach GJ, Tolin DF, Hannan S, et al. Trichotillomania: impact on psychosocial functioning and quality of life. Behav Res Ther 2005;43:869–84.

[12] Diefenbach GJ, Mouton-Odum S, Stanley MA. Affective correlates of trichotillomania. Behav Res Ther 2002;40:1305–15.

[13] Woods DW, Friman PC, Teng E. Physical and social functioning in persons with repetitive behavior disorders. In: Woods DW, Miltenberger RG, editors. Tic disorders, trichotillomania, and other repetitive behavior disorders: behavioral approaches to analysis and treatment. Norwell (MA): Kluwer Academic Publishers; 2001. p. 33–52.

[14] O'Sullivan RL, Keuthen NJ, Jenike MA, et al. Trichotillomania and carpal tunnel syndrome. J Clin Psychiatry 1996;57:174.

[15] Bouwer C, Stein DJ. Trichobezoars in trichotillomania: case report and literature overview. Psychosom Med 1998;60:658–60.

[16] Wetterneck CT, Woods DW, Norberg MM, etal. The social and economic impact of trichotillomania. Behavioral Interventions, in press.

[17] Stemberger RMT, Thomas AM, Mansueto CS, et al. Personal toll of trichotillomania: behavioral and interpersonal sequelae. J Anxiety Disord 2000;14:97–104.

[18] Schlosser S, Black DW, Blum N, et al. The demography, phenomenology, and family history of 22 persons with compulsive hair pulling. Ann Clin Psychiatry 1994;6:147–52.

[19] Friman PC, Blum N, Rostain A. Is hair pulling benign? J Am Acad Child Adolesc Psychiatry 1992;31:991–2.

[20] Greer JM, Capecchi MR. Hoxb8 is required for normal grooming behavior in mice. Neuron 1994;33:23–34.

[21] Lenane MC, Swedo SE, Rapoport JL, et al. Rates of obsessive compulsive disorder in first degree relatives of patients with trichotillomania: a research note. J Child Psychiatry 1992;33:925–33.

[22] Swedo SE, Leonard HL, Rapoport JL, et al. A double-blind comparison of clomipramine and despramine in the treatment of trichotillomania (hair pulling). N Engl J Med 1989;321:497–501.

[23] Stein DJ, Hollander E. Low-dose pimozide augmentation of serotonin reuptake blockers in the treatment of trichotillomania. J Clin Psychiatry 1992;53:123–6.

[24] Christenson GA, Crow SJ, MacKenzie TB, et al. A placebo controlled double-blind study of naltrexone for trichotillomania [abstract]. In: New Research Program and Abstracts of the 150th Annual Meeting of the American Psychiatric Association. Philadelphia, May 23, 1994.

[25] Christenson GA, Raymond NC, Faris PL, et al. Pain thresholds are not elevated in trichotillomania. Biol Psychiatry 1994;36:347–9.

[26] Frecska E, Arato M. Opiate sensitivity test in patients with stereotypic movement disorder and trichotillomania. Prog Neuropsychopharmacol Biol Psychiatry 2002;26:909–12.

[27] Breiter HC, Rauch SL, Kwong KK, et al. Functional magnetic resonance imaging of symptom provocation in obsessive-compulsive disorder. Arch Gen Psychiatry 1996;53:595–606.

[28] Jenike MA, Breiter HC, Baer L, et al. Cerebral structural abnormalities in obsessive-compulsive disorder: a qualitative morphometric magnetic resonance imaging study. Arch Gen Psychiatry 1996;53:625–32.

[29] Robinson D, Wu H, Munne RA, et al. Reduced caudate nucleus volume in obsessive-compulsive disorder. Arch Gen Psychiatry 1995;52:393–8.

[30] Swedo SE, Rapoport JL, Loenard HL, et al. Regional cerebral glucose metabolism of women with trichotillomania. Arch Gen Psychiatry 1991;48:828–33.

[31] Stein DJ, van Heerden B, Hugo C, van et al. Functional brain imaging and pharmacotherapy in trichotillomania single photon emission computed tomography before and after treatment with the selective serotonin reuptake inhibitor citalopram. Prog Neuropsychopharmacol Biol Psychiatry 2002;26:885–90.

[32] Begotka AM, Woods DW, Wetterneck CT. The relationship between experiential avoidance and the severity of Trichotillomania in a nonreferred sample. J Behav Ther Exp Psychiatry 2004;35:17–24.

[33] Hayes SC, Strosahl KD, Wilson KG. Acceptance and commitment therapy: an experiential approach to behavior change. New York: Guilford Press, Inc; 1999.

[34] Woods DW, Miltenberger RG. Are persons with nervous habits nervous? A preliminary examination of habit function in a nonreferred population. J Appl Behav Anal 1996;29: 259–61.

[35] O'Connor K, Brisebois H, Brault M, et al. Behavioral activity associated with onset in chronic tic and habit disorder. Behav Res Ther 2003;41:241–9.

[36] Miltenberger RG, Long ES, Rapp JT. Evaluating the function of hair pulling: a preliminary investigation. Behav Ther 1998;29:211–9.

[37] Rapp JT, Dozier CL, Carr JE, et al. Functional analysis of hair manipulation: a replication and extension. Behavioral Interventions 2001;15:121–33.

[38] Rapp JT, Miltenberger RG, Galensky TL, et al. A functional analysis of hair pulling. J Appl Behav Anal 1999;32:329–37.

[39] Christenson GA, Mackenzie TB, Mitchell J. Adult men and women with trichotillomania: a comparison of male and female characteristics. Psychosomatics 1994;35:365–70.

[40] Du Toit PL, van Kradenburg J, Niehaus DJH, et al. Characteristics and phenomenology of hair-pulling: an exploration of subtypes. Compr Psychiatry 2001;42:247–56.

[41] Azrin NH, Nunn RG, Frantz SE. Treatment of hairpulling (trichotillomania): a comparative study of habit reversal and negative practice training. J Behav Ther Exp Psychiatry 1980;11: 13–20.

[42] Winchell RM, Jones JS, Molcho A, et al. Rating the severity of trichotillomania: methods and problems. Psychopharmacol Bull 1992a;28:457–62.

[43] Rapp JT, Miltenberger RG, Long ES, et al. Simplified habit reversal treatment for chronic hair pulling in three adolescents: a clinical replication with direct observation. J Appl Behav Anal 1998;31:299–302.

[44] Mackenzie TB, Ristvedt SL, Christenson GA, et al. Identification of cues associated with compulsive, bulimic, and hair-pulling symptoms. J Behav Ther Exp Psychiatry 1995;26: 9–16.

[45] Byrd MR, Richards DF, Hove G, et al. Treatment of early onset hair pulling as a simple habit. Behav Modif 2002;26:400–11.

[46] Stanley MA, Prather RC, Wagner AL, et al. Can the Yale-Brown Obsessive Compulsive Scale be used to assess trichotillomania? A preliminary report. Behav Res Ther 1993;31: 171–7.

[47] Winchell RM, Jones JS, Molcho A, et al. The psychiatric institute trichotillomania scale (PITS). Psychopharmacol Bull 1992b;28:463–76.

[48] Keuthen NJ, O'Sullivan RL, Ricciardi JN, et al. The Massachusetts General Hospital (MGH) Hairpulling Scale: 1. Development and factor analyses. Psychother Psychosom 1995;64:141–5.

[49] Diefenbach GJ, Tolin DF, Franklin ME, et al. The trichotillomania scale for children (TSC): a new self-report measure to assess pediatric hair pulling. Presented at the meeting of the Association for the Advancement of Behavior Therapy. Boston, November 20–23, 2003.

[50] Stanley MA, Breckenridge JK, Snyder AG, et al. Clinician rated measure of hairpulling: a preliminary psychometric evaluation. Journal of Psychopathology & Behavioral Assessment 1999;21:157–82.

[51] Diefenbach GJ, Tolin DF, Crocetto J, et al. Assessment of trichotillomania: a psychometric evaluation of hair-pulling scales. Journal of Psychopathology & Behavioral Assessment 2005;27:169–78.

[52] O'Sullivan RL, Keuthen NJ, Hayday CF, et al. The Massachusetts Hospital (MGH) Hair-pulling Scale: 2. Reliability and validity. Psychother Psychosom 1995;64:146–8.

[53] Marcks BA, Wetterneck CT, Woods DW. Investigating health care providers' knowledge about trichotillomania and its treatment. Cogn Behav Ther 2006;35:19–27.

[54] Elliot AJ, Fuqua RW. Trichotillomania: conceptualization, measurement, and treatment. Behav Ther 2000;31:529–45.

[55] Swedo SE, Lenaine MC, Leonard HL. Long-term treatment of trichotillomania (hair pulling) [letter]. N Engl J Med 1993;329:141–2.

[56] Christenson GA, Mackenzie TB, Mitchell JE, et al. A placebo-controlled, double-blind crossover study of fluoxetine in trichotillomania. Am J Psychiatry 1991;148:1566–71.

[57] Streichenwein SM, Thornby JI. A long-term, double-blind, placebo-controlled crossover trial of the efficacy of fluoxetine for trichotillomania. Am J Psychiatry 1995;152:1192–6.

[58] Ninan PT, Rothbaum BO, Marsteller FA, et al. A placebo-controlled trial of cognitive-behavioral therapy and clomipramine in trichotillomania. J Clin Psychiatry 2000;61:47–50.

[59] van Minnen A, Hoogduin K, Keijsers G, et al. Treatment of trichotillomania with behavioral therapy or fluoxetine: a randomized, waiting-list controlled study. Arch Gen Psychiatry 2003;60:517–22.

[60] Woods DW, Wetterneck CT, Flessner CA. A controlled evaluation of acceptance and commitment therapy plus habit reversal as a treatment for trichotillomania. Behav Res Ther 2006;44:639–56.

[61] Woods DW, Miltenberger RG. A review of habit reversal with childhood habit disorders. Education and Treatment of Children 1996;19:197–214.

[62] Franklin ME, Ledley DA, Cardona D, et al. Cognitive-behavioral therapy for pediatric trichotillomania: a randomized controlled trial. Presented at the meeting of the Association for Behavioral and Cognitive Therapies. Washington, DC, November 17–20, 2005.

[63] Iancu I, Weizman A, Kindler S, et al. Serotonergic drugs in trichotillomania: treatment results in 12 patients. J Nerv Ment Dis 1996;184:641–4.

[64] Keuthen NJ, Fraim C, Deckersbach TD, et al. Longitudinal follow-up of naturalistic treatment outcome in patients with trichotillomania. J Clin Psychiatry 2001;62:101–7.

[65] Lerner J, Franklin ME, Meadows EA, et al. Effectiveness of a cognitive-behavioral treatment program for trichotillomania: an uncontrolled evaluation. Behav Ther 1998;29:157–71.

[66] Mouton SG, Stanley MA. Habit reversal training for trichotillomania: a group approach. Cognitive & Behavioral Practice 1996;3:159–82.

[67] Pollard CA, Ibe IO, Krojanker DN, et al. Clomipramine treatment of trichotillomania: a follow-up report on four cases. J Clin Psychiatry 1991;52:128–30.

[68] Foa EB, Kozak MJ. Beyond the efficacy ceiling? Cognitive behavior therapy in search of theory. Behav Ther 1997;28:601–11.

ELSEVIER
SAUNDERS

PSYCHIATRIC
CLINICS
OF NORTH AMERICA

Psychiatr Clin N Am 29 (2006) 503–519

Hypochondriasis: Conceptualization, Treatment, and Relationship to Obsessive-Compulsive Disorder

Jonathan S. Abramowitz, PhD[a],*,
Autumn E. Braddock, PhD[b]

[a]OCD/Anxiety Disorders Program, Department of Psychiatry and Psychology,
Mayo Clinic, 200 First Street SW, Rochester, MN 55905, USA
[b]Department of Psychiatry and Psychology, Mayo Clinic, 200 First Street SW,
Rochester, MN 55905, USA

Diagnosis and clinical features

According to the *Diagnostic and Statistical Manual of Mental Disorders*, fourth edition, text revised (DSM-IV-TR) [1], the essential feature of hypochondriasis (HC) is a preoccupation with the (inaccurate) belief that one has, or is in danger of developing, a serious medical illness. In many instances, the fear of illness disrupts social, occupational, and family functioning. Moreover, it persists despite appropriate medical evaluation and reassurance of good health. Patients' preoccupation may be symptom based, with a focus on (1) certain specific bodily functions (eg, swollen lymph nodes, vestibular sensations), (2) actual physical abnormalities that are not typically dangerous (eg, a small sore, postural orthostatic tachycardia syndrome), or (3) vague and ambiguous physical sensations (eg, "tired lungs," "foggy brain"). The person ascribes these generally innocuous signs and sensations to a feared malignant disease (eg, cancer, an unexplained heart condition) and becomes highly engrossed with determining their meaning, authenticity, and underlying etiology. The case of Greg illustrates the features of HC:

> Greg, a 28-year-old student, was referred to the Mayo Clinic by his primary care doctor for psychologic assessment and treatment because of Greg's unrelenting fear that his recent episodes of tachycardia, dizziness, and chest pain meant that he was suffering from a serious heart condition. A comprehensive medical evaluation, including a complete cardiac work-up, revealed

---

* Corresponding author.
E-mail address: abramowitz.jonathan@mayo.edu (J.S. Abramowitz).

no evidence of a medical condition that might account for his complaints. Despite these results, Greg was intent on determining the exact nature and cause of his symptoms, believing that a serious undetected medical illness was present.

Fears of and preoccupations with illness in HC are typically accompanied by safety behaviors—activities performed with the aim of reducing fear and protecting one's personal health. Common safety behaviors in HC include excessive seeking reassurance of good health (eg, through medical tests), checking one's body (eg, frequent breast self-examinations for cancer), reviewing other sources of information on the feared disease (eg, searching the Internet), and exploring various remedies such as herbal preparations [2]. Phobic avoidance of situations and stimuli perceived to be associated with the feared malady (eg, avoidance of old buildings for fear of asbestos) often occur within HC, as well.

> Greg reported a number of safety behaviors that he believed would reduce the risks he associated with his feared condition. First, he had moved from his home in Florida to Rochester, MN to be closer to the Mayo Clinic— the only place he believed that could accurately detect and save him from his "misunderstood" heart problem. He required that his fiancée, Jody, stay with him at all times in case he needed to be transported to the hospital. Because of his fear that physical exertion would strain his "delicate" heart, Greg abstained from many athletic activities he previously enjoyed, including jogging, biking, and playing basketball. He used a portable heart-rate monitor for checking his heart rate and blood pressure to determine whether immediate medical attention was needed. He reported spending hours searching the Internet for information about cardiovascular and other medical diseases that might account for his symptoms.

Individuals who have HC are often reluctant to view their complaints as anything other than physical and therefore often take offense at the suggestion that they seek consultation from mental or behavioral health professionals (eg, psychologists or psychiatrists). Because of this reluctance, they rarely present self-referred to mental health clinics, preferring consultation from primary and specialty medical settings. Additionally, although individuals who have HC may admit to being overly concerned about their feared illness, they are likely to remain dissatisfied until they receive a medical diagnosis. For this reason, many individuals who have HC "shop" for physicians who will provide them with such an answer. The negative implications of this behavior are numerous and include straining the doctor–patient relationship, obtaining multiple health care providers, and undergoing potentially harmful testing procedures when ostensibly healthy.

> Greg had been told by various physicians that the "symptoms" he feared were "not serious" and that he "had nothing to worry about." Greg was not satisfied with these doctors because they were not interested in trying to determine what was causing his symptoms. He believed he was not being

taken seriously enough and that his doctors thought his problems were "all in his head." When it was initially suggested to Greg that he seek consultation with a psychologist, Greg became angry and felt cast off. He strongly believed that his symptoms were "real," not imaginary.

Reluctance to seek behavioral health consultation among individuals who have HC renders it difficult to determine its prevalence. Available estimates of the lifetime prevalence rate vary widely and range from 0.8% to 8.5% depending on the setting [3,4]. According to the DSM-IV-TR, HC may begin at any age, but the most common age of onset is thought to be in early adulthood. Symptoms often arise during periods of increased stress but may be more directly influenced by recovery from a serious illness, diagnosis of an illness in a loved one, or the death of a close friend or relative [5]. Exposure to illness-related information in the media also probably influences the onset and focus of HC.

Differential diagnosis

The symptoms of HC are similar to those of several other mental disorders; thus a brief discussion of differential diagnosis is in order. Both HC and panic disorder involve fears related to bodily sensations, and panic attacks can occur in both conditions. Panic attacks and panic disorder, however, are marked by the fear of imminent physical catastrophe (eg, "I am having a heart attack, losing control, dying") that will occur before help can be obtained. In contrast, the fears in HC often concern more latent threats (eg, "I may have a brain tumor or lung cancer") that could be treated with the appropriate medical attention. Both HC and generalized anxiety disorder can include worries about illness, but individuals who have generalized anxiety disorder evidence additional areas of worry (eg, relationships, finances, world affairs), and the content of their health-related worries often shifts. In addition, patients who have generalized anxiety disorder tend to ruminate more and engage in less safety-seeking behavior than those who have HC. Finally, as in HC, obsessive-compulsive disorder (OCD) can involve preoccupation with illness and seeking of assurances from medical professionals (ie, checking rituals). Patients who have OCD typically have varied themes of obsessions and compulsions (eg, contamination, scrupulosity, sex), whereas those who have HC are singly obsessed with their health. The potential relationship between HC and OCD in the context of a putative spectrum of OCDs is discussed later.

Conceptual approaches to hypochondriasis

Traditional approaches

There are numerous psychodynamic hypotheses of HC, each proposing that unconscious conflicts underlie the disorder [6]. One model proposes that hostile and aggressive feelings are transformed subconsciously into physical complaints. Another holds that HC symptoms arise from traumatic or frustrating childhood experiences that are reawakened in adult life by similar stress or frustration. Still other dynamic models propose that HC symptoms represent a defense against guilt or low self-esteem. Although numerous, these psychodynamic theories have not been supported by research, nor has the idea that HC behavior is maintained by interpersonal rewards (ie, "secondary gain" for playing the "sick role"). This last view, although perhaps intuitively appealing, has pejorative connotations and can result in the simple (for the clinician) but disparaging (for the patient) dismissal of the patient's problems as "made up" or a manifestation of an underlying "personality disorder." Not only does such a formulation lack empiric support; it overlooks the need for a more careful patient-specific analysis of symptoms, which has proven highly useful in the management of HC.

The cognitive-behavioral approach: hypochondriasis as health anxiety

In contrast to early traditional approaches to understanding HC, the cognitive-behavioral model is an empirically grounded biopsychosocial approach that leads to effective treatment. Within this model, HC is viewed as an excessive and persistent manifestation of anxiety focused upon a perceived threat to one's own health. In general, anxiety (often termed the "fight-or-flight response") represents a normal and adaptive response to perceived threat; with the importance and imminence of the perceived threat influencing the intensity of the anxiety. Because most people would consider a threat to their own physical health as vitally important, it is not surprising that health-focused anxiety is a common phenomenon in the population at large [7,8]. In HC, then, the central problem is a chronic pattern of misinterpreting essentially harmless bodily symptoms as suggesting the presence of a malignant disease.

How does HC develop? The cognitive-behavioral model of HC is based on Beck's cognitive theory of psychopathology, which proposes that emotional disorders are caused by particular sorts of fundamental ("core") dysfunctional beliefs that people hold about themselves and the world [9]. For example, overly negative beliefs about the self, world, and future (eg, "I am a failure") underlie depression, whereas core beliefs about social incompetence and negative evaluation (eg, "If people knew the real me, they wouldn't approve") underlie social phobia. In HC, the habitual tendency to misinterpret health-relevant information as highly threatening is thought to arise from pan-situational but erroneous assumptions about health and illness (eg, "good health means having no symptoms" or "I am especially vulnerable to illnesses"). Research supports the hypothesis that such dysfunctional assumptions underlie HC symptoms: individuals who have HC have been shown to hold overly narrow concepts of good health, such as the belief that good health means being 100% free of symptoms and therefore that any symptoms are indicative of serious medical illnesses [10–12]. Such overly rigid or otherwise dysfunctional assumptions probably originate from personal experiences, such as living through a parent's bout with serious illness (eg, multiple myeloma). Such an experience could lead to dysfunctional health-related core beliefs, (eg, "multiple myeloma runs in my family"). As a result, the person feels especially vulnerable and might misinterpret unexpected bodily sensations as indicating the presence of the anticipated malady. Information gleaned from media sources can also increase the probability of misinterpreting benign signs and symptoms. Following extensive media coverage of an outbreak of the bird flu in the fall of 2005, authors evaluated several individuals who had HC who were concerned that their symptoms could be caused by bird flu.

According to the cognitive-behavioral hypothesis, threatening appraisals of essentially benign bodily perturbations is thought to trigger anxiety and worry, as well as urges to escape this affective distress by seeking assurance of good health (ie, safety behaviors). To illustrate, whereas most people would consult a doctor if they experienced chronic headaches over the course of a few weeks that did not respond to aspirin, a person prone to developing HC would assume that any head pain is always a sign of serious illness. Whereas the former assumption leads to appropriate medical consultation or intervention, the latter will evoke apprehension, continuous monitoring of symptoms, and urges to seek medical consultation. Thus, according to the cognitive-behavioral model, HC develops when dysfunctional health-related core beliefs lead to misinterpreting benign physical signs and symptoms as indicating a serious illness. The misinterpretations evoke distress as well as efforts to reduce this distress through safety behaviors, as described previously.

Why does HC persist? When concerned about their health, most people who do not have HC are relieved to be reassured by their doctors that they are in fact healthy, and any rumination about serious illness ceases. Thus, an important phenomenon that any theory of HC must explain is why, despite being told by their doctors that they are not ill, people with HC persist in their misinterpretations of innocuous bodily sensations and remain preoccupied with their health. Several processes that occur in HC interfere with patients' ability to recognize that their health anxiety is unfounded.

Research suggests that the normal physiologic correlates of anxiety and stress probably contribute to the persistence of health-focused anxiety despite lack of evidence of serious illness [13]. When anxiety is evoked (ie, when a threat is anticipated), adrenalin and noradrenalin are released from the adrenal glands, producing a noticeable increase in physiologic arousal (part of the body's normal fight-or-flight response and therefore in reality aimed at protecting the organism). Such bodily sensations can seem ominous if they happen to occur unexpectedly, have rapid onset, or are especially intense. In addition to an increase in heart rate, arousal can

include the following sets of sensations: numbness and tingling from the reduced blood flow to the extremities; feelings of breathlessness (sometimes
extending to dryness in the mouth and throat); muscle tension and pain (often head, neck, and chest pain); increased sweating, nausea, and constipa-
tion; dizziness, blurred vision, confusion, unreality; hot flashes; and
trembling, shaking, or general tiredness. Not surprisingly, individuals who
have HC often misinterpret these benign and temporary sensations as indicating the presence of severe illnesses [13,14]. Thus, at the very point that
one is becoming anxious or stressed over one's health, additional threatening "symptoms" seem to appear. The result is intensified anxiety, increased
arousal, and a vicious cycle leading to urges to seek medical attention for
a suspected illness.

Another factor in the persistence of HC is body vigilance—the tendency
to monitor and pay excessive attention to one's body for threatening signs
and symptoms [15]. Many physicians unintentionally reinforce body vigilance by suggesting that patients monitor their symptoms. Indeed such vigilance is wise if a physical threat is actually present (eg, a diabetic must
monitor glucose levels). For individuals who have HC, however, in which
actual threats to health are not present, body vigilance results in a learned
sensitivity to normal "body noise" (ie, slight perturbations and fluctuations
that occur normally within the human body, often serving a homeostatic
function). Thus, the opportunities for noticing and misinterpreting possible
signs of illness are increased. Additionally, body vigilance can explain why
external sources of stress and anxiety are not necessary to evoke episodes of
HC. Indeed, many patients argue that their condition is not stress related
because they do not feel anxious when they experience body sensations
that trigger HC concerns. If such individuals are body vigilant, however, even subtle internal triggers (ie, normal "body noise") can cue HC
episodes. Research from the authors' laboratory suggests that body vigilance plays a key role in HC [16,17].

A confirmation bias in which anxious people attempt to confirm their
fears also implicated in the maintenance of HC. This attempt to confirm
fears is a normal and adaptive response to actual threat. In HC, however,
it results in selective attention toward information erroneously considered
suggestive of illness and away from accurate information suggestive of
good health. Such selective attention biases the impact of information provided by doctors during medical consultations. That is, someone with health
concerns who is given a clean bill of health from 10 physicians might dis-
count all of this evidence if one additional doctor even hints otherwise
(eg, "I think you're OK, but we might run one more test just to be
sure"). Thus, for individuals who have HC, evidence of illness strengthens
the belief that one is ill, whereas information that is inconsistent with illness
is overlooked as either inadequate or immaterial. This bias explains the urge
of patients who have HC to "doctor shop" when told that there is no sign of
medical illness.

Finally, safety-seeking behavior serves to preserve HC symptoms and underlying beliefs and (mis)interpretations [7,8,16]. Indeed, any responses that result in avoidance, escape, or reassurance about potential threat are adaptive if the perceived threat is realistic. If the situation poses no real danger, however, safety-seeking behavior prevents the person from noticing that the fear was groundless in the first place. This proclivity is most clear in the case of avoidance behavior. Consider Greg—introduced at the beginning of this article—who avoided physical exertion because of his erroneous beliefs that such activity would exacerbate his heart troubles. By never engaging in such activities, Greg is robbed of the opportunity to correct his mistaken beliefs about his health and find out that he is healthy.

Reassurance seeking can have similar detrimental effects. After receiving assurance of good health, some individuals who have HC experience a temporary reduction in distress. This immediate relief, however, strengthens the urge to use such strategies when doubts related to health arise in the future, explaining the seemingly "compulsive" nature of reassurance seeking in HC. Furthermore, the person comes to view such reassurances as the "only" way of managing health anxiety; for example, "hearing Dr. Smith say I do not have cancer is the only way to get me to stop worrying about it." This attitude in turn strengthens inaccurate beliefs about illness and about one's ability to cope (eg, "I couldn't cope with having a serious illness"). Reassurance seeking can maintain dysfunctional illness-related doubts and beliefs if patients receive inconsistent information from different sources or, worse, inconsistent information from the same source on different occasions.

Body checking, another common safety-seeking behavior in HC, often serves inadvertently to increase patients' feared bodily sensations. For example, a patient the authors evaluated complained of neck soreness and was concerned that his "inflamed" lymph nodes indicated the presence of cancer (as opposed to a simple infection). This individual habitually manipulated the sides of his neck with his fingers to "check" continually on the suspected inflammation. After a medical evaluation it was concluded that the patient's lymph nodes were not abnormally swollen, and that the neck soreness was the result of the patient's constant manipulation. Thus, the frequent body checking augmented the patient's physical discomfort, which was subsequently misinterpreted as a sign of serious illness.

Many individuals who have HC repeatedly check their own vital signs (eg, heart rate, blood pressure, body temperature, balance) as a way of gaining reassurance of safety. In fact, some invest in expensive devices for accurately measuring such variables. There are two problems with such behavior. First, the more precise the measuring device, the more likely the individual is to notice normal body noise. Indeed, vital processes ordinarily fluctuate as the body maintains itself. Although such shifts in heart rate, blood pressure, temperature, vestibular functioning, and visual acuity (to name a few) are perfectly normal and are not harmful, persons who have HC might misinterpret these fluctuations as highly significant. This misinterpretation gives rise to health-related concern, increased physiologic arousal, and additional health anxiety. The second, more surreptitious problem is that individuals who have HC are *most* compelled to measure their vital signs during times of emotional distress (ie, to see if something really is wrong). Thus, they tend to "tune in" to their bodies when there is increased, but still normal, bodily noise. One man who was referred to the authors reported measuring his heart rate and blood pressure whenever he felt tachycardic or anxious about his health. He used his findings of elevated heart rate and blood pressure as evidence that he had a serious circulatory disease. Thus, it was no surprise that he strongly believed he had a problem with his heart. This circular reasoning illustrates an important way in which body checking serves to maintain HC symptoms and beliefs.

In summary, according to the cognitive-behavioral framework, HC symptoms persist because of the physiologic, cognitive, and behavioral responses to patients' erroneously perceived threats to their own health. As discussed later, this conceptual model leads to effective treatment of HC that aims to correct misinterpretations of benign bodily sensations and reduce the use of behaviors that interfere with the natural correction of such misinterpretations.

Assessment and treatment

Assessment

Proper medical evaluation

If not recently completed, the patient should have a comprehensive physical examination and thorough review of medical records to rule out any medical condition that could confound the diagnosis of HC. Information from this examination should be considered as evidence of good health to confirm the diagnosis. Additionally, because severe depression may interfere with response to cognitive-behavioral therapy (CBT), comorbid mood disorders should be assessed, and, if they are present, pharmacologic management should be considered.

Functional assessment

Although structured diagnostic interviews for HC exist, an individualized functional assessment of HC symptoms best reveals the nature of the patient's problems. The emphasis in functional assessment is on collecting highly detailed patient-specific information about health-anxiety triggers and the types of safety behaviors used in response to these triggers. It involves understanding what the patient considers as evidence of a serious illness and why evidence to the contrary fails to reduce the patient's health concerns. The assessment should be an open, as opposed to secretive, process, and the clinician should convey a genuine interest in understanding the patient's discomfort. Because formal rating scales for determining the severity of HC symptoms have not been developed or psychometrically validated, the authors assess symptom severity using simple 0 (none) to 10 (extreme) ratings of health anxiety and urges to perform safety behaviors.

Pharmacologic treatment

The use of antidepressant medications to treat HC derives from the traditional view that HC exists primarily in the context of depression [18]. Subsequent research, however, indicates that it is not necessary for a person to have depression to have HC or to benefit from antidepressants. Such agents (including tricyclics and selective serotonin reuptake inhibitors) show effects for a variety of emotional disorders, including mood, anxiety, and eating disorders, and thus might be useful in reducing HC symptoms. Several case studies and a small number of outcome studies suggest that the medications in Table 1 can be effective for HC.

Studies indicate that these medications can reduce fear of disease, dysfunctional beliefs, anxiety, somatic complaints, phobic avoidance, and reassurance-seeking behavior [19]. Little is known, however, about the long-term effects of these agents. As in other disorders (eg, OCD), clinical observations and case reports suggest that patients typically relapse if medications are discontinued [20]. Another limitation of medication treatment is that no medication seems to be universally effective. Furthermore, there are reports of HC symptoms worsening during drug treatment because patients become alarmed by side effects such as headaches and stomach distress [19].

A final issue with medications concerns the degree to which the observed effects are caused by specific properties of the medications, as opposed to nonspecific (placebo) factors, such as expectations for improvement. In the only placebo-controlled medication trial for HC, Fallon and colleagues [21] randomly assigned 20 patients to receive either fluoxetine or placebo. After the 12-week medication period, 80% of the fluoxetine group and 60% of the placebo group was classified as responders. The difference in responder rate between groups was not significant. This finding suggests that improvement with medication was largely attributable to placebo effects.

Table 1
Medications with initial empirical support for hypochondriasis

Medication	Recommended dose based on study findings	Studies
Clomipramine	25–225 mg/d	Kamlana & Gray, 1988; Stone, 1993
Imipramine	125–150 mg/d	Lippert, 1986; Wesner & Noyes, 1991
Fluoxetine	20–80 mg/d	Fallon, 1999; Fallon et al, 1991, 1993, 1996
Fluvoxamine	300 mg/d	Fallon, 2001; Fallon et al, 1996
Paroxetine	up to 60 mg/d	Oosterbaan et al, 2001
Nefazodone	200–500 mg/d	Kjernisted et al, 2002

Often physicians have to "talk patients into" using psychotropic medications for HC because these patients refuse to view their symptoms as psychiatric in nature. Some individuals who have HC perceive that prescribing these medications is merely the doctor's way of "getting rid" of a difficult patient. Consequently, many patients do not follow up with pharmacologic recommendations. To reduce rates of dropout and poor adherence to pharmacotherapy, the authors recommend the patient be given a clear and logical explanation for the use of an antidepressant. Specifically, this rationale should convey that HC involves real body sensations that the patient is responding to in unhelpful ways that can increase the uncomfortable sensations as well as the concern with these sensations. The purpose of the medication, therefore, is to reduce the patient's sensitivity to these sensations. Potential side effects should be carefully discussed in advance so that their misinterpretation is limited.

Psychological treatment: cognitive-behavioral therapy

Traditionally, the psychological treatments offered to individuals with HC have included psychodynamic psychotherapy aimed at helping the patient identify unconscious motivational factors and supportive therapy focusing on symptom management rather than amelioration. Although no research has formally evaluated the effectiveness of these interventions, the widely accepted view of HC as a treatment-resistant condition speaks to the inability of such interventions to produce long-lasting effects [2]. Moreover, because, as a rule, patients who have HC are reluctant to regard their symptoms as psychologic in nature, they often reject psychotherapy in favor of seeking further medical attention.

In contrast to the "talk therapies," CBT for HC is a skills-based approach that has been logically derived from the empirically consistent conceptual framework reviewed earlier. Specifically, the conceptual model suggests that patients who have HC experience actual physical sensations that they incorrectly perceive as threatening, leading to anxiety about health and the use of maladaptive strategies for reducing anxiety, which paradoxically complete a vicious cycle. Therefore treatment for HC must (1) help patients recognize and modify faulty beliefs concerning their health, and (2) eliminate safety behaviors and other barriers to the correction of such faulty beliefs [8]. As described later, CBT involves the use of specific procedures empirically demonstrated to weaken maladaptive thinking and behavioral patterns.

Formulation of an idiosyncratic model

A strength of CBT is that it is guided by a patient-specific "blue-print" that is formulated collaboratively with the patient. This blue-print diagrams how the patient's health anxiety is influenced by erroneous illness-related beliefs and how the physiologic, cognitive, and behavioral processes described previously maintain such beliefs. Because the typical experience for such patients is to feel discounted by their doctors, a thorough and open consideration of their feelings, thoughts, and behaviors often leads to an acceptance of the conceptual model and the treatment itself [22]. To illustrate, Fig. 1 displays an idiosyncratic model of Greg's HC symptoms. This model was derived from a functional assessment, as discussed previously.

Psychoeducation

Education is an important part of CBT for HC. In light of the cognitive-behavioral conceptualization, patients are helped view their problem as one in which uncomfortable but benign bodily sensations and perturbations have become the focus of excessive concern. This concern evokes certain maladaptive behavioral and physiologic responses that paradoxically serve to increase the health concerns. Patients are taught that anxiety is a normal and adaptive reaction to a perceived threat to one's health which involves behavioral, mental, and physiologic responses aimed at preparing the individual for fight or flight. Time is spent identifying feared bodily sensations, providing physiologic explanations where applicable (eg, vestibular functioning might vary depending on when one last ate), and explaining the detrimental effects of safety behaviors (eg, checking leads to increased preoccupation).

Modifying erroneous beliefs

Cognitive restructuring helps the patient identify evidence for and against faulty beliefs about health and illness [9,23]. The therapist helps the patient

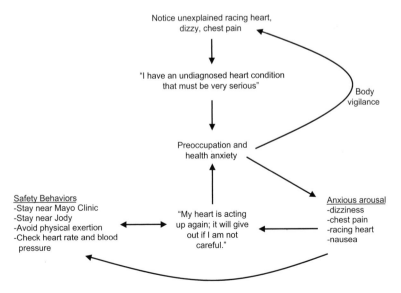

Fig. 1. An idiosyncratic model of health anxiety.

(1) identify the basis for these beliefs; (2) recognize contradictory events or experiences; and (3) understand the significance of contradictory evidence. The goal is to help the patient adopt rational responses to normal physiologic sensations. For example, Greg found that when he sat down and relaxed after being tachycardic, his heart rate slowed, his dizziness went away, and his fear subsided. The therapist helped Greg view this experience in a new light in the following exchange:

> THERAPIST: Would a cardiologist treat a serious heart condition just by having the patient sit down and relax?
> GREG: Of course not. You need medical interventions to treat heart troubles.
> THERAPIST: I agree. So, if trying to relax is not the right treatment, but relaxing makes your heart symptoms go away, and makes you feel better, is there a better explanation for what is happening in light of what you have learned about your physiologic response to threat?
> GREG: I never looked at it that way before. Maybe the feelings in my chest are there because of how much I am worried about my heart.

After his faulty cognitions were challenged, Greg learned to interpret his tachycardia and chest pain as normal bodily reactions to stress rather than as symptoms of a serious heart problem.

Exposure and response prevention

Exposure therapy, a CBT technique in which patients practice directly confronting their fears, is the most essential component of effective psychological treatment of anxiety. There are three methods of conducting exposure: (1) in vivo exposure, or confronting the actual feared situations and stimuli (eg, hospitals, TV shows about people with cancer), (2) imaginal exposure, or confronting feared thoughts and image, in one's imagination (eg, doubts about illnesses, thoughts of dying), and (3) interoceptive exposure, confronting feared body sensations (eg, dizziness, rapid heart rate). Interoceptive exposures might be produced by having the patient use caffeine, exercise vigorously, or by spinning in an office chair, for example. To benefit from exposure, the patient must be motivated to reduce health anxiety and be willing to tolerate an elevated degree of temporary anxiety. Put another way, exposure requires patients to invest anxiety now for a calmer future. An exposure hierarchy of Greg's feared situations and stimuli was developed collaboratively with the therapist (Table 2). Greg rated the experiences on a Subjective Units of Distress Scale (SUDS) of 1 to 10 in which 1 indicated no anxiety and 10 indicated very severe anxiety. He agreed to confront these situations during subsequent graduated exposure sessions, first beginning with those eliciting moderate symptoms of anxiety (SUDS = 4–5) and gradually building up to his most feared situations (SUDS = 10).

Exposure works for a number of reasons. First, and most importantly, patients realize that the disastrous consequences they fear do not occur

Table 2
Greg's exposure hierarchy

Situation/Stimulus	Type of exposure	Difficulty (0–10)
Dizziness	Interoceptive (spinning)	4
Racing heart	Interoceptive (running in place)	4
Visiting cardiac unit in hospital	In vivo	5
Reading sad stories about people who have heart disease	In vivo	6
Picturing living with a heart condition	Imaginal	7
Not knowing for sure about cardiac health	Imaginal	7
Going to the store without Jody	In vivo	8
Driving alone to a rural area 50 miles from Mayo Clinic	In vivo	10
Staying over night alone and far from Mayo	Imaginal	10

(eg, "If I don't go to the doctor, my 'illness' will go undetected and I will die"). Second, anxiety naturally decreases with prolonged and uninterrupted exposure to a feared situation, a process known as habituation. Patients learn that whether or not they seek reassurance from the doctor or the Internet, their anxiety will remit eventually. Third, patients gain self-efficacy and learn to master their fear without having to rely on avoidance or safety behaviors. For exposure to be successful, the patient must refrain from safety behaviors and other strategies designed to protect from unrealistically feared illnesses (ie, response prevention). Taylor and Asmundson [2] describe the details of implementing these treatment strategies with patients.

Effectiveness of cognitive-behavioral therapy

Despite early doubts about the effectiveness of psychological treatments, there is now clear evidence that HC can be managed using CBT [24]. Three controlled studies demonstrate that fewer than 20 sessions of this treatment can produce clinically significant and lasting improvement. In a wait-list–controlled study, Warwick and colleagues [25] found that CBT significantly decreased the need for reassurance, overall health anxiety, and checking frequency. General anxiety was reduced on average by about 70%, whereas depressive symptoms were reduced by 53%. Moreover, CBT was acceptable to patients: only 6% of patients recruited for this study refused to begin therapy, and only 6% discontinued prematurely. In a subsequent controlled study, a regimen of 16 weekly sessions of CBT was shown to have both short- and long-term (1-year) efficacy in reducing fears of illness as well as unnecessary medical visits [26]. In addition, CBT was more effective than stress management techniques, which also produced improvement. This finding suggests that the specific procedures of CBT (ie, psychoeducation, cognitive restructuring, exposure-response prevention), as opposed to non-specific factors (attention from a therapist, relaxation techniques), are the active ingredients for improvement of HC symptoms. Again, refusal and dropout rates were low (4%), suggesting acceptability and tolerability. Finally, in a large study ($N = 187$), Barsky and Ahern [27] found that relative to medical care as usual, six group CBT sessions focusing on education and modifying dysfunctional health-related beliefs produced significant decreases in health anxiety, HC-related beliefs, and functional impairment.

Is hypochondriasis a form of obsessive-compulsive disorder?

At various points, authors have considered that HC might be related to OCD [28]. The following discussion presents the basis for this notion and considers the similarities and differences between the two conditions.

OCD is an anxiety disorder characterized by (1) intrusive, unacceptable thoughts, ideas, or images (obsessions) that evoke anxiety and (2) efforts to resist or neutralize obsessional anxiety by engaging in some other thought or action (compulsive rituals). There is a clear phenomenologic link between the occurrence of obsessions and the performance of rituals or neutralizing behaviors. For example, obsessions about germs lead to washing and cleaning rituals. Some writers have proposed that there exists a spectrum of obsessive-compulsive disorders that incorporates numerous conditions with diagnostic criteria of repetitive behaviors, including some neurologic disorders (eg, Tourette's syndrome), impulse-control disorders (eg, trichotillomania), and disorders involving preoccupations with bodily sensations or appearance (eg, HC) [29]. In some sense, these disorders are assumed to have a common underlying etiology [29].

Similarities between OCD and other disorders may be found on two levels. The first, and less compelling, is at the level of symptom form or topography. A great number of mental disorders with repetitive behaviors in their diagnostic criteria fall into this category, including Tourette's syndrome, trichotillomania, and HC. Indeed, tics, hair pulling, and reassurance seeking about one's health are repetitive in much the same way that compulsive rituals in OCD are repetitive. The problem with using the presence of repetitive thinking and behavior to determine the boundaries of an OCD spectrum, however, is that vastly different factors might motivate the repetitive behaviors in OCD and in, for instance, Tourette's syndrome. A strong case has been made that such an approach leads to an illusion of relationships among unrelated disorders because of the high base rates of overlapping features with poor sensitivity and specificity (eg, repetition) [30].

In contrast, examining phenomenology at the functional level provides a more specific and fine-grained approach to understanding the nature of behavior disorders and determining whether a disorder might be related to OCD. To this end, disorders characterized by behaviors that are similarly motivated will be expected to converge. For example, in addition to being repetitive, both safety behaviors in HC and rituals in OCD are performed in response to threat-relevant triggers (eg, they are motivated by unrealistic threats of illness in HC and unrealistic threats of responsibility for harm in OCD). These behaviors (1) serve the function of preventing some feared outcome, (2) result in the desired reduction in distress and are thereby reinforced, and (3) maintain the perception of threat because of the nonoccurrence of the feared outcome. Thus, HC and OCD are functionally similar. Repetitive behaviors in trichotillomania and in Tourette's syndrome do not share these functional characteristics, however. In fact, research demonstrates that hair pulling is performed in response to boredom (as opposed to threat) and that it results in pleasurable feelings (as opposed to a reduction in anxiety) [31]; tics are performed to satisfy a sensory urge rather than as a means of reducing anxiety [32]. Thus, at a functional level, these disorders are quite dissimilar to OCD.

This functional approach leads to the conclusion that the fundamental nature of HC is similar to that of OCD. Empiric research demonstrates that stimuli that trigger thoughts about illness in patients who have HC evoke anxiety in much the same way that obsessional stimuli do in OCD and that safety behaviors in HC (eg, checking, asking for assurance from doctors) serve the function of reducing health anxiety in HC much as compulsive rituals reduce fears of catastrophes in OCD (Abramowitz JS, Moore EL. An experimental analysis of hypochondriasis, unpublished manuscript). There are important differences between these two disorders, however. In particular, individuals who have HC evidence more fears of bodily sensations and less insight into the senselessness of their fears than do individuals who have OCD. Nevertheless, on the basis of their overlapping functional properties, the authors conclude that HC most likely represents a form of OCD.

Summary

Once considered exclusively as a problem secondary to other mental disorders (ie, mood disorders), HC is now known to occur quite often as a primary diagnosis. A frequent drain on medical resources, patients who have HC can be viewed as suffering essentially from an anxiety disorder in which intense fear is focused on the possibility that they might be seriously physically ill or that such illness is imminent. The processes that contribute to the development and maintenance of such health anxiety consist largely of beliefs, assumptions, and behavioral responses that, although internally consistent with the perception of health-related threat, are erroneous and highly maladaptive in that they prevent the correction of erroneous perceptions of threat. There is growing evidence that this conceptualization leads to effective reduction in HC symptoms through cognitive-behavioral and pharmacologic treatments.

By far the main obstacle to successful treatment of HC is the patient's reluctance to view the problem as anything other than physical. The authors have found, however, that patients appreciate their care providers showing a genuine understanding of their concerns and taking the time to offer a logical, coherent explanation and rationale for the need for psychological and psychiatric services.

References

[1] American Psychiatric Association. Diagnostic and statistical manual of mental disorders. 4th editon, text revision. Washington (DC): American Psychiatric Association; 2000.

[2] Taylor S, Asmundson G. Health anxiety. New York: Guilford; 2004.

[3] Faravelli C, Salvatori S, Galassi F, et al. Epidemiology of somatoform disorders: a community survey in Florence. Soc Psychiatry Psychiatr Epidemiol 1997;32:24–9.

[4] Barsky AJ, Wyshak G, Klerman GL. et al. The prevalence of hypochondriasis in medical outpatients. Soc Psychiatry Psychiatr Epidemiol 1990;25:89–94.

[5] Barsky AJ, Klerman GL. Overview: hypochondriasis, bodily complaints, and somatic styles. Am J Psychiatry 1983;140:273–83.

[6] Starevic V, Lipsett D, editors. Hypochondriasis: modern perspectives on an ancient malady. New York: Oxford University Press; 2001.

[7] Warwick HA, Salkovskis PM. Hypochondriasis. Behav Res Ther 1990;28:105–17.

[8] Abramowitz J, Schwartz S, Whiteside S. A contemporary conceptual model of hypochondriasis. Mayo Clin Proc 2002;77:1323–30.

[9] Beck AT, Emery G, Greenberg R. Anxiety disorders and phobias: a cognitive perspective. New York: Basic Books; 1985.

[10] Barsky AJ, Coeytaux RR, Sarnie MK, et al. Hypochondriacal patients' beliefs about good health. Am J Psychiatry 1993;150:1085–9.

[11] MacLeod A, Haynes C, Sensky T. Attributions about common bodily sensations: their associations with hypochondriasis and anxiety. Psychol Med 1998;28:225–8.

[12] Reif W, Hiller W, Margraf J. Cognitive aspects of hypochondriasis and the somatization syndrome. J Abnorm Psychol 1998;107:587–95.

[13] Hiller W, Leibbrand R, Rief W, et al. Differentiating hypochondriasis from panic disorder. J Anx Dis 2005;19:29–49.

[14] Deacon BJ, Abramowitz JS. Anxiety sensitivity and its dimensions across the anxiety disorders. J Anxiety Disord, in press.

[15] Schmidt NB, Lerew DR, Trakowski JH. Body vigilance in panic disorder: evaluating attention to bodily perturbations. J Consult Clin Psychol 1997;65:214–20.

[16] Abramowitz JS, Deacon BJ, Valenteiner DP. The short health anxiety inventory in an undergraduate sample: implications for a cognitive-behavioral model of hypochondriasis. Cognit Ther Res, in press.

[17] Abramowitz JS, Olatunji BO, Deacon BJ. Health anxiety, hypochondriasis, and the anxiety disorders. Behavior Therapy, in press.

[18] Lesse S. Hypochondriasis and psychosomatic disorders masking depression. Am J Psychother 1967;21:607–20.

[19] Fallon B. Pharmacologic strategies for hypochondriasis. In: Starcevic V, Lipsett D, editors. Hypochondriasis: modern perspectives on an ancient malady. New York: Oxford University Press; 2001. p. 329–51.

[20] Viswnathan R, Paradis C. Treatment of cancer phobia with fluoxetine. Am J Psychiatry 1991;148:1090.

[21] Fallon BA, Schneier FR, Marshall R, et al. The pharmacotherapy of hypochondriasis. Psychopharmacol Bull 1996;32:607–11.

[22] Walker J, Vincent N, Furer P, et al. Treatment preference in hypochondriasis. J Behav Ther Exp Psychiatry 1999;30:251–8.

[23] Beck AT. Cognitive therapy and the emotional disorders. New York: International Universities Press; 1976.

[24] Taylor S, Asmundson G, Coons M. Current directions in the treatment of hypochondriasis. Journal of Cognitive Psychotherapy 2005;19:285–304.

[25] Warwick HM, Clark DM, Cobb AM, et al. A controlled trial of cognitive-behavioral treatment of hypochondriasis. Br J Psychiatry 1996;169:189–95.

[26] Clark DM, Salkovskis PM, Hackman A, et al. Two psychological treatments for hypochondriasis: a randomized controlled trial. Br J Psychiatry 1998;173:218–25.

[27] Barsky A, Ahern D. Cognitive-behavior therapy for hypochondriasis: a randomized controlled trial. JAMA 2004;291:1464–70.

[28] Fallon BA, Javitch JA, Hollander E, et al. Hypochondriasis and obsessive-compulsive disorder: overlaps in diagnosis and treatment. J Clin Psychiatry 1992;52:457–60.

[29] Hollander E, Friedberg JP, Wasserman S, et al. The case for the OCD spectrum. In: Abramowitz JS, Hours AC, editors. Concepts and controversies in obsessive-compulsive disorder. New York: Springer; 2005. p. 95–118.

[30] Abramowitz JS, Deacon BJ. The OC spectrum: a closer look at the arguments and the data. In: Abramowitz JS, Hours AC, editors. Concepts and controversies in obsessive-compulsive disorder. New York: Springer; 2005. p. 141–9.

[31] Stanley M, Swann A, Bowers T, et al. A comparison of clinical features in trichotillomania and obsessive-compulsive disorder. Behav Res Ther 1993;30:39–44.

[32] Miguel E, Coffee B, Baer L, et al. Phenomenology of intentional repetitive behaviors in obsessive-compulsive disorder and Tourette's disorder. J Clin Psychiatry 1995;56:246–55.

ELSEVIER
SAUNDERS

Psychiatr Clin N Am 29 (2006) 521–538

PSYCHIATRIC
CLINICS
OF NORTH AMERICA

Body Dysmorphic Disorder

David J. Castle, MSc, MD, MRCPsych[a,b,]*,
Susan Rossell, PhD[c], Michael Kyrios, PhD[d]

[a]*University of Melbourne, Melbourne, Australia*
[b]*St. Vincent's Hospital, Melbourne, Australia*
[c]*Mental Health Research Institute of Victoria, 155 Oak Street,*
Parkville, Victoria 3052, Australia
[d]*Department of Psychology, Faculty of Life & Social Sciences, Swinburne University*
of Technology, P.O. Box 218, Hawthorn 3122, Australia

Humans are visual beings, with a long history of self-adornment and attempts to change appearance to conform with social or religious ideals, to try to stand out from the crowd, or simply to look "good." Indeed, few could deny some degree of preoccupation with appearance. For some, however, dissatisfaction with appearance reaches an intensity that is pathologic in that it causes significant distress or impairs functioning in vocational or social domains. This psychiatric disorder, initially termed "dysmorphophobia," was described by the Italian physician Morselli in the late nineteenth century and has subsequently been labeled, inter alia, "dermatologic hypochondriasis," "beauty hypochondria," and "worry about being ugly" [1]. In 1987 it entered the official United States psychiatric nosology in the *Diagnostic and Statistical Manual of Mental Disorders III-revised* (DSM-IIIR) under the label "body dysmorphic disorder" (BDD) [2]. Its relevance to this issue of the *Psychiatric Clinics of North America* lies in its links with obsessive-compulsive disorder (OCD) and the consideration being given to its being part of the obsessive-compulsive (OC) spectrum.

BDD is characterized by an obsession with some aspect of physical appearance that is, to objective viewers, quite normal; if there is indeed some objective defect in appearance, the sufferer's concern is considered excessive. Almost any aspect of appearance can be the focus of concern [3]. The most common are the head and face (too big, too small, asymmetrical), skin (too red, too pale, blotchy, pimply, scarred), hair (too much, too little,

* Corresponding author. St. Vincent's Hospital and the University of Melbourne, Level 2, 46 Nicholson Street, Fitzroy 3065, Australia.
E-mail address: david.castle@svhm.org.au (D.J. Castle).

0193-953X/06/$ - see front matter © 2006 Elsevier Inc. All rights reserved.
doi:10.1016/j.psc.2006.02.001

too fine, too coarse, wrong color), or nose (too big, crooked, too small, nostrils too prominent). Some individuals are concerned by areas, such as the genitalia, that are not usually exposed to public scrutiny.

The extent to which this "imagined ugliness" [1] affects the individual's everyday life can be marked. For example, some sufferers refuse to be seen by others unless their perceived defect is covered up in some way, with make-up, wigs,. dark glasses, clothing and hats, or even with bandages and plasters. In some cases, the camouflaging is performed in a very ritualized and stereotyped manner and can take large amounts of time, impairing the individual's ability to get to appointments on time and generally impeding daily life.

People who have BDD tend to focus almost exclusively on their perceived defect in appearance rather than seeing the entirety of themselves. Many find glimpsing themselves in a mirror or other reflecting surface very distressing, and they avoid mirrors altogether or allow themselves to see themselves only bit by bit (eg, to apply make-up). Many can face the mirror only under certain specified and predictable conditions, for example in a darkened room and at a certain angle. Others must check themselves in the mirror repeatedly, ostensibly to reassure themselves that their appearance actually is acceptable, but mostly with the opposite effect, so that the mirror gazing merely confirms how "repulsive" they are and makes them feel even worse about themselves [3].

Certain situations are avoided where possible, for example when lights are too intense, sunshine is too bright, or there are too many mirrors. Social avoidance is particularly common, and there is a significant overlap between social anxiety disorder and BDD, although the cognition in social anxiety disorder usually is related more to the belief that one will act in a way that others will judge negatively rather than, as in BDD, being an object of derision solely because of how one looks. It is not surprising that people who have BDD are significantly disabled in terms of social as well as occupational adjustment. Phillips [4] reported on 62 patients who had BDD who completed the Short Form-36 schedule of disability and found their ratings were higher (more impaired) than those for the general population in the United States and also were higher than those for groups of patients who had depression, diabetes, or a recent myocardial infarct.

Etiology

Little is known about what causes BDD. There is some evidence for familial aggregation and genetic links with obsessive-compulsive disorder (OCD) [5]. Other links with OCD have been suggested through neuropsychologic and neuroimaging studies, although the literature is limited and inconsistent. A clear role for the serotonin system is evidenced by the specificity of therapeutic response to serotonergic antidepressants.

Some patients report a family background that prioritized appearance, but there is little specificity. Some individuals recall their BDD having been precipitated by a particular incident such as teasing, but many patients do not report a precipitating event, and the reported events probably merely precipitated the overt manifestation of an underlying predisposition.

Epidemiology

Rates of BDD in the general population are difficult to ascertain accurately, given the degree to which people tend to be ashamed of and hide their concerns. Also, self-reported and clinician-determined rates may differ, different rating scales may produce different results, and screening for a relatively rare disorder is notoriously inaccurate. Published studies in the general population tend to aggregate between 0.7% [6,7] and 2.3% [8], with the lower figure possibly more accurate.

Certain groups of individuals have much higher rates of BDD, although again exact rates vary. In plastic surgery settings, rates of 6% to 15% have been reported [9], and in two cosmetic dermatology clinics, the rate was 12% [10].

There is little information about cross-cultural comparisons of rates of BDD, although, as stated previously, there are historical descriptions from a number of settings in different cultures. It seems that in some cultures there is a variation in the cognition associated with the perceived ugliness and its impact on others. For example, in Japan the sufferer might be concerned mostly with the distress that their imagined ugliness causes the observer [3].

What is less contentious is that BDD seems to afflict as many males as females. This finding is in strong contrast to the eating disorders, which are essentially disorders of females. The focus of concern does differ between the sexes: males are more likely to obsess about thinning hair, genitalia, and physique; females are unhappy with skin, hips, and weight and are more likely to suffer from comorbid bulimia nervosa [11].

One form of BDD is particularly common in males. This variant, known variably as "bigorexia," "reverse anorexia," "Adonis complex," or "muscle dysmorphia" [12] is characterized by a belief that the sufferer is too thin and puny, even in the face of objective evidence to the contrary. There are, as in anorexia nervosa, both a distortion in the perception of the individual's own weight and shape and an overinvestment in the importance of weight and shape in determining self worth. These false perceptions lead sufferers to go to extreme lengths to gain muscle mass in an attempt to achieve their perceived ideal. Special diets, many hours in the gym, and even the use of anabolic steroids are part of the lives of people who have muscle dysmorphia. Some avoid being seen unclothed, and others use padded clothing to enhance a muscular appearance.

Most clinical series of patients who have BDD describe an onset in the teens, but many sufferers describe having been sensitive about appearance throughout their lives.

Unless treated, the condition is usually lifelong, but the outlook for those who do receive treatment is much more favorable. For example, Phillips and colleagues [13] reported on a mean 1.7-year (range, 0.5–6.4 years) retrospective follow-up of 95 outpatients who had BDD, all of whom had received at least one medication trial and a third of whom had received additional psychotherapy. At 12 months, approximately one fourth of patients had achieved remission, and the rate rose to nearly 60% at 4 years. The inclusion of partially remitted patients raised these proportions to nearly 58% at 12 months and to more than 80% at 4 years. Of those who did achieve remission, 29% subsequently relapsed, however. A worse overall outcome was associated with greater severity of baseline BDD symptoms and comorbid depression or social anxiety disorder.

Nosologic issues

An area of contention is the classification of BDD. In the DSM-IV [14], BDD is subsumed under the somatoform disorders, but it sits uneasily there and has little in common with other members of that heterogeneous group. Indeed, the whole somatoform disorder grouping has been criticized, and it has been suggested that the grouping be abandoned in favor of a multiaxial formulation [15].

BDD shows substantial overlap in symptomatology with both OCD and social anxiety disorder, and arguments could be made for classifying BDD with either of those disorders. The inclusion of BDD in the putative OC spectrum has gained particular currency, with the demonstration of some familial aggregation of the two disorders as well as a shared treatment response to serotonergic antidepressant medications. Anorexia nervosa is another disorder with symptomatic similarities with BDD (most obviously in the case of muscle dysmorphia), and some commentators would include anorexia nervosa, BDD, and a number of other disorders in the OC spectrum [16]. This approach has its detractors, however [17,18].

Another area of nosologic contention in the BDD literature is how to classify those patients who have BDD and hold their belief with delusional intensity. This situation is common in BDD, with most clinical samples showing that around 50% of sufferers have a delusional form of the illness [3,19]. Under DSM rules, people who have delusional BDD must be ascribed another, additional diagnostic label, namely that of delusional disorder, somatic subtype. This additional diagnosis makes little sense, because the degree of delusional conviction with which beliefs are held is considered more usefully on a spectrum rather than categorically, and this approach has been shown to be applicable in BDD. Thus, Phillips [20] recently reported on ratings using the Brown Assessment of Beliefs Scale [21] in 129 patients who had BDD. This scale gives ratings of delusionality both categorically and dimensionally. Total scores showed 68 patients had delusional belief about their appearance; only 25 had excellent, good, or fair insight. On subscale scores, 60 subjects (47%) were completely convinced their beliefs were true, but only 36 (28%) were completely certain others thought their beliefs were realistic, and 44 (34%) absolutely refused to consider the possibility that their beliefs were wrong. Eighty-eight subjects (60%) at least occasionally attempted to disprove their beliefs, and there was a gradation of insight into whether they had a psychiatric/psychologic problem; only 39 subjects (30%) were absolutely certain this was not the case. Thus, various categories of delusionality can be rated dimensionally in people who have BDD, making a categorical distinction between deluded and nondeluded very tenuous.

Furthermore, in a comparison between 52 patients who had delusional BDD and 48 patients who had the nondelusional form (categorization based on degree of conviction about their view of their "defect"), Phillips and colleagues [19] found few differences in demographic and clinical variables. Neither group responded favorably to antipsychotic medication alone, suggesting a failure of pharmacologic dissection between the putative groups and suggesting that the delusional patients merely have a more severe form of the same illness.

Comorbid anxiety, mood, and related disorders in body dysmorphic disorder

Because of similarities in phenomenology or high rates of comorbidity, BDD has been associated with a range of mood, anxiety, substance use, eating, and personality disorders. With respect to depression, patients who have BDD commonly report symptoms such as low self-esteem, a lack of worth, a sense of personal defectiveness, guilt, depressed mood, and suicidal ideation. Although the association of BDD with major depression has been reported frequently [7], this finding has not been consistent. A particular association has been noted between BDD and so-called "atypical" depression; in a cohort of 80 such patients, 14% had BDD [22]. Not all studies have found consistently high rates of BDD in people who have depression, however. For instance, Brawman-Mintzer and colleagues [23] did not find comorbid BDD in patients who had a primary diagnosis of major depression, although patients who have BDD are commonly depressed [21], suggesting the causal influence of BDD on the experience of depression.

Studies with clinical and nonclinical cohorts have shown the association of BDD with anxiety disorders, particularly OCD and social phobia, more consistently. Phillips and colleagues [24] observed the intrusive, recurrent, and persistent nature of BDD preoccupations and their similarities with features of DSM-defined obsessions. Furthermore, BDD is associated with compulsive behaviors such as frequent mirror checking and excessive hair combing. Numerous researchers have reported on the clinical, demographic, and treatment response similarities between BDD and OCD [3,25]. Moreover, as do people who have social phobia, patients who have BDD exhibit avoidance in social and occupational contexts [1,24], excessive self-focused attention [26], and concerns about other's judgments of them [27].

Early research indicated comorbid lifetime prevalence rates for OCD and social phobia of up to 50% in patients who had BDD [19,28]. In investigating the prevalence and phenomenology of BDD in patients who participated in the DSM-IV field trial for OCD, however, Simeon and colleagues [29] found only 12% of patients who had OCD had a lifetime comorbid diagnosis of BDD. Although individuals who had and those who did not have BDD did not differ in demographic characteristics, those who had comorbid OCD and BDD had more anxious, impulsive, and schizotypal features than those who had OCD alone. There was also significantly less insight in BDD cohorts than in OCD cohorts. The authors concluded that, although the two disorders are strongly related, there are also notable differences; thus, BDD is not merely a subtype of OCD.

Conducting a cross-sectional interview survey of 50 volunteers from a range of sources who satisfied DSM-IV criteria for BDD as their primary disorder, Veale and colleagues [27] found high degrees of comorbidity. The most common additional Axis I diagnoses were mood disorder (26%), social phobia (16%), and OCD (6%); on Axis II, 72% of patients had features of at least one personality disorder, the most common being paranoid, avoidant, and OC behavior.

Studies of the prevalence of BDD in anxious patients have also been conducted. Brawman-Mintzer and colleagues [23] examined the frequency of BDD in patients who had a primary diagnosis of depression or an anxiety disorder. They found that 5% of clinical and 0% of healthy control subjects met DSM-IV criteria for BDD. They found differences within specific clinical groups, with 11% of patients who had social phobia and 8% of patients who had OCD presenting with comorbid BDD, in contrast to only 2% of patients suffering from panic; no patients who had generalized anxiety disorder or major depression met criteria for BDD. In general, compared with the normal control subjects, the difference in prevalence was statistically significant for patients who had social phobia and approached significance for patients who had OCD. The authors concluded that BDD might share aspects of etiology with social phobia and OCD.

Similar findings regarding comorbidity have been reported from studies of BDD in children and adolescents. For instance, Albertini and Phillips [30] found that the most common comorbid disorder was major depression, followed by OCD and social phobia. In most cases, the onset of social phobia preceded that of BDD by at least 1 year (80%), whereas OCD preceded the onset of BDD by at least 1 year in 40% of cases, and major depression preceded the onset of BDD by at least 1 year in only 17% of cases. Again these findings suggest that depression is mostly a consequence of living with BDD.

Otto and colleagues [7] examined the prevalence and correlates of BDD in a large population-based, cross-sectional sample of depressed and nondepressed women. Similar to findings from clinical studies, the presence of BDD was significantly associated with the presence of major depression and anxiety disorders. The authors estimated the overall point prevalence of BDD as 0.7% in women in this age range in the community. Biby [31] investigated the relationship of depression, self-esteem, somatization, and OCD to BDD concerns in undergraduates controlling for eating disorders. Lower body-esteem scores were linked with lower levels of self-esteem but with higher levels of OC tendencies, depressive tendencies, and somatization tendencies.

Given common concerns about body image and aspects of appearance, Grant and colleagues [32] examined the prevalence of BDD in patients who had anorexia nervosa. Sixteen of 41 patients (39%) who had anorexia nervosa were diagnosed as having comorbid BDD unrelated to weight concerns. Comorbid anorexia nervosa and BDD were associated with significantly lower overall functioning and higher levels of delusionality than seen in anorexia without BDD. In a review of similarities and differences between anorexia nervosa and BDD, however, Grant and Phillips [17] concluded that the disorders should be differentiated clinically because they seem to respond differently to treatment and have different psychiatric comorbidities, familial patterns, and different gender ratios.

Gender differences in comorbidities within BDD have also been reported. Perugi and colleagues [33] examined 58 consecutive outpatients who had DSM-III-R BDD. Women who had BDD had significantly higher lifetime comorbidity with panic, generalized anxiety, and bulimia, whereas men who had BDD had higher lifetime comorbidity with bipolar disorder. They concluded that gender tends to influence the nature and extent of comorbidity in BDD. Although Phillips and Diaz [11] found that men and women who had BDD did not differ significantly in terms of rates of major depression, men were more likely to have alcohol abuse or dependence. The relationship between BDD and substance use may be relevant across BDD presentations, however. Grant and colleagues [34] found 49% of BDD subjects reported a lifetime substance use disorder, and 36% reported lifetime substance dependence, most commonly with alcohol. More than two thirds (68%) reported that the BDD contributed significantly to their substance-use problem although, with the exception of a higher rate of suicide attempts, there were few differences between those subjects who had BDD and a substance-use problem and those who had BDD but did not have a substance-use problem.

Some interesting findings have emerged from familial studies of prevalence in BDD. In a study examining OCD cases and control probands, as well as case and control first-degree relatives, Bienvenu and colleagues [5] found that BDD occurred more frequently in case probands and case relatives, whether or not case probands also had the same diagnosis. Overall,

BDD was four times as prevalent in first-degree relatives of case probands with than in relatives of probands that did not have BDD. The authors concluded that BDD is part of the familial OC spectrum. Supporting a broader conceptualization of BDD, Frare and colleagues [35] concluded that BDD is not just a clinical variant of OCD but also is related to mood disorders, social anxiety disorder, and eating disorders. Comparing patients who had BDD, OCD, and both disorders, they found that the OCD group was older, had a later onset of illness, and was less likely to be unemployed and unmarried than the cohorts who had BDD. The comorbid cohort that had both BDD and OCD exhibited the highest rates of bulimia, social phobia, bipolar disorder, and substance use problems; the group that had OCD showed the lowest levels of comorbidity.

In summary, high rates of comorbidity have been found between BDD and a range of psychiatric disorders. BDD commonly co-presents with social phobia, OCD, eating disorders, substance-use disorders, and major depression. In men, there also seem to be high rates of bipolar disorder. Similarities have been observed consistently between the clinical features of BDD and many of these disorders, and there seems to be a strong familial pattern in BDD and some of the other putative OC-spectrum disorders. Nonetheless, BDD is not merely a clinical variant of OCD, although it may share aspects of etiology with a range of OC-spectrum disorders.

Body dysmorphic disorder and cognition

The clinical presentation of BDD suggests a primary and significant impairment of somatosensory and perceptual processing, as well as memory and attentional disturbances. Surprisingly, however, there have been few cognitive investigations in patients who have BDD. The authors are aware of only nine published studies in this area [36–45]. The data so far indicate that a range of cognitive deficits is present, including executive function, memory, facial emotion perception, and attributional bias or self-discrepancy.

Overall, cognitive research in BDD has suggested that selective information processing might be important in the origin and maintenance of symptoms. Using an emotional Stroop paradigm, Buhlmann and colleagues [37], for example, demonstrated that, in contrast to healthy controls, a group of patients who had BDD selectively attended to words related to body image, such as "attractive" and "ugly." Lim and Kim [46] similarly established that somatoform patients showed bias toward physical-threat words on an Emotional Stroop task.

To date, most research concerning selective attention in BDD has used words as stimuli. Ecologically valid stimuli, which could include photographs of objects or faces, might be more useful. Recently, there have been two investigations of the perception of facial affect in BDD. Buhlmann and colleagues [38] investigated the ability of patients who had BDD, patients who had OCD, and healthy control participants (1) to discriminate single facial features (using the Short Form of the Benton Facial Recognition Test [47], which required matching a target face with up to three pictures of the same person in a six-stimuli array of faces that vary in terms of angles and lighting), and (2) to identify facial expressions of emotion using 42 photographs of emotional expressions from Ekman and Friesen [48] (ie, six models displaying seven emotions: angry, disgusted, happy, neutral, sad, scared, or surprised). Patients who had BDD did not have any difficulty identifying facial features. They were less accurate than the normal controls but were more accurate than the patients who had OCD in identifying overall facial expressions of emotion. Patients who had BDD , however, were more likely to misidentify emotional expressions as anger when errors were made.

In a follow-up experiment, Buhlmann and colleagues [40] asked patients who had BDD and controls to identify facial expressions within two scenarios: (1) self-referent (eg, "Imagine that the bank teller is looking at you. What is his expression like?") or (2) other-referent (eg,"Imagine that the bank teller is looking at a friend. What is his expression like?"). Patients who had BDD had difficulty identifying the correct emotional expression in the self-referent condition; they misinterpreted more expressions as angry than did the controls. Poor insight and ideas of reference were related to this deficit in both these studies.

Alternatively, Buhlmann and colleagues [36] have shown that patients who have BDD have a negative interpretive bias during the presentation of physically related and social situation–related information. An individual who has BDD, for example, is more likely to interpret someone behind them laughing as a negative response to their appearance, an interpretation not found in patients who have OCD or in controls. The results of these four studies suggest that individuals who have BDD have a selective bias toward perceiving anger in others. This bias confirms their recognition of others as rejecting, which in turn might reinforce their concerns about personal ugliness and social desirability, leading to social isolation as a coping strategy.

Osman and colleagues [43] have shown that a bias in selective attention can result in the collection of negative memories or images with regard to self. These authors used a semistructured interview to investigate spontaneously occurring images in BDD. The patients who had BDD were found to have appearance-related images that were significantly more negative, recurrent, and viewed from an observer perspective than those of control participants. These images were linked to stressful memories. Veale and colleagues [44] explored self-discrepancy biases and found that patients who have BDD have an unrealistic ideal for appearance and thus frequently fail to achieve their own (internal) aesthetic standard. Veale [26] has recently used such findings to develop a cognitive-behavioral model of BDD, in which he argues that the core of BDD is an excessive self-focused attention on negative body-related information. This model informs a cognitive-behavioral treatment approach to the disorder.

Selective information processing and attentional biases may also result in impairments in tasks requiring cognitive flexibility and adaptive behavior, for example, executive-functioning tasks. Hanes [42] reported poor performance in subjects who had BDD on two executive-functioning tasks, Stroop and the New Tower of London. Their deficits on these tasks paralleled those of patients who had OCD. Thus, it was suggested that the pathophysiology of BDD might involve the prefrontal region, because in normal controls prefrontal structures commonly are reported to be involved in both these cognitive measures.

Alternatively, it may be argued that an abnormality in selective information processing may be the result of difficulties in perceptual organization. Deckersbach and colleagues [41] reported that patients who had BDD differed significantly from controls on verbal and nonverbal learning and memory indices using the California Verbal Learning Test and the Rey Complex Figure Test. The patients who had BDD engaged in inappropriate scanning and categorization strategies. During both tasks, impaired performance in the group who had BDD was the result of the patients recalling specific isolated details rather than larger organizational design features. Deckersbach and colleagues [41] argued their perceptual organization might also explain deficits in patients who have BDD on facial emotion recognition tasks. That is, the patients who have BDD recall and focus on specific facial features instead of seeing the face as a whole and thus have insufficient information to interpret emotional expressions adequately. Yaryura-Tobias and colleagues [45] further established that patients who have BDD and OCD are impaired at detecting distortions of their computerized facial images, whereas healthy individuals show no problems performing this task. A perceptual organization approach, however, does not explain why impairments were not found in BDD during Buhlmann and colleagues' [38] study requiring nonreferential/nonemotional discrimination of single facial features. Thus, further research examining this distinction is required.

The cognitive data to date suggest that abnormal perception and emotional processing deficits are part of a neurobiologic paradigm of BDD. To process information efficiently, interdependence exists between cerebral regions through integrated neural networks. The involvement of cerebral structure therefore seems logical, because faulty beliefs and misperceptions characterize the disorder. This structural involvement may correlate with sensorial and higher cortical functions; and an imbalance in this loop may provoke false beliefs or overvalued ideas and body misperceptions. To date there have been no cognitive neuroimaging studies in BDD; consequently, little is understood about its neurobiologic underpinnings. In the only study that has investigated neuroanatomy in BDD, Rauch and colleagues [49] used morphometric MRI to show, in comparison with a healthy control group, that participants who have BDD have a leftward shift in caudate nucleus asymmetry similar to that in patients who have OCD. The caudate has many connections with the frontal lobes, and its function is to regulate, organize, and filter information. Caudate abnormalities may therefore explain why participants who had BDD had selective attentional biases: because incoming information may be reduced. Caudate abnormalities, however, do not explain why this bias is toward body-related information. Caution is needed in interpreting the results of the Rauch study, because the sample size was extremely small. Replication is recommended using more advanced image-analysis techniques and further focused region-of-interest measurements (ie, the frontal regions, especially the orbito-frontal lobe and amygdala).

In summary, nine studies have investigated cognitive processing in BDD. The authors speculate that these studies are suggestive of selective information processing of somatosensorial information and toward the facial emotional expression of "angry." Further empiric testing of this hypothesis is required.

Treatment of body dysmorphic disorder

There are pharmacologic and psychologic treatments that have had some success in the treatment of BDD. There can, however, be a major problem in engaging in a psychiatric/psychologic treatment a person who believes their problem is physical and can only be "cured" by a cosmetic procedure. Patients who have BDD are much more likely to seek the help of a cosmetic specialist than of a mental health professional. Cosmetic interventions for such people are highly unlikely to be successful and lead all too often to such individuals seeking redress through legal or even violent means. For example, in the study of Phillips and Diaz [11], 109 of 131 patients who had BDD had received surgical, dermatologic, or other nonpsychiatric treatments, resulting in a worsening or at best no change in BDD symptoms in 83%.

Thus, cosmetic specialists need to be aware of those at risk of a poor psychosocial outcome from cosmetic procedures, despite a good cosmetic result. Honigman and colleagues [50] reviewed all published psychosocial outcomes studies of plastic surgical procedures and identified minimal defect as a risk factor for a poor outcome. Thus, the cosmetic specialist needs to be wary about individuals seeking procedures for perceived defects that are not objectively evident. Other warning signs include an excessive amount of distress and disability associated with the perceived defect and unrealistic expectations for outcome either in cosmetic or psychosocial terms. Individuals who have such risk factors should be engaged in a discussion about their problem in broad terms such as "distress" and "disability," and they should be referred to a suitable mental health professional.

Psychologic treatment of body dysphoric disorder

As detailed previously, recent neurocognitive models of etiology have focused on the tendency for those who have BDD to self-focus attention excessively on distorted body image, with negative appraisals of such images leading to rumination, changes in mood, and the use of reassurance seeking and other maladaptive safety behaviors such as mirror checking [26]. The most widely used and generally effective psychologic interventions for BDD target such etiologically relevant phenomena and include behavior therapy aiming to change maladaptive behavior patterns and avoidance, cognitive therapy aiming to change specific beliefs and assumptions thought to underlie BDD [39], and the combination of cognitive therapy and behavior therapy strategies in the form of cognitive-behavior therapy (CBT).

Behavior therapy primarily involves prolonged, graded exposure to distressing stimuli or situations together with the prevention of associated compulsive overt and covert responses (eg, rituals or safety and avoidance behaviors) [51]. Exposure is particularly useful in dealing with avoidance and anxiety, whereas response-prevention techniques deal effectively with the prevention or limiting of maladaptive behaviors such as reassurance seeking, inspecting assumed deformities, and mirror checking. Cognitive therapy strategies principally aim to challenge dysfunctional thinking and replace it with more adaptive cognitive styles. Cognitive therapists often use behavioral experiments to disprove unsubstantiated thinking or to provide evidence for more rational thinking styles. For instance, someone who has BDD who believes that others will notice some imagined flaw in their appearance if they do not hide their face by wearing a hat may be asked to undertake an activity without a hat to see if their catastrophic predictions are realized. The implications of their experiences during such a behavioral experiment are then discussed in therapy. When cognitive therapy is used alone, it is detailed and direct in the way it deals with the cognitive features of BDD and is more likely to rely on behavioral experiments rather than on systematic, graded exposure and response prevention techniques. Nonetheless, the extent to which behavior and cognitive therapists use techniques from the alternative therapy modality varies, and many combine both types of strategies in CBT.

Additional components of CBT relevant to BDD can include skills training, particularly social skills, psychoeducation, and reverse role-playing, which requires patients to research and debate beliefs that are contrary to their overvalued ideas [52]. Furthermore, because the risk of relapse is high in BDD, the inclusion of a relapse-prevention or maintenance component to treatment can be effective in preventing symptom relapse and assisting in patients self-managing such lapses [53]. Finally, given similarities in phenomenology, enhanced developments in cognitive therapy for social phobia (eg, self-focused interventions [54,55]) could be of particular relevance to BDD, as could developments in mindfulness training to deal with ruminations and obsessions [56].

Relatively little research has been conducted to examine the efficacy of psychologic treatments for BDD. Early support for cognitive and behavioral treatments was found in a number of individual case reports [57,58] as well as in case series [59,60]. Wait-list–controlled trials lent further support to this approach [61], indicating that CBT was associated with better outcomes than no treatment or wait-list control. A recent meta-analysis of randomized trials and case series of pharmacologic and psychologic treatments for BDD supported the effectiveness of both modalities but concluded that CBT was the most useful [62]. Specifically, both pharmacologic and psychologic treatments were associated with large effect sizes, although outcomes from psychologic treatments were associated with significantly larger effect sizes than those from the pharmacologic studies. There were no differences in effect sizes between CBT and behavior therapy, or between behavior therapy and pharmacotherapy, although CBT was significantly more effective than medication treatments. It was not possible to tease out the effects of combined treatments. Retention rates for the psychologic treatments ranged from 44% to 100%, with half the studies reporting no dropouts. Psychologic treatment periods ranged from 7 to 30 sessions, whereas pharmacologic treatments were of relatively short duration (4–16 weeks).

Nonetheless, the published literature on the treatment of BDD is characterized by a paucity of randomized, controlled trials, with few studies directly comparing different treatments. Moreover, combined psychologic and pharmacologic treatments have not been evaluated rigorously [25]. A number of additional challenges remain in the evaluation of psychologic treatments for BDD. For instance, are group treatments and self-management as effective as individual treatment? How and when should one combine psychologic and pharmacologic treatments? What patient characteristics are good predictors of outcome for particular treatment modalities? What nonspecific factors (eg, therapist characteristics) influence treatment outcome for BDD? Such issues require further research.

Pharmacologic approaches

Most early data on the pharmacologic treatment of BDD came from retrospective clinical case series. Despite variations inherent in day-to-day clinical practice, the striking finding from reviews of pharmacologic treatments is the efficacy of serotonergic antidepressants, notably clomipramine and the selective serotonin reuptake inhibitors (SSRIs). For example, Hollander and colleagues [28] reported on 50 patients who had BDD, 35 of whom had been treated with SSRIs or clomipramine (SRIs), with a mean clinical global impression (CGI) improvement score of 1.9 (much improved); the 18 patients treated with tricyclics other than clomipramine showed much less robust improvement. Similarly, Phillips' [22] review of 130 patients who had BDD showed that 42% of 65 SRI trials resulted in much or very much improvement on the CGI, in contrast to only 30% of 23 trials of monoamine oxidase inhibitors, 15% of 48 trials of non-SRI antidepressants, 3% of trials of antipsychotics, and 6% of trials of other medications.

The crossover study of Hollander and colleagues [63] established the superiority of serotonergic over nonserotonergic antidepressants in the treatment of BDD. In this study, 29 patients were treated blindly with either clomipramine or desipramine (a noradrenergic reuptake inhibitor) and then were crossed over to the other agent. Clomipramine showed clear superiority for BDD symptoms, functional disability, and overall illness severity.

Medication trials involving adults who have BDD have recently been subjected to meta-analysis by Williams and colleagues [62]. Apart from the crossover trial of Hollander and colleagues [63], these authors identified three case series (range, 15–30 subjects; one 10-week and one 16-week study of fluvoxamine, and one 12-week trial of citalopram); and one randomized controlled trial (67 subjects; 12 weeks of fluoxetine versus placebo). The weighted mean effect size for the combined pharmacologic studies was 0.92, significantly superior to zero ($z = 8.55$; $P < .01$). Drops-outs for the medication treatments ranged from 16% to 40%. Of interest is that psychologic studies reviewed in the same meta-analysis showed a greater effect size (1.63), significantly better than the pharmacotherapy trials ($P < .01$). Of course direct comparisons between these two types of interventions potentially are confounded by, inter alia, differing severity of included patients. The authors are not aware of any direct comparison study, nor are there robust data on combined treatment with medication and psychologic treatment.

A particularly contentious issue is the role of antipsychotic medications in patients who have delusional BDD. In their work on monosymptomatic hypochondriacal delusions, Riding and Munro [64] included patients who had BDD and claimed they, like the rest of their patients, responded to the antipsychotic pimozide. Clinical case series, however, do not seem to support the efficacy of antipsychotics alone for BDD, even if the beliefs are held with delusional conviction [19].

The use of antipsychotics, expressly atypical antipsychotics such as olanzapine and quetiapine, as augmenting agents for patients who show only modest response to an SRI, has currency in clinical practice but has little support from the literature. For example, an 8-week placebo-controlled trial of pimozide (mean endpoint dose, 1.7 mg/d) augmentation of fluoxetine in 28 patients failed to show benefit even for delusional patients [65], and an 8-week open trial of olanzapine augmentation (mean dose, 4.6 mg/d) of fluoxetine showed slight benefit in two patients and no benefit in a further four [66]. These studies suffer the methodological problems of small sample sizes, a relatively restricted range of antipsychotic dose, and a short duration of treatment.

In clinical practice [3] and supported by the available literature, SRIs are seen as the first-line pharmacologic treatment for BDD. Often rather high doses are required (eg, up to 400 mg of fluvoxamine, 80 mg of fluoxetine, or equivalent), and a treatment trial should be of at least 12 weeks' duration.

If one SRI fails, the suggestion is to try another, and then another, because some patients seem to respond to particular agents. Clomipramine should be tried, although the higher doses required often carry an unacceptable side-effect burden.

Overall, very few data support any particular pharmacologic strategy for patients who do not respond to consecutive trials of a variety of SRIs. The authors' experience is that low doses of the antipsychotic quetiapine (25–100 mg/d) are well tolerated and can be of great additive benefit in such scenarios, expressly to reduce the distress associated with intrusive thoughts. This approach is supported by the literature on antipsychotic augmentation of SRIs in OCD [67] but requires formal study in BDD. Other augmenting agents with some evidence in OCD (such as lithium, clonazepam, and buspirone) should also be studied in patients who have refractory BDD [68].

Summary

BDD remains an understudied psychiatric disorder. Further research is required to establish its etiopathology and neurocognitive underpinnings. Its relationship to other psychiatric disorders requires clarification. Also needed is a much better understanding of the best treatments to adopt should conventional approaches (eg, SRIs, CBT) fail.

References

[1] Phillips KA. Body dysmorphic disorder: the distress of imagined ugliness. Am J Psychiatry 1991;148:1138–49.

[2] American Psychiatric Association. Diagnostic and statistical manual of mental disorders. 3rd edition, revised. Washington (DC): American Psychiatric Association; 1987.

[3] Phillips KA, Castle DJ. Body dysmorphic disorder. In: Castle DJ, Phillips KA, editors. Disorders of body image. Petersfield (UK): Wrightson Biomedical; 2002. p. 101–20.

[4] Phillips KA. Quality of life for patients with body dysmorphic disorder. J Nerv Ment Dis 2000;188:170–5.

[5] Bienvenu OJ, Samuels JF, Riddle MA, et al. The relationship of obsessive-compulsive disorder to possible spectrum disorders: results from a family study. Biol Psychiatry 2000;48: 287–93.

[6] Faravelli C, Salvatori S, Galassi F, et al. Epidemiology of somatoform disorders: a community survey in Florence. Soc Psychiatry Psychiatr Epidemiol 1997;32:24–9.

[7] Otto MW, Wilhelm S, Cohen LS, et al. Prevalence of body dysmorphic disorder in a community sample of women. Am J Psychiatry 2001;158:2061–3.

[8] Mayville S, Katz RC, Gipson MT, et al. Assessing the prevalence of body dysmorphic disorder in an ethnically diverse group of adolescents. J Clin Fam Stud 1999;8:357–62.

[9] Sarwer DB, Wadden TA, Pertschuk MJ, et al. Body image dissatisfaction and body dysmorphic disorder in 100 cosmetic surgery patients. Plast Reconstr Surg 1998;101:1644–9.

[10] Phillips KA, Dusfresne RG Jr, Wilkel C, et al. Rate of body dysmorphic disorder in dermatology patients. J Am Acad Dermatol 2000;42:436–41.

[11] Phillips KA, Diaz S. Gender differences in body dysmorphic disorder. J Nerv Ment Dis 1997; 185:570–7.

[12] Pope HG, Phillips KA, Olivardia R. The Adonis complex: the secret crisis of male body obsession. New York: The Free Press; 2000.

[13] Phillips KA, Grant JE, Siniscalchi JM, et al. A retrospective follow-up study of body dysmorphic disorder. Compr Psychiatry 2005;46:315–21.

[14] American Psychiatric Association. Diagnostic and statistical manual of mental disorders. 4th edition. Washington (DC): American Psychiatric Association; 1994.

[15] Mayou R, Kirmayer LJ, Simon G, et al. Somatoform disorders: time for a new approach in DSM-V. Am J Psychiatry 2005;162:847–55.

[16] Hollander E. Introduction. In: Hollander E, editor. Obsessive-compulsive related disorders. Washington (DC): American Psychiatric Press; 1993.

[17] Grant JE, Phillips KA. Is anorexia nervosa a subtype of body dysmorphic disorder? Probably not, but read on. Harv Rev Psychiatry 2004;12:123–6.

[18] Castle DJ, Phillips KA. The obsessive compulsive spectrum of disorders: a defensible construct? ANZ J Psychiatry 2006;40:114–20.

[19] Phillips KA, McElroy SL, Keck PE Jr. A comparison of delusional and nondelusional body dysmorphic disorder in 100 cases. Psychopharmacol Bull 1994;30:179–86.

[20] Phillips KA. Psychosis in body dysmorphic disorder. J Psychiatr Res 2004;38:63–72.

[21] Eisen JL, Phillips KA, Baer L, et al. The Brown Assessment of Beliefs Scale: reliability and validity. Am J Psychiatry 1998;155:102–8.

[22] Phillips KA, Nierenberg AA, Brendel G, et al. Prevalence and clinical features of body dysmorphic disorder in atypical major depression. J Nerv Ment Dis 1996;184:125–9.

[23] Brawman-Mintzer O, Lydiard RB, Phillips KA, et al. Body dysmorphic disorder in patients with anxiety disorders and major depression: a comorbidity study. Am J Psychiatry 1995;152:1665–7.

[24] Phillips KA, McElroy SL, Keck PE, et al. Body dysmorphic disorder: 30 cases of imagined ugliness. Am J Psychiatry 1993;150:302–8.

[25] Castle DJ, Rossell SL. Body dysmorphic disorder. Curr Opin Psychiatry 2006;19:74–8.

[26] Veale D. Advances in a cognitive behavioural model of body dysmorphic disorder. Body Image 2004;1:113–25.

[27] Veale D, Boocock A, Gournay K, et al. Body dysmorphic disorder: a survey of fifty cases. Br J Psychiatry 1996;169:196–201.

[28] Hollander E, Cohen LJ, Simeon D. Body dysmorphic disorder. Psych Ann 1993;23:359–64.

[29] Simeon D, Hollander E, Stein DJ, et al. Body dysmorphic disorder in the DSM-IV Field Trial for Obsessive-Compulsive Disorder. Am J Psychiatry 1995;152:1207–9.

[30] Albertini RS, Phillips KA. Thirty-three cases of body dysmorphic disorder in children and adolescents. J Am Acad Child Adolesc Psychiatry 1999;38:453–9.

[31] Biby EL. The relationship between body dysmorphic disorder and depression, self-esteem, somatization, and obsessive-compulsive disorder. J Clin Psychol 1998;54:489–99.

[32] Grant JE, Kim SW, Eckert ED. Body dysmorphic disorder in patients with anorexia nervosa: prevalence, clinical features, and delusionality of body image. Int J Eat Disord 2002;32:291–300.

[33] Perugi G, Akiskal HS, Giannotti D, et al. Gender-related differences in body dysmorphic disorder (dysmorphophobia). J Nerv Ment Dis 1997;185:578–82.

[34] Grant JE, Menard W, Pagano ME, et al. Substance use disorders in individuals with body dysmorphic disorder. J Clin Psychiatry 2005;66:309–16.

[35] Frare F, Perugi G, Ruffolo G, et al. Obsessive-compulsive disorder and body dysmorphic disorder: a comparison of clinical features. Eur Psychiatry 2004;19:292–8.

[36] Buhlmann U, Wilhelm S, McNally RJ, et al. Interpretive biases for ambiguous information in body dysmorphic disorder. CNS Spectr 2002;7:435–43.

[37] Buhlmann U, McNally RC, Wilhelm S, et al. Selective processing of emotional information in body dysmorphic disorder. J Anxiety Disord 2002;16:289–98.

[38] Buhlmann U, McNally RJ, Etcoff NL, et al. Emotion recognition deficits in body dysmorphic disorder. J Psychiatr Res 2004;38(2):201–6.

[39] Buhlmann U, Wilhelm S. Cognitive factors in body dysmorphic disorder. Psychiatr Ann 2004;34:922–6.

[40] Buhlmann U, Etcoff NL, Wilhelm S. Emotion recognition bias for contempt and anger in body dysmorphic disorder. J Psychiatr Res 2006;40:105–11.

[41] Deckersbach T, Savage CR, Phillips KA, et al. Characteristics of memory dysfunction in body dysmorphic disorder. J Int Neuropsychol Soc 2000;6:673–81.

[42] Hanes KR. Neuropsychological performance in body dysmorphic disorder. J Int Neuropsychol Soc 1998;4:167–71.

[43] Osman S, Cooper M, Hackmann A, et al. Spontaneously occurring images and early memories in people with body dysmorphic disorder. Memory 2004;12:428–36.

[44] Veale D, Kinderman P, Riley S, et al. Self-discrepancy in body dysmorphic disorder. Br J Clin Psychol 2003;42:157–69.

[45] Yaryura-Tobias JA, Neziroglu F, Torres-Gallegos M. Neuroanatomical correlates and somatosensorial disturbance in body dysmorphic disorder. CNS Spectrums 2002;7:432–4.

[46] Lim S, Kim J. Cognitive processing of emotional information in depression, panic and somatoform disorder. J Abnorm Psychol 2005;114:50–61.

[47] Benton AL, Hamsher KdeS, Varyney NR, et al. Facial recognition: stimulus and multiple-choice pictures. New York: Oxford University Press; 1983.

[48] Ekman P, Friesen WV. Measuring facial movement. Environmental Psychology and Nonverbal Behavior 1976;1:56–75.

[49] Rauch SL, Phillips KA, Segal E, et al. A preliminary morphometric magnetic resonance imaging study of regional brain volumes in body dysmorphic disorder. Psychiatry Res 2003; 122:13–9.

[50] Honigman R, Phillips K, Castle DJ. A review of psychosocial outcomes for patients seeking cosmetic surgery. Plast Reconstr Surg 2004;113:1229–37.

[51] Meyer V, Levy R, Schnurer A. The behavioral treatment of obsessive-compulsive disorders. In: Beech HR, editor. Obsess ional states. London: Methuen; 1974. p. 233–58.

[52] Cororve MB, Gleaves DH. Body dysmorphic disorder: a review of conceptualizations, assessment, and treatment strategies. Clin Psychol Rev 2001;21:949–70.

[53] McKay D. Two-year follow-up of behavioral treatment and maintenance for body dysmorphic disorder. Behav Modif 1999;23:620–9.

[54] Wells A. Cognitive therapy of anxiety disorders: practical manual and conceptual guide. Wiley; 1997.

[55] Clark DM, Ehlers A, McManus F, et al. Cognitive therapy vs fluoxetine plus self-exposure in the treatment of generalised social phobia (social anxiety disorder): a randomized controlled trial. J Consult Clin Psychol 2003;71:1058–67.

[56] Segal ZV, Williams JM, Teasdale JD. Mindfulness-based cognitive therapy for depression: a new approach to preventing relapse. New York: Guilford Press; 2001.

[57] Giles TR. Distortion of body image as an effect on conditioned fear. Journal of Behav Ther Exper Psychiatry 1988;19:143–6.

[58] Schmidt NB, Harrington P. Cognitive behavioral treatment of body dysmorphic disorder, a case report. J Behav Ther Exper Psychiatry 1995;26:161–7.

[59] Neziroglu FA, Yaryura-Tobias JA. Exposure, response prevention and cognitive therapy in the treatment of body dysmorphic disorder. Behav Ther 1993;24:431–8.

[60] Wilhelm S, Otto MW, Lohr B, et al. Cognitive behavior group therapy for body dysmorphic disorder: a case series. Behav Res Therapy 1999;37:71–5.

[61] Veale D, Gournay K, Dryden W, et al. Body dysmorphic disorder: a cognitive behavioural model and pilot randomised controlled trial. Behav Res Therapy 1996;34:717–29.

[62] Williams J, Hadjistavropoulos T, Sharpe D. A meta-analysis of psychological and pharmacological treatments for Body Dysmorphic Disorder. Behav Res Therapy 2006;44:99–111.

[63] Hollander E, Allen A, Kwon J, et al. Clomipramine vs desipramine crossover trial in body dysmorphic disorder: selective efficacy of a serotonin reuptake inhibitor in imagined ugliness. Arch Gen Psychiatry 1999;56:1033–42.

[64] Riding J, Munro A. Pimozide in the treatment of monosymptomatic hypochondriacal psychosis. Acta Psychiatr Scand 1975;52:23–30.

[65] Phillips KA. Placebo-controlled trial of pimozide augmentation of fluoxetine in body dysmorphic disorder. Am J Psychiatry 2005;162:377–9.

[66] Phillips KA. Olanzapine augmentation of fluoxetine in body dysmorphic disorder. Am J Psychiatry 2005;162:1022–3.
[67] Keuneman R, Pokos V, Weerasundera R, et al. Antipsychotics in the treatment of obsessive-compulsive disorder: a literature review. ANZ J Psychiatry 2005;39:336–43.
[68] Hadley SJ, Newcorn JH, Hollander E. The neurobiology and psychopharmacology of body dysmorphic disorder. In: Castle DJ, Phillips KA, editors. Disorders of body image. Petersfield (UK): Wrightson Biomedical; 2002. p. 139–55.

ELSEVIER
SAUNDERS

PSYCHIATRIC
CLINICS
OF NORTH AMERICA

Psychiatr Clin N Am 29 (2006) 539–551

Compulsive Aspects of Impulse-Control Disorders

Jon E. Grant, JD, MD, MPH[a],*,
Marc N. Potenza, MD, PhD[b]

[a]Department of Psychiatry, University of Minnesota Medical School,
2450 Riverside Avenue Minneapolis, MN 55454, USA
[b]Department of Psychiatry, Yale University School of Medicine,
New Haven, CT 06510, USA

Case vignette

Anna, a 32-year-old married woman, described herself as being "compulsive." She reported a history, beginning in late adolescence, of uncontrollable shoplifting. She reports that over the course of a few months she became "obsessed" with stealing, thinking about it "all day." She reports that her shoplifting started when she stole candy with friends and, over a period of a few months, developed into an almost daily ritual, which she did by herself. Anna reports that she currently shoplifts one to two times each week. She reports a "high" or a "rush" each time she steals. She primarily steals hygiene products, such as shampoo and soap. She usually steals multiple versions of the same item. Anna reports that she has boxes of the same shampoo and soap hidden in her closet. She steals shampoo and soap that she does not use and buys her preferred shampoo and soap at another store. When asked why she does not discard the shampoo, Anna reports that having these products "comforts" her. Anna's shoplifting may consume 2 to 3 hours at a time. Anna also describes daily thoughts and urges to shoplift that preoccupy her for 3 to 4 hours each day. She may even leave work early, with projects unfinished, so that she can get to a store and steal something. In addition, she lies to her husband, telling him that she buys the items she steals. Anna reports feeling "compelled" to shoplift items.

The work was supported by a grant from the National Institute of Mental Health (K23 MH069754-01A1) to Dr. Grant.

* Corresponding author.
E-mail address: grant045@umn.edu (J.E. Grant).

doi:10.1016/j.psc.2006.02.002
psych.theclinics.com

Does Anna suffer from obsessive-compulsive disorder (OCD) or klepto-mania? Is her behavior compulsive, impulsive, or both? How might concep-tualization of her behavior influence the treatment of Anna's behavior? Might Anna benefit most from a high dose of a selective serotonin reuptake inhibitor, or would a mood stabilizer or naltrexone be more effective options?

Impulsivity has been defined as a predisposition toward rapid, unplanned reactions to either internal or external stimuli without regard for negative consequences [1]. Although certain disorders are formally classified as im-pulse-control disorders (ICDs), impulsivity is a key element of many psychi-atric disorders (eg, substance-use disorders, bipolar disorder, personality disorders, attention-deficit hyperactivity disorder).

The American Psychiatric Association defines compulsivity as the perfor-mance of repetitive behaviors with the goal of reducing or preventing anx-iety or distress, not to provide pleasure or gratification [2]. Although OCD may be the most apparent disorder with compulsive features, compul-sivity is often a prominent symptom in a number of psychiatric disorders (eg, substance-use disorders, personality disorders, schizophrenia) [3].

Some have considered the domains of impulsivity and compulsivity to be diametrically opposed, but the relationship seems to be more intricate. Com-pulsivity and impulsivity may co-occur simultaneously in the same disorders or at different times within the same disorders, thereby complicating both the understanding and treatment of certain behaviors. ICDs, disorders clas-sically characterized by impulsivity, have more recently been found to have features of compulsivity. A central aim of this article is to explore how com-pulsivity pertains to ICDs. In this process, the article also explores the rela-tionship between OCD and ICDs.

Historically, one conceptualization of ICDs has been as part of an obses-sive-compulsive spectrum [4]. This initial understanding of ICDs was based on available data on the clinical characteristics of these disorders, patterns of familial transmission, and responses to pharmacologic and psychosocial treatments. In the Diagnostic and Statistical Manual of Mental Disorders, edition four, text revised (DSM-IV-TR), the category of ICDs not elsewhere classified currently includes intermittent explosive disorder, kleptomania, pyromania, pathological gambling (PG), and trichotillomania. Other disor-ders have been proposed for inclusion based on perceived phenomenologic, clinical, and possibly biologic similarities: psychogenic excoriation (skin picking), compulsive buying, compulsive Internet use, and non-paraphilic compulsive sexual behavior. The extent to which these ICDs share clinical, genetic, phenomenologic, and biologic features is incompletely understood. Although ICDs are still relatively understudied, research in these disorders has increased recently. Data from these studies suggest a complex relation-ship between ICDs and OCD, heterogeneity within the ICDs, and a compli-cated overlap between impulsivity and compulsivity. Because rigorous research on most ICDs is limited, this article focuses largely on PG and trichotillomania, the two ICDs that have received the most research attention. It also reviews kleptomania, which, although less studied than other psychiatric disorders, is receiving increasing attention from clinicians and researchers. The article reviews the relationships between these ICDs and OCD, the compulsive aspects of the ICDs, and the clinical implications for assessing compulsivity in ICDs.

Pathological gambling

PG, characterized by persistent and recurrent maladaptive patterns of gambling behavior, is associated with impaired functioning, reduced quality of life, and high rates of bankruptcy, divorce, and incarceration [5]. PG usually begins in early adulthood, with males tending to start at an earlier age [6]. If left untreated, PG seems to be a chronic, recurring condition.

Compulsivity refers to repetitive behaviors performed according to certain rules or in a stereotyped fashion, and PG is associated with many features of compulsivity. PG is characterized by the repetitive behavior of gambling and impaired inhibition of the behavior. People who have PG often describe gambling as difficult to resist or control, and in this respect PG seems similar to the frequently excessive, unnecessary, and unwanted rituals of OCD. Additionally, individuals who have PG often have specific rituals associated with their gambling (eg, wearing certain clothes when gambling or gambling on particular slot machines). Another putative link between PG and OCD is the propensity of individuals who have PG to engage in excessive, possibly harmful behavior that leads to significant impairment in social or occupational functioning and causes personal distress [7]. As in OCD, the compulsive behavior of PG-gambling-is often triggered by aversive or stressful stimuli [8]. Individuals who have PG often report that their urges to gamble are triggered by feelings of anxiety, sadness, or loneliness [9,10].

Studies consistently find that individuals who have PG have high rates of lifetime mood (60%–76%), anxiety (16%–40%), and other (23%) ICDs [5,11,12]. Rates of co-occurrence between PG and OCD have been largely inconsistent, however. For example, in samples of subjects who have PG, rates of co-occurring OCD have ranged from 1% to 20% [5], with some, but not all, studies finding higher rates of OCD (approximately 2%) than found in the general population. The St. Louis Epidemiologic Catchment Area study, however, found no significant relationship between problem gambling and OCD (an odds ratio of 0.6 for OCD in problem gamblers as compared with non-gamblers) [13]. Although this study collected data in the 1980s, it is the only study published to date in which a community sample was assessed for DSM-based diagnoses for both OCD and PG.

Studies of PG among individuals who have OCD have reported little, if any, relationship between PG and OCD. Although studies of small OCD samples have reported PG rates ranging from 2.2% to 2.6% [14,15], a recently completed study of a large sample of subjects who had primary OCD (n = 293) found rates of current (0.3%) and lifetime (1.0%) PG [16] that were no greater than those in the general population (0.7–1.6%) [13]. These recent findings are consistent with those from a sample of more than 2000 individuals who had OCD in which both current and past rates of PG were lower than 1% [17]. Similarly, a family study of OCD probands did not find evidence of a significant relationship between OCD and PG or OCD and ICDs in general (with the exception of grooming and eating disorders) [18].

Family-history studies of subjects who have PG are limited. Black and colleagues [19] examined 17 subjects who had PG and 75 of their first-degree relatives. The study found that 1% of the first-degree relatives had OCD (similar to rates in the community), compared with none in the control group. Although the sample was small, the study used a control group as well as structured interviews for the subjects and first-degree relatives. As in the study of OCD probands, the family study of subjects who had PG and their relatives failed to find a link between PG and OCD.

Although on the surface PG shares many phenomenologic features with OCD, the majority of data suggests that the co-occurrence between these disorders is not elevated. Thus it seems that PG has multiple compulsive features but is not associated with high rates of OCD. One reason for this observation may involve limitations of categorical diagnoses. An alternate, not mutually exclusive explanation is that although compulsive features are observed in each disorder, the underlying biologies of the disorders differ. Another consideration is that aspects of compulsivity may differ between the disorders.

Assessing compulsivity in OCD and in PG and other ICDs might clarify the role of compulsivity in each disorder. Although many studies have assessed impulsivity and related constructs (eg, sensation seeking) in PG [5,20], relatively few have explored the construct of compulsivity in PG. In one study (the Padua Inventory), pathologic gamblers scored higher than normal controls on a measure of compulsivity [21]. A recent study attempting to understand the compulsive and impulsive dimensions of PG used the Padua Inventory to examine 38 subjects before and after 12 weeks of treatment with paroxetine [22]. The Padua Inventory measures obsessions and compulsions and contains four factors [23]:

1. Impaired control over mental activities, which assesses ruminations and exaggerated doubts
2. Fear of contamination
3. Checking
4. Impaired control over motor activities which measures urges and worries related to motor behavior, such as violent impulses

At baseline, the severity pf PG symptoms was associated with features of both impulsivity and compulsivity (specifically, factors 1 and 4 of the Padua

Inventory). During treatment, overall scores on measures of impulsivity and compulsivity diminished, with significant decreases seen in factor 1 of the Padua Inventory and the impulsiveness subscales of the Eysenck Impulsivity Questionnaire [22]. This study suggests that compulsivity and impulsivity in PG interact in a complex fashion, and that measures of impulsivity and compulsivity have relevance with respect to treatment outcome. A corollary of this finding is that compulsivity or impulsivity (or specific aspects of each) might represent treatment targets for PG.

Although pathogenesis is arguably the most valid indicator of whether disorders are related, only a sparse amount of research has investigated possible neurobiologic correlates of PG, and the evidence suggests a different pathology from that seen in OCD. A functional MRI study of gambling urges in male pathologic gamblers suggests that PG has neural features (relatively decreased activation within cortical, basal ganglionic, and thalamic brain regions in subjects who have PG as compared with controls) distinct from the brain activation pattern observed in cue-provocation studies of OCD (relatively increased cortico-basal-ganglionic-thalamic activity) [24,25]. Whereas research on the neurobiology of PG is increasing, the neurobiologic relationship of PG to OCD remains to be qualified. More systematic studies of PG and OCD (eg, those that directly compare and contrast subjects using the same paradigm) are needed.

Treatment of pathological gambling

Originally it was suggested that PG, like OCD, may demonstrate a preferential response to serotonin reuptake inhibitors (SRIs). Data from double-blinded, randomized pharmacotherapy trials of SRIs in the treatment of PG, have been inconclusive, however [7], with medication showing a significant advantage over placebo in some but not in other trials of SRIs [26–29]. In addition, PG has demonstrated responses to opioid antagonists [30,31], drugs that have not been shown to be effective in treating OCD. The response of PG to pharmacologic treatment has been studied insufficiently to determine clearly the choice of treatment. The extent to which measures of compulsivity may be used to match specific treatments with specific individuals who have PG or used to assess or predict treatment outcome remains to be examined.

Cognitive and behavioral treatments that address the compulsive aspect of PG have shown early benefit [32]. Cognitive-behavioral therapy for PG, however, differs from the exposure and response prevention treatment used for OCD [33]. Cognitive therapy focuses on changing the patient's beliefs regarding perceived control over randomly determined events. Cognitive therapy helps the patient understand that the laws of probability, not ritualistic behavior, control the outcome of gambling. In one study, individual cognitive therapy resulted in reduced gambling frequency and increased perceived self-control over gambling when compared with wait-list controls

[34]. A second study that included relapse prevention also produced improvement in gambling symptoms compared with wait-list controls [35].

Cognitive-behavioral therapy has also been used to treat PG. The behavioral element addresses substituting alternative behaviors for gambling. One randomized trial compared four types of treatment: (1) individual stimulus control and in vivo exposure with response prevention, (2) group cognitive restructuring, (3) a combination of methods 1 and 2, and (4) a wait-list control. At 12 months, rates of abstinence or minimal gambling were higher in the individual treatment (69%) group than in the group cognitive restructuring (38%) and the combined treatment (38%) groups [36]. An independent, controlled trial, based upon cognitive-behavior therapies used in the treatment of substance-use disorders and including relapse-prevention strategies, is currently under way; initial results suggest the efficacy of manually driven cognitive-behavioral therapy [37].

One study of a brief intervention in the form of a workbook (which included cognitive-behavioral and motivational enhancement techniques) was compared with the use of the workbook plus one clinician interview [38]. Both groups reported significant reductions in gambling at a 6-month follow-up. Similarly, a separate study assigned gamblers to use of a workbook, use of a workbook plus a telephone motivational enhancement intervention, or a wait list. Compared with those using the workbook alone, the gamblers assigned to the motivational intervention plus workbook reduced gambling throughout a 2-year follow-up period [39].

Two studies have also tested aversion therapy and imaginal desensitization in randomized designs. In the first study, both treatments resulted in improvement in a small sample of patients [40]. In the second study, 120 pathologic gamblers were assigned randomly to aversion therapy, imaginal desensitization, in vivo desensitization, or imaginal relaxation. Participants receiving imaginal desensitization reported better outcomes at 1 month and up to 9 years later [41].

Trichotillomania

Trichotillomania has been defined as repetitive, intentional hair pulling that causes noticeable hair loss and results in clinically significant distress or functional impairment [2]. A discussed elsewhere in this issue, trichotillomania seems to be relatively common, with an estimated prevalence between 1% and 3% [42]. The mean age at onset for trichotillomania is approximately 13 years [43].

The repetitive motor behavior of hair pulling with perceived diminished control bears a striking resemblance to OCD. In contrast to OCD, in which compulsions occur in a variety of situations, individuals who have trichotillomania tend to pull most often when engaged in sedentary activities [44]. Although the hair pulling in trichotillomania decreases anxiety, as do compulsions in OCD, it may also produce feelings of pleasure, whereas OCD compulsions typically do not.

Trichotillomania traditionally has been considered a disorder predominantly affecting females [45] and frequently is associated with depression (39%–65%), generalized anxiety disorder (27%–32%), and substance abuse (15%–20%). In particular, rates of co-occurring OCD are significantly higher (13%–27%) [43] than found in the community (1%–3%) [46], and this comorbidity raises the possibility of an underlying common neurobiologic pathway for the compulsivity seen in these two disorders. Trichotillomania is not associated with higher rates of obsessive-compulsive symptoms, with scores generally in the normal range [44].

Rates of trichotillomania among individuals who have OCD are inconsistent across studies. Three studies of small samples of OCD subjects have reported rates ranging from 4.6% to 7.1% [14,15,47]. One larger study of 293 subjects who had OCD reported lifetime and current rates of trichotillomania of 1.4% and 1.0%, respectively [16]. As with PG, the question remains whether examining the domain of compulsivity across these disorders would provide insight into possible pathophysiology.

A relationship between trichotillomania and OCD is supported partially by findings that OCD is common in relatives of subjects who have trichotillomania. Although family-history studies of trichotillomania are limited, one study has suggested a familial relationship with OCD. The study involved 22 subjects who had trichotillomania and 102 first-degree relatives. When compared with a control group (n = 33, with 182 first-degree relatives), significantly more relatives of the trichotillomania probands had OCD (2.9%) compared with the control group [48]. A family study of OCD probands found a higher proportion of case subjects than control subjects had trichotillomania (4% versus 1%), although the difference was not statistically significant given the sample size [18].

Treatment of trichotillomania

Treatments evaluated for trichotillomania include pharmacologic and behavioral interventions. It is well established that the pharmacologic first-line treatment for OCD is an SRI (eg, clomipramine, fluvoxamine, or fluoxetine). The data regarding the efficacies of SRIs for trichotillomania are less convincing, however. One study compared clomipramine with desipramine in a 10-week double-blinded, cross-over design (5 weeks for each agent after 2 weeks of single-blind placebo lead-in) [49]. Twelve of 13 subjects had significant improvement when receiving clomipramine. Although SRIs are effective for OCD, these medications have demonstrated mixed results in three randomized trials of trichotillomania [50–52]. In addition, individuals who have trichotillomania and who are successfully treated with an SRI tend to have higher rates of symptom relapse than do SRI-treated people who have OCD [51].

Other pharmacologic agents that have shown benefit for trichotillomania have not been effective for OCD. This lack of efficacy raises questions about the overlap between these disorders. Christenson and colleagues [51] compared the opioid antagonist naltrexone with placebo in a 6-week randomized, double-blinded, parallel study. Significant improvement was noted for the naltrexone group on one measure of trichotillomania symptoms. In an open-label study of lithium, 8 of 10 subjects reported decreases in pulling frequency, amount of hair pulled, and extent of hair loss [53] Lithium has often been beneficial in treating individuals who have disorders characterized by impaired impulse control [54]. The positive results from the open-label trial of lithium [53] raise the possibility that impulsive rather than compulsive features represent an important treatment target in some individuals who trichotillomania. Direct testing of this hypothesis is needed before this claim can be verified.

Both OCD and trichotillomania respond to behavioral interventions; however, the modes of behavioral treatment differ quite substantially. Azrin and colleagues [55] randomly assigned 34 subjects to habit-reversal therapy or negative practice (in which subjects were instructed to stand in front of a mirror and act out motions of hair-pulling without actually pulling). Habit reversal reduced hair pulling by more than 90% for 4 months, compared with a 52% to 68% reduction for negative practice at 3 months. No control group was included, and therefore time and therapist attention could not be assessed.

A recent study examined 25 subjects randomized to 12 weeks (10 sessions) of either acceptance and commitment therapy/habit reversal or wait list [56]. Subjects assigned to the therapy experienced significant reductions in hair-pulling severity and impairment compared to those assigned to the wait list, and improvement was maintained at 3-month follow-up.

Kleptomania

The core features of kleptomania include (1) a recurrent failure to resist an impulse to steal unneeded objects; (2) an increasing sense of tension before committing the theft; (3) an experience of pleasure, gratification, or release at the time of committing the theft; and (4) stealing not performed out of anger, vengeance, or because of psychosis [2].

Like OCD, kleptomania usually appears first during late adolescence or early adulthood [57]. The course is generally chronic with waxing and waning of symptoms. Unlike OCD, however, women are two times more likely than men to suffer from kleptomania [57]. In one study, all participants reported increased urges to steal when trying to stop stealing [57]. The diminished ability to stop often leads to feelings of shame and guilt, reported by most subjects (77.3%) [57].

Although people who have kleptomania often steal various items from multiple places, most steal from stores. In one study, 68.2% of patients reported that the value of stolen items had increased over time [57]. Many (64%–87%) have been apprehended at some time because of their behavior [58], and 15% to 23% report having been jailed [57]. Although most of the patients who were apprehended reported that their urges to steal were diminished after the apprehension, the symptom remission generally lasted only for a few days or weeks [58]. Together, these findings demonstrate a continued engagement in the problematic behavior despite adverse consequences.

This repetitive behavior seen in kleptomania is suggestive of a compulsion, as in the case vignette that opened this article. In addition, most individuals who have kleptomania (63%) hoard particular items that they steal [57]. Personality examinations of individuals who have kleptomania suggest, however, that they are generally sensation seeking [59] and impulsive [60] and thereby differ from individuals who have OCD, who are generally harm avoidant with a compulsive risk-aversive endpoint to their behaviors [4]. Unlike individuals who have OCD, people who have kleptomania may report an urge or craving before engaging in the stealing and a hedonic quality during the performance of the thefts [7].

High rates of other psychiatric disorders have been found in patients who have kleptomania. Rates of lifetime comorbid affective disorders range from 59% [61] to 100% [58]. Studies have also found high lifetime rates of comorbid anxiety disorders (60% to 80%) [58,62] and substance-use disorders (23% to 50%) [58,61].

The extent to which OCD and kleptomania co-occur is not well understood. Rates of co-occurring OCD in samples of individuals who have kleptomania have ranged from 6.5% [61] to 60% [63]. Conversely, rates of kleptomania in OCD samples suggest a higher rate of co-occurrence than found in the community (2.2%–5.9%) [14,15]. A recent study of 293 subjects who had OCD reported current and lifetime rates of kleptomania (0.3% and 1.0%) [16] that were lower than rates found in a population of general psychiatric inpatients (7.8% and 9.3%, respectively) [64]. Large psychiatric epidemiologic studies have typically excluded measures of kleptomania, thus limiting the available knowledge regarding its prevalence and patterns of co-occurrence with other psychiatric disorders.

A family history study compared 31 individuals who had kleptomania and 152 of their first-degree relatives with 35 control subjects and 118 of their first-degree relatives [61]. The study found that 0.7% of the relatives of the kleptomania proband suffered from OCD compared with 0% in families of the controls.

Treatment of kleptomania

Only case reports, two small case series, and one open-label study of pharmacotherapy have been performed for kleptomania. Various medications have been studied in case reports or case series, and several have been found effective: fluoxetine, nortriptyline, trazodone, clonazepam, valproate, lithium, fluvoxamine, paroxetine, and topiramate [65]. Unlike the treatment of OCD, there does not seem to be a preferential response of kleptomania to serotonergic medications. The only formal trial of medication for kleptomania involved 10 subjects in a 12-week, open-label study of naltrexone. At a mean dose of 150 mg/d, medication resulted in a significant decline in the intensity of urges to steal, thoughts about stealing, and stealing behavior [66].

Although multiple types of psychotherapies have been described in the treatment of kleptomania, no controlled trials exist in the literature. Forms of psychotherapy described in case reports as demonstrating success include psychoanalytic, insight-oriented, and behavioral techniques [58,67]. Because no controlled trials of therapy for kleptomania have been published, the efficacies of these interventions are difficult to evaluate, but the range of psychosocial interventions, as with medications, suggests that kleptomania is heterogeneous.

Summary

As seen in the introductory case vignette, ICDs are characterized by repetitive behaviors and impaired inhibition of these behaviors. The difficult-to-control behaviors characteristic of ICDs suggest a similarity to the frequently excessive, unnecessary, and unwanted rituals of OCD. There are, however, differences between ICDs and OCD (eg, the urge or craving state seen in ICDs, the hedonic quality during the performance of the ICD behavior, and the sensation-seeking personality type often seen in individuals who have ICD) [7]. Despite the differences between ICDs and OCD, features of compulsivity have been observed in association with ICDs, and preliminary data suggest that features of compulsivity, as well as impulsivity, might represent important treatment targets in some ICDs.

Future directions

Because research is limited, and findings are varied, it seems premature to identify ICDs too closely with OCD. The extent to which there exist specific ICDs or subtypes of ICD that are more closely associated with OCD remains to be investigated more systematically. In addition, the construct of compulsivity as related to ICDs and OCD warrants additional investigation to identify the similarities and differences and to examine the implications for prevention and treatment strategies. For example, given that the treatment of ICDs with SRIs has demonstrated mixed results, future investigations are needed to determine whether specific subgroups (eg, individuals who have PG with specific features of compulsivity or impulsivity) respond better or worse to specific treatments (eg, SRIs). Similarly, specific aspects of compulsivity might represent targets for behavioral interventions for ICDs.

Future biologic studies of ICDs (eg, genetic, neuroimaging) should also include measures of compulsivity to understand better its relevance to the OC spectrum disorders.

References

[1] Moeller FG, Barratt ES, Dougherty DM, et al. Psychiatric aspects of impulsivity. Am J Psychiatry 2001;158:1783–93.

[2] American Psychiatric Association. Diagnostic and statistical manual of mental disorders. 4th edition text revision. Washington (DC): American Psychiatric Association Press; 2000.

[3] Godlstein RZ, Volkow ND. Drug addiction and its underlying neurobiological basis: neuroimaging evidence for the involvement of the frontal cortex. Am J Psychiatry 2002;159: 1642–52.

[4] Hollander E. Obsessive-compulsive spectrum disorders: an overview. Psychiatr Ann 1993; 23:355–8.

[5] Argo TR, Black DW. Clinical characteristics. In: Grant JE, Potenza MN, editors. Pathological gambling: a clinical guide to treatment. Washington (DC): American Psychiatric Publishing, Inc.; 2004. p. 39–53.

[6] Ibanez A, Blanco C, Moreryra P, et al. Gender differences in pathological gambling. J Clin Psychiatry 2003;64:295–301.

[7] Grant JE, Potenza MN. Impulse control disorders: clinical characteristics and pharmacological management. Ann Clin Psychiatry 2004;16:27–34.

[8] Potenza MN, Leung HC, Blumberg HP, et al. An fMRI Stroop task study of ventromedial prefrontal cortical function in pathological gamblers. Am J Psychiatry 2003;160:1990–4.

[9] Grant JE, Kim SW. Demographic and clinical features of 131 adult pathological gamblers. J Clin Psychiatry 2001;62:957–62.

[10] Ladd GT, Petry NM. Gender differences among pathological gamblers seeking treatment. Exp Clin Psychopharmacol 2002;10:302–9.

[11] Black DW, Moyer T. Clinical features and psychiatric comorbidity of subjects with pathological gambling behavior. Psychiatr Serv 1998;49:1434–9.

[12] Crockford DN, el-Guebaly N. Psychiatric comorbidity in pathological gambling: a critical review. Can J Psychiatry 1998;43:43–50.

[13] Cunningham-Williams RM, Cottler LB, Compton WM III, et al. Taking chances: problem gamblers and mental health disorders—results from the St. Louis Epidemiologic Catchment Area study. Am J Public Health 1998;88:1093–6.

[14] Fontenelle LF, Mendlowicz MV, Versiani M. Impulse control disorders in patients with obsessive-compulsive disorder. Psychiatr Clin Neurosci 2005;59:30–7.

[15] Matsunaga H, Kiriike N, Matsui T, et al. Impulsive disorders in Japanese adult patients with obsessive-compulsive disorder. Compr Psychiatry 2005;46:43–9.

[16] Grant JE, Mancebo MC, Pinto A, et al. Impulse control disorders in adults with obsessive compulsive disorder. J Psychiatr Res, in press.

[17] Hollander E, Stein DJ, Kwon JH, et al. Psychosocial function and economic costs of obsessive-compulsive disorder. CNS Spectr 1997;2:16–25.

[18] Bienvenu OJ, Samuels JF, Riddle MA, et al. The relationship of obsessive-compulsive disorder to possible spectrum disorders: results from a family study. Biol Psychiatry 2000;48: 287–93.

[19] Black DW, Moyer T, Schlosser S. Quality of life and family history in pathological gambling. J Nerv Ment Dis 2003;191:124–6.

[20] Tavares H, Zilberman ML, Hodgins DC, et al. Comparison of craving between pathological gamblers and alcoholics. Alcohol Clin Exp Res 2005;29:1427–31.

[21] Blaszczynski A. Pathological gambling and obsessive compulsive spectrum disorders. Psychol Rep 1999;84:107–13.

[22] Blanco C, Grant J, Potenza MN, et al. Impulsivity and compulsivity in pathological gambling [abstract]. San Juan (Puerto Rico): College on Problems of Drug Dependence; 2004.

[23] Sanavio. Obsessions and compulsions: the Padua Inventory. Behav Res Ther 1988;26: 169–77.

[24] Potenza MN, Steinberg MA, Skudlarski P, et al. Gambling urges in pathological gambling: a functional magnetic resonance imaging study. Arch Gen Psychiatry 2003;60:828–36.

[25] Saxena S, Rauch SL. Functional neuroimaging and the neuroanatomy of obsessive-compulsive disorder. Psychiatr Clin North Am 2000;23:563–86.

[26] Hollander E, DeCaria CM, Finkell JN, et al. A randomized double-blind fluvoxamine/placebo crossover trial in pathologic gambling. Biol Psychiatry 2000;47:813–7.

[27] Kim SW, Grant JE, Adson DE, et al. A double-blind placebo-controlled study of the efficacy and safety of paroxetine in the treatment of pathological gambling. J Clin Psychiatry 2002; 63:501–7.

[28] Blanco C, Petkova E, Ibanez A, et al. A pilot placebo-controlled study of fluvoxamine for pathological gambling. Ann Clin Psychiatry 2002;14:9–15.

[29] Grant JE, Kim SW, Potenza MN, et al. Paroxetine treatment of pathological gambling: a multi-center randomized controlled trial. Int Clin Psychopharmacol 2003;18:243–9.

[30] Grant JE, Potenza MN, Hollander E, et al. A multicenter investigation of the opioid antagonist nalmefene in the treatment of pathological gambling. Am J Psychiatry 2006;163:303–12.

[31] Kim SW, Grant JE, Adson DE, et al. Double-blind naltrexone and placebo comparison study in the treatment of pathological gambling. Biol Psychiatry 2001;49:914–21.

[32] Hodgins DC, Petry NM. Cognitive and behavioral treatments. In: Grant JE, Potenza MN, editors. Pathological gambling: a clinical guide to treatment. Washington (DC): American Psychiatric Publishing, Inc.; 2004. p. 169–87.

[33] Simpson HB, Fallon BA. Obsessive-compulsive disorder: an overview. J Psychiatr Pract 2000;6:3–17.

[34] Sylvain C, Ladouceur R, Boisvert JM. Cognitive and behavioral treatment of pathological gambling: a controlled study. J Consult Clin Psychol 1997;65:727–32.

[35] Ladouceur R, Sylvain C, Boutin C, et al. Cognitive treatment of pathological gambling. J Nerv Ment Dis 2001;189:774–80.

[36] Eucheburua E, Baez C, Fernandez-Montalvo J. Comparative effectiveness of three therapeutic modalities in psychological treatment of pathological gambling: long term outcome. Behav Cog Psychother 1996;24:51–72.

[37] Petry NM. Pathological gambling: etiology, comorbidity, and treatment. Washington, DC: American Psychological Association; 2005.

[38] Dickerson M, Hinchy J, England SL. Minimal treatments and problem gamblers: a preliminary investigation. J Gambl Stud 1990;6:87–102.

[39] Hodgins DC, Currie SR, el-Guebaly N. Motivational enhancement and self-help treatments for problem gambling. J Consult Clin Psychol 2001;69:50–7.

[40] McConaghy N, Armstrong MS, Blaszczynski A, et al. Controlled comparison of aversive therapy and imaginal desensitization in compulsive gambling. Br J Psychiatry 1983;142: 366–72.

[41] McConaghy N, Blaszczynski A, Frankova A. Comparison of imaginal desensitization with other behavioral treatments of pathological gambling: a two to nine year follow-up. Br J Psychiatry 1991;159:390–3.

[42] Christenson GA, Pyle RL, Mitchell JE. Estimated lifetime prevalence of trichotillomania in college students. J Clin Psychiatry 1991;52:415–7.

[43] Christenson GA, Mansueto CS. Trichotillomania: descriptive characteristics and phenomenology. In: Stein DJ, Christenson GA, Hollander E, editors. Trichotillomania. Washington (DC): American Psychiatric Publishing, Inc; 1999. p. 1–42.

[44] Stanley MA, Cohen LJ. Trichotillomania and obsessive-compulsive disorder. In: Stein DJ, Christenson GA, Hollander E, editors. Trichotillomania. Washington (DC): American Psychiatric Publishing, Inc; 1999. p. 225–61.

[45] Swedo SE, Leonard HL. Trichotillomania: an obsessive compulsive spectrum disorder? Psychiatr Clin North Am 1992;15:777–90.

[46] Regier DA, Kaelber CT, Roper MT, et al. The ICD-10 clinical field trial for mental and behavioral disorders: results in Canada and the United States. Am J Psychiatry 1994;151:1340–50.

[47] Du Toit PL, van Kradenburg J, Niehaus D, et al. Comparison of obsessive-compulsive disorder in patients with and without comorbid putative obsessive-compulsive spectrum disorders using a structured clinical interview. Compr Psychiatry 2005;42:291–300.

[48] Schlosser S, Black DW, Blum N, et al. The demography, phenomenology, and family history of 22 persons with compulsive hair pulling. Ann Clin Psychiatry 1994;6:147–52.

[49] Swedo SE, Leonard HL, Rapoport JL, et al. A double-blind comparison of clomipramine and desipramine in the treatment of trichotillomania (hair pulling). N Engl J Med 1989; 321:497–501.

[50] Christenson GA, Mackenzie TB, Mitchell JE, et al. A placebo-controlled, double-blind crossover study of fluoxetine in trichotillomania. Am J Psychiatry 1991;148:1566–71.

[51] O'Sullivan RL, Christenson GA, Stein DJ. Pharmacotherapy of trichotillomania. In: Stein DJ, Christenson GA, Hollander E, editors. Trichotillomania. Washington (DC): American Psychiatric Publishing, Inc; 1999. p. 93–123.

[52] Streichenwein SM, Thornby JI. A long-term, double-blind, placebo-controlled crossover trial of the efficacy of fluoxetine for trichotillomania. Am J Psychiatry 1995;152: 1192–6.

[53] Christenson GA, Popkin MK, Mackenzie TB, et al. Lithium treatment of chronic hair pulling. J Clin Psychiatry 1991;52:116–20.

[54] Corrigan PW, Yudofsky SC, Silver JM. Pharmacological and behavioral treatments for aggressive psychiatric inpatients. Hosp Community Psychiatry 1993;44:125–33.

[55] Azrin NH, Nunn RG, Frantz SE. Treatment of hairpulling (trichotillomania): a comparative study of habit reversal and negative practice training. J Behav Ther Exp Psychiatry 1980;11: 13–20.

[56] Woods DW, Wetterneck CT, Flessner CA. A controlled evaluation of acceptance and commitment therapy plus habit reversal for trichotillomania. Behav Res Ther 2006;44:639–56.

[57] Grant JE, Kim SW. Clinical characteristics and associated psychopathology of 22 patients with kleptomania. Compr Psychiatry 2002;43:378–84.

[58] McElroy SL, Pope HG, Hudson JI, et al. Kleptomania: a report of 20 cases. Am J Psychiatry 1991;148:652–7.

[59] Grant JE, Kim SW. Temperament and early environmental influences in kleptomania. Compr Psychiatry 2002;43:223–9.

[60] Bayle FJ, Caci H, Millet B, et al. Psychopathology and comorbidity of psychiatric disorders in patients with kleptomania. Am J Psychiatry 2003;160:1509–13.

[61] Grant JE. Family history and psychiatric comorbidity in persons with kleptomania. Compr Psychiatry 2003;44:437–41.

[62] McElroy SL, Hudson JI, Pope HG, et al. The DSM-III-R impulse control disorders not elsewhere classified: clinical characteristics and relationship to other psychiatric disorders. Am J Psychiatry 1992;149:318–27.

[63] Presta S, Marazziti D, Dell'Osso L, et al. Kleptomania: clinical features and comorbidity in an Italian sample. Compr Psychiatry 2002;43:7–12.

[64] Grant JE, Levine L, Kim D, et al. Impulse control disorders in adult psychiatric inpatients. Am J Psychiatry 2005;162:2184–8.

[65] Grant JE. Kleptomania. In: Hollander E, Stein DJ, editors. A clinical manual of impulse control disorders. Washington (DC): American Psychiatric Publishing, Inc.; 2005.

[66] Grant JE, Kim SW. An open label study of naltrexone in the treatment of kleptomania. J Clin Psychiatry 2002;63:349–56.

[67] Goldman MJ. Kleptomania: making sense of the nonsensical. Am J Psychiatry 1991;148: 986–96.

ELSEVIER
SAUNDERS

PSYCHIATRIC
CLINICS
OF NORTH AMERICA

Psychiatr Clin N Am 29 (2006) 553–584

Pharmacotherapy of Obsessive-compulsive Disorder and Obsessive-Compulsive Spectrum Disorders

Damiaan Denys, MD, PhD*

Department of Anxiety Disorders, Rudolf Magnus Institute of Neuroscience, Department of Psychiatry, University Medical Center, Utrecht, The Netherlands

In one of the first articles addressing pharmacotherapy for obsessive-compulsive disorder (OCD) published in 1969, intravenous clomipramine unexpectedly proved effective for 11 of 13 patients [1]. The authors offered the following hypotheses to explain the improvement:

1. OCD symptoms remitted spontaneously
2. Clomipramine relieved the depression, and OCD symptoms subsequently receded
3. OCD patients are all hysterics who would respond to any dramatic method of treatment
4. OCD patients habitually employ magical mental mechanisms and are therefore more susceptible than most to "magical" treatment methods such as intravenous treatment
5. Clomipramine induced sleep, which is an anxiety-reducing form of deconditioning similar to pentothal injections
6. OCD symptoms may be symptoms of disturbed brain chemistry

In addition to the open-mindedness of the authors, the surprising content of these hypotheses illustrates how dramatically the attitude towards OCS has shifted in a few decades, from obsessional neurosis rooted in psychoanalysis to OCD embedded in neurobiology. In 2006, the hypothesis of disturbed brain chemistry and potential improvement with drugs in OCD seems self-evident.

* Correspondence. University Medical Center (B.01.206), P.O. Box 85500, GA Utrecht 3508, The Netherlands.
E-mail address: d.a.j.p.denys@umcutrecht.nl

0193-953X/06/$ - see front matter © 2006 Elsevier Inc. All rights reserved.
doi:10.1016/j.psc.2006.02.013
psych.theclinics.com

During the past 25 years a large number of controlled studies have established the efficacy of pharmacologic treatment for OCD. Thanks to pharmacotherapy, as many as 90% of OCD patients eventually have a clinically meaningful response. Nonetheless, a recent survey at the author's institution revealed that a large proportion of OCD patients still fail to receive adequate pharmacotherapy. On admission, 35% of patients declared that they never had received pharmacotherapy, 16% had received inappropriate drugs, and 50% never had taken the maximal effective dose of serotonin-reuptake inhibitors (SRIs) during the course of their treatment [2]. Despite current evidence of disturbed brain pathophysiology and apparent efficacy of pharmacotherapy, for some mental health professionals, OCD still carries an association with obsessional neurosis.

This article reviews pharmacologic approaches to the treatment of OCD and obsessive-compulsive spectrum disorders. The first section is devoted to OCD and discusses developments of pharmacotherapy during the past 5 years since the publication of the last review of pharmacotherapy in OCD in the *Psychiatric Clinics of North America*. For comprehensive reviews of earlier literature on pharmacotherapy of OCD, the reader should see Fineberg and colleagues [3], Kaplan and colleagues [4], Hollander and colleagues [5], and Jenike and colleagues [6]. The second section reviews pharmacologic treatment studies in obsessive-compulsive spectrum disorders such as skin picking, nail biting, compulsive buying disorder, and compulsive non-paraphilic sexual disorders.

OCD

Developments in pharmacotherapy of OCD during the past 5 years primarily involve (1) the extension of evidence of efficacy of SRIs as treatment for drug-naïve patients, (2) the use of atypical antipsychotics in addition to SRIs for patients who have treatment-refractory OCD, (3) an expansion of studies examining the combination of pharmacotherapy and behavior therapy, and (4) studies assessing predictors of response.

Treating drug-naïve OCD patients

Placebo-controlled studies of SRIs

The cornerstone of pharmacotherapy for OCD is inhibition of serotonin reuptake, either with clomipramine or with selective serotonin-reuptake inhibitors (SSRIs). During the past 25 years, a number of double-blind, randomized, placebo-controlled studies in OCD have confirmed the efficacy of clomipramine and the SSRIs: fluvoxamine, paroxetine, sertraline, and fluoxetine. Novel placebo-controlled trials of SSRIs include two paroxetine studies, a large multicenter citalopram study, and a study of controlled-release (CR) formulation of fluvoxamine. The efficacy of drug trials is expressed in absolute changes in scores on the Yale-Brown Obsessive Compulsive

Scale (Y-BOCS). The Y-BOCS is a clinician-rated 10-item scale with a total range of 0 to 40 that measures severity of obsessions and compulsions [7,8]. In many cases, patients are classified as responders when their scores on the Y-BOCS decrease by 25% to 35%. A recent paper reported that a Y-BOCS reduction of 30% is optimal for predicting improvement on the clinical global impression rating scale (CGI) [9].

Clomipramine. The efficacy of clomipramine was established in more than 10 placebo-controlled trials. In a recent meta-analysis, clomipramine shows a net improvement (difference) compared with placebo of 8.20 points on the Y-BOCS [10]. Responder rates to clomipramine vary from 40% to 50% of patients. Although in some cases low doses of clomipramine over a short period of time may result in significant improvement of symptoms, clomipramine treatment should last at least 10 to 12 weeks in a dose of 250 to 300 mg/d to demonstrate a full effect. Clomipramine has never been tested in a controlled fixed-dose study to assess optimal doses.

Fluvoxamine. Fluvoxamine was superior to placebo in four placebo-controlled trials and was equipotent to clomipramine in five comparison trials [11]. The pooled difference of fluvoxamine compared with placebo in these trials was 4.8 points on the Y-BOCS [10]. Fluvoxamine has never been examined in a fixed-dose trial but seems to be efficacious at dosages from 150 to 300 mg/d. Recently, Hollander and colleagues [12] assessed the CR formulation of fluvoxamine in a 12-week placebo-controlled study (Table 1). At end point, the mean Y-BOCS score decreased 8.5 in the fluvoxamine CR treatment group versus 5.6 in the placebo group. Thirty-two percent of patients treated with fluvoxamine CR were responders, compared with 21% given placebo. Of particular interest is the early onset of therapeutic effect: fluvoxamine CR was superior to placebo as early as week 2.

Table 1
Recent placebo-controlled studies of SRIs for OCD

Author	Drug	N	Weeks	Dose (mg/day)	Baseline*	End Point*	Change*
Hollander [12]	fluvoxamine CR	127	12	200	26.8	18.3	8.5
	placebo	126	12		26.4	21.0	5.4
Kamijima [17]	paroxetine	94	12	40–50	24.3	14.8	8.1
	placebo	94	12		23.4	18.6	3.5
Hollander [18]	paroxetine	88	12	20	25.9	22.0	3.9
	paroxetine	86	12	40	25.4	18.7	6.7
	paroxetine	85	12	60	25.3	17.5	7.8
	placebo	89	12		25.6	22.0	3.6
Montgomery [19]	citalopram	102	12	20	25.1	16.7	8.4
	citalopram	98	12	40	26.0	17.1	8.9
	citalopram	100	12	60	25.9	15.5	10.4
	placebo	101	12		25.4	19.8	5.6

* Absolute Y-BOCS scores

Fluoxetine. Fluoxetine was effective in three placebo-controlled trials and was equipotent to clomipramine in two comparison trials. The pooled difference on the Y-BOCS of fluoxetine compared with placebo was 1.6 points [10]. Responder rates to fluoxetine vary from 25% to 30% of patients. Two fixed-dose studies examined efficacy of 20-, 40-, and 60-mg/d doses of fluoxetine in OCD. The 60-mg/d dose was significantly more effective than the 20-mg/d dose, which in the study of Montgomery and colleagues [13] was not superior to placebo. Anecdotal evidence suggests that 80 mg/d is even more effective in OCD.

Sertraline. Sertraline was effective in four placebo-controlled trials and was equipotent to clomipramine in one comparison trial. The pooled difference of sertraline compared with placebo in these trials was 2.5 points on the Y-BOCS [10]. Although no correlation was found between sertraline plasma levels and treatment outcome, in a large multicenter trial, sertraline 50 mg/d and 200 mg/d were superior to placebo, whereas 100 mg/d was not. Bogetto and colleagues [14] compared efficacy of rapid-titration regimens of sertraline (150 mg/d reached at day 5 from the beginning of therapy) versus slow-titration regimens (150 mg/d reached at day 15) [14]. Rapid-titration regimens may have a faster onset of response but are equally well tolerated and at end point are as effective in reducing OCD symptoms as slow-titration regimens.

Paroxetine. For a long time, paroxetine was shown to be effective in only one published placebo-controlled trial and was equipotent to clomipramine in the same trial [10,15,16]. The difference in paroxetine and placebo was 3.1 points on the Y-BOCS. Doses of 40 and 60 mg/d were significantly better than placebo, whereas 20 mg/d was not. A recent placebo-controlled study in Japanese patients confirmed the efficacy of paroxetine with a mean decrease in Y-BOCS score of 8.1 points in the active group versus a decrease of 3.5 points in the placebo group (Table 1) [17]. Hollander and colleagues [18] assessed paroxetine in a fixed-dose, placebo-controlled trial. The mean reduction in Y-BOCS score was 16% at a dosage of paroxetine of 20 mg/d; 25% at a dosage of 40 mg/d; and 29% at a dosage of 60 mg/d, compared with a reduction of 13% with placebo. Paroxetine at a dosage of 20 mg/d was not significantly more effective than placebo on any measure (Table 1).

Citalopram. The efficacy of citalopram in OCD recently was established in a placebo-controlled study including 401 patients who were randomly assigned to receive citalopram, 20 mg/d, 40 mg/d, 60 mg/d, or placebo for 12 weeks (Table 1) [19]. The difference of citalopram compared with placebo was 3.6 points on the Y-BOCS. The highest responder rate (65%), defined as 25% improvement in Y-BOCS entry score, was observed in the group receiving citalopram, 60 mg/d, compared with 52% in the group receiving

40 mg/d and 57.4% in the group receiving 20 mg/d. Surprisingly, the responder rate on placebo was 36.6% with a mean decrease on the Y-BOCS score of 5.6 points. This high improvement rate on placebo, uncommon in OCD, has been explained as resulting from the inclusion of milder, atypical cases, in which spontaneous remission is more frequent. OCD patients of longer duration, more severe OCD symptoms, or previous SRI use were less likely to respond to citalopram, whereas patients who received adequate medication doses for sufficient periods of time were more likely to respond [20]. In a small study, clinical response does not seem to be related to citalopram plasma concentrations [21].

Meta-analyses of placebo-controlled trials of selective serotonin-reuptake inhibitors

The efficacy of clomipramine and five SSRIs has been established with placebo-controlled trials, but what is the best drug for OCD? Are clomipramine, fluvoxamine, paroxetine, sertraline, citalopram, and fluoxetine equally effective? Meta-analyses using statistical methods to pool samples from different studies may answer this question, offering a precise estimate of the treatment effect from separate drug trials.

Consistent with previous meta-analyses, Ackerman and colleagues [10] recently confirmed that clomipramine is more effective than SSRIs in placebo-controlled trials. The net decrease in Y-BOCS score compared with placebo was 8.19 for seven clomipramine trials, 4.84 for four fluvoxamine trials, 1.61 for three fluoxetine trials, and 2.47 for four sertraline trials. It is worth noting, however, that the largest effect sizes for clomipramine were found in early studies and have not been as clearly replicated in more recent studies comparing clomipramine with SSRIs. Moreover, over the long term, drop-out rates of clomipramine-treated patients are higher than those of SSRI-treated patients.

In another meta-analysis, which included 32 studies involving 3588 patients who had OCD, clomipramine again had the largest effect size, 1.55 versus 0.81 for fluoxetine and 1.36 for sertraline [22]. This meta-analysis also demonstrated that two thirds of the patients who completed a medication trial improved. Across all active treatments, the mean decrease Y-BOCS score was 7.1 resulting in a mean posttreatment Y-BOCS score of 17.9. For placebo conditions the decrease in Y-BOCS score was 1.8.

Clearly, in effectiveness, clomipramine is superior to all the SSRIs. In practice, however, the choice of a drug also depends on side-effect profile and potential for drug interactions. Clomipramine has the most anticholinergic side-effect profile, potential cardiotoxicity, and is the most noxious in an overdose. In contrast, SSRIs may be associated with more complaints of headaches, nausea, insomnia, or agitation but are safer and less prone to drug interactions. Considering side effects, toxicity, and potential drug interactions, SSRIs usually are the first treatment of choice.

Active-controlled comparison studies of serotonin-reuptake inhibitors

Because combining data from disparate groups is problematic, meta-analyses usually are considered more suggestive than definitive. Another way to assess superior or equivalent efficacy of drugs is the use of active-controlled trials comparing one active investigational drug with another drug known to be effective in a parallel design. Contrary to meta-analytic studies, in active-controlled comparison studies clomipramine often has been found to be equally effective as SSRIs. Until 2000, no controlled study had compared the mutual efficacy of SSRIs. Novel active-controlled comparison studies include fluvoxamine versus clomipramine, sertraline versus fluoxetine and desipramine, and venlafaxine versus clomipramine and paroxetine.

Fluvoxamine versus clomipramine. Mundo and colleagues [23] compared fluvoxamine with clomipramine in a double-blind, parallel 10-week study (Table 2). Fluvoxamine and clomipramine had similar efficacy, but fluvoxamine was better tolerated: five patients receiving fluvoxamine withdrew because of intolerable side effects compared with nine patients receiving clomipramine. In view of the superior safety profile of fluvoxamine compared with clomipramine, Mundo and colleagues [23] concluded that fluvoxamine would be advantageous for OCD (Table 2).

Sertraline versus fluoxetine and sertraline versus desipramine. Bergeron and colleagues [24] compared sertraline with fluoxetine in a 24-week double-blind trial (Table 2). By the end of the study at week 24, improvement was equivalent for both drugs. At week 12, however, the mean change in Y-BOCS score was 8.4 for sertraline and 6.1 for fluoxetine; 49.2% of patients receiving sertraline were rated on the CGI-S scale as being "mildly ill" or "not ill," compared with 24.6% of those receiving fluoxetine. Sertraline treatment also resulted in a higher proportion of remissions than fluoxetine (defined as a CGI-I $\leq$ 2 and a Y-BOCS score $\leq$ 11) both at week 12

Table 2
Recent active-controlled comparison studies of SRIs for OCD

Author	Drug	N	Weeks	Dose (mg/day)	Baseline*	End Point*	Change*
Mundo [23]	fluvoxamine	115	10	150–300	26.5	14.3	12.2
	clomipramine	112	10	150–300	25.4	13.4	12.0
Hoehn-Saric [25]	desipramine	85	12	300	25.6	19.6	6.0
	sertraline	79	12	200	26.1	17.7	8.4
Bergeron [24]	fluoxetine	73	24	20–80	26.1	16.4	9.7
	sertraline	77	24	50–200	25.3	15.7	9.6
Albert [29]	venlafaxine	26	12	225–300	25.0	18.7	6.3
	clomipramine	47	12	150–225	25.7	17.3	8.4
Denys [30]	venlafaxine	75	12	300	26.9	19.7	7.2
	paroxetine	75	12	60	25.3	17.5	7.8

* Absolute Y-BOCS scores

(20% versus 8%) and week 24 (36% versus 22%). In conclusion, fluoxetine and sertraline demonstrated significant and similar efficacy, but sertraline-treated patients show an earlier improvement and a greater likelihood of remission on some, but not all, efficacy measures.

Hoehn-Saric and colleagues [25] examined the efficacy of sertraline and desipramine, a non-SRI antidepressant, in the treatment of OCD with concurrent major depressive disorder (MDD) (Table 2). Patients assigned to sertraline responded significantly better on OCD symptoms at end point than did patients assigned to desipramine. Also, a significantly greater number of sertraline-treated patients achieved a "robust" improvement in OCD symptoms ($\geq$ 40% reduction) compared with patients receiving desipramine. In a concomitant study using single-photon emission computed tomography (SPECT), patients receiving sertraline showed significantly reduced regional cerebral blood flow (rCBF) in the right prefrontal and temporal regions, whereas patients receiving desipramine showed more diffuse rCBF reductions in frontal and temporal regions, more so in the left side [26]. This finding substantiates and extends results from previous studies comparing SRIs and non-SRIs for OCD. Serotonergic antidepressants have greater efficacy than the noradrenergic antidepressants for both OCD and MDD symptoms.

Venlafaxine versus clomipramine and venlafaxine versus paroxetine. In a recent review on the role of venlafaxine in OCD, Phelps and colleagues [27] concluded that, although the scarcity of data precludes definitive conclusions, available data suggest that venlafaxine is effective in OCD (Table 2). As present, because of limited evidence, no clear conclusions can be drawn regarding the efficacy of venlafaxine in OCD. The only placebo-controlled study available showed no significant difference between venlafaxine, 225 mg/d, and placebo [28]. Recently, one study compared the efficacy of venlafaxine with clomipramine, and another study used paroxetine as the active comparator drug.

Albert and colleagues [29] compared venlafaxine with clomipramine (Table 2). By the end of the study, mean reductions in Y-BOCS total score of 6.3 for venlafaxine and 8.4 for clomipramine were observed. The mean responder rates were 36% for venlafaxine and 50% for clomipramine. Nevertheless, the authors concluded that venlafaxine might be as efficacious as clomipramine in the acute treatment of OCD and had fewer side effects. Denys and colleagues [30] compared venlafaxine with paroxetine in 150 patients (Table 2). The mean decrease in the Y-BOCS score was 7.2 in the venlafaxine group and 7.8 in the paroxetine group. In both treatment groups, a responder rate (decrease > 35% on the Y-BOCS) of approximately 40% was found. The incidence of adverse events for venlafaxine and paroxetine was comparable. These results suggest that venlafaxine is equally effective as paroxetine in treating OCD patients. Additional data, including a placebo-controlled trial, are needed to confirm efficacy of venlafaxine in OCD.

*Long-term treatment and relapse prevention studies
of serotonin-reuptake inhibitors*

The optimal time to maintain a patient who has OCD and who has responded to pharmacotherapy on medication is unclear. Although it is believed that many responders require ongoing maintenance pharmacotherapy, placebo-controlled studies examining the relapse-prevention efficacy of maintenance therapy are sparse. Recently, the efficacy of sertraline, fluoxetine, and paroxetine has been investigated in placebo-controlled, long-term treatment trials.

Sertaline. Koran and colleagues [31] randomly assigned 223 patients who responded to a 52-week single-blind trial of sertraline to a subsequent 28-week double-blind trial of 50 to 200 mg/d of sertraline or placebo (Table 3). Sertraline had significantly greater efficacy than placebo in regard to dropout because of relapse or insufficient clinical response (9% versus 24%, respectively) and in acute exacerbation of symptoms (12% versus 35%) but was not superior in relapse prevention. According to the authors, relapse was defined too stringently as requiring (1) an increase of 5 points on the Y-BOCS score, (2) a total of 20 or more points on the Y-BOCS score, and (3) an increase of 1 point on the CGI during at least three consecutive visits. Ongoing treatment with sertraline was associated with continued improvement, supporting the usefulness of continuous treatment.

Fluoxetine. To evaluate continuation of pharmacotherapy for relapse prevention, Romano and colleagues [32] assessed the efficacy and safety of fluoxetine versus placebo in preventing relapse of OCD during a 52-week period in patients who had responded to fluoxetine, 20, 40, or 60 mg/d, in a previous single-blind, 20-week study (Table 3). Of the responders, 36 patients received fluoxetine, and 35 received placebo. Only patients receiving 60 mg of fluoxetine per day showed significantly lower rates of relapse than those who were switched to placebo (Kaplan-Meier 1-year relapse rates: fluoxetine, 17.5%; placebo, 38.0%), suggesting that higher doses are needed to protect against relapse.

Table 3
Placebo-controlled long-term studies of SRIs for OCD

Author	Drug	N	Weeks	Dose (mg/day)	Baseline*	End Point*	Change*	Relapse (%)
Koran [31]	sertraline	109	28	150–300	10.1	11.4	+ 1.3	10.9
	placebo	114	28		10.1	14.2	+ 4.1	27.2
Romano [32]	fluoxetine	36	52	20–60	10.5	12.0	+ 1.5	20.6
	placebo	35	52		10.9	13.4	+ 2.5	31.9
Hollander [18]	paroxetine	53	24	20–60	11.3	9.5	1.9	37.7
	placebo	52	24		11.4	11.0	0.4	58.8

* Absolute Y-BOCS scores

Paroxetine. Hollander and colleagues [16] assessed the long-term efficacy and impact on relapse prevention of paroxetine in OCD (Table 3). One hundred five responders to an open-label paroxetine trial were randomly assigned to 6-month double-blind, fixed-dose, parallel paroxetine/placebo treatment. Long-term treatment with paroxetine seemed to be effective: 38% of paroxetine-treated patients relapsed, versus 59% of placebo-treated patients.

Based on these data, pharmacotherapy at maximal effective dose should be maintained for a minimum of 12 months after acute treatment. Some expert consensus guidelines recommend continuation for a minimum of 3 to 6 months, whereas others propose a minimum of 1 to 2 years [33,34].

Open studies with other drugs

Connor and colleagues [35] investigated aripiprazole, an atypical antipsychotic with dopamine-serotonin stabilizing properties, in eight patients who had OCD (Table 4). The mean Y-BOCS score decreased by 6.3 points with improvement more pronounced in compulsive symptoms. Two patients discontinued treatment within 1 week because of akathisia and nausea, and a mean weight gain of 1.8 kg was observed. Sixteen patients responded to mirtazapine (up to 60 mg/d) in a 12-week trial by Koran and colleagues [36]. In an 8-week double-blind, placebo-controlled discontinuation phase, the mirtazapine group's mean Y-BOCS score fell a mean of 2.6 points, whereas the placebo group's mean score rose a mean of 9.1 points. Ondansetron, a serotonin ($5-HT_3$) receptor antagonist, at a fixed dose of 3 mg/d, showed a mean reduction of 28% on the Y-BOCS in eight patients [37]. Bupropion at a maximum dose of 300 mg/d failed to be effective in an 8-week trial: four patients improved with a mean decrease in Y-BOCS score of 31%, whereas eight patients got worse, with a mean increase in Y-BOCS scale of 21% [38]. Four of five patients receiving nicotine treatment (chewing gum 1–4 mg/d) displayed a favorable response with reductions of three to five points on the Y-BOCS score [39]. The authors suggest that the effectiveness of nicotine might be attributed to an improvement of memory. Because OCD has been associated with serotonin dysfunction, Taylor and colleagues [40] postulated that St. John's Wort (*Hypericum perforatum*) inhibiting the

Table 4
Recent open studies in monotherapy for OCD

Author	Drug	N	Weeks	Dose (mg/day)	Baseline*	End Point*	Change*
Connor [35]	aripiprazole	8	8	10–30	23.9	17.6	6.3
Koran [36]	mirtazapine	12	12	30–60	28.3	20.3	8.0
Hewlett [37]	ondansetron	8	8	3	23.8	17.2	6.6
Vulink [38]	bupropion	12	8	300	25.8	24.7	1.1
Pasquini [39]	nicotine	5	15	1–4	19.4	17.7	1.7
Taylor [40]	St. John's Wort	12	12	450	21.4	14.0	7.4

* Absolute Y-BOCS scores

synaptosomal uptake of serotonin may be effective. Twelve patients were treated for 12 weeks with a fixed dose of 450 mg of 0.3% hypericin twice daily. The Y-BOCS score decreased 7.4 points from week 1 on, and continued to decrease throughout the trial.

Treating patients who have drug-refractory obsessive-compulsive disorder

Nonresponse to treatment in OCD is common. In spite of the success of SRIs, 20% to 40% of OCD patients do not respond adequately to treatment [41]. Defining and managing nonresponse in OCD is a considerable challenge. Patients who do not respond are difficult to characterize because of ambiguities in diagnostic criteria, high comorbidity rates, lack of clear definitions of response, and most of all because a substantial number of patients who do respond still have significant residual OCD symptoms. Pallanti and colleagues [41] recently have discussed procedural issues involved in managing nonresponse in OCD. Although a discussion on managing nonresponse in OCD requires a separate section, treatment options consist of (1) adding another drug, (2) increasing the dose, (3) switching drugs, or (4) changing the mode of delivery.

Placebo-controlled addition studies with antipsychotics

Following the successful combination of haloperidol and pimozide plus SRIs for patients who have treatment-refractory OCD, a number of studies combining atypical antipsychotics with SRIs have been published during the past 5 years. There have been two open studies and five placebo-controlled trials of risperidone, seven open and two placebo-controlled studies of olanzapine, and five open and four placebo-controlled trials of quetiapine. The addition of atypical antipsychotics to SRIs for treatment of OCD has been reviewed recently by Sareen and colleagues [42] and by Keuneman and colleagues [43], and two meta-analyses by Fineberg and colleagues and Bloch and colleagues are in press.

Risperidone. McDougle and colleagues [44] performed the first placebo-controlled trial with the addition of risperidone to an SRI for treatment of OCD (Table 5). Thirty-six patients who had OCD refractory to a 12-week SRI treatment were randomly assigned in a double-blind manner to 6 weeks of risperidone (n = 20) or placebo (n = 16) addition. Nine of 18 risperidone-treated patients responded, compared with none of the 15 in the placebo-addition group. There was no difference in response between patients who had OCD with or without comorbid diagnoses of chronic tic disorder or schizotypal personality disorder. Other than mild, transient sedation, risperidone was well tolerated. In the study by Hollander and colleagues [45] 16 patients who did not respond to at least two SRI trials subsequently received either risperidone or placebo for 8 weeks. Four patients

Table 5
Placebo-controlled addition studies with atypical antipsychotics for patients who have therapy-refractory OCD

Author	Drug	N	Weeks	Dose (mg/day)	Baseline*	End Point*	Change*
McDougle [44]	risperidone	20	6	2.2	27.4	18.7	8.7
	placebo	16			27.6	25.0	2.6
Hollander [45]	risperidone	10	8	2.3	NA	NA	NA
	placebo	6					
Erzegovesi [46]	risperidone	10	6	0.5	30.9	23.0	7.9
	placebo	10			26.4	24.6	1.8
Li [47]	risperidone	12	9	1	24.3	15.1	9.2
	placebo	12			24.3	17.8	6.5
Shapira [48]	olanzapine	22	6	6.1	20.0	14.9	5.1
	placebo	22			20.0	16.2	3.8
Bystritsky [49]	olanzapine	13	6	11.2	24.2	20.0	4.2
	placebo	13			25.2	25.7	+ 0.5
Atmaca [50]	quetiapine	14	8	50–200	24.1	13.4	10.7
	placebo	14			23.8	21.4	2.4
Denys [51]	quetiapine	20	8	300	28.2	19.2	9.0
	placebo	20			26.4	24.6	1.8
Carey [52]	quetiapine	20	6	168	26.4	19.3	7.1
	placebo	21			27.7	20.5	7.2
Fineberg [53]	quetiapine	11	16	215	24.5	21.1	3.4
	placebo	10			24.1	22.7	1.4

* Absolute Y-BOCS scores

receiving risperidone and none receiving placebo responded. A better Y-BOCS insight score at baseline correlated significantly with a greater CGI-I score at end point on risperidone augmentation. In a study by Erzegovesi and colleagues [46], 20 patients who did not respond to 12 weeks of fluvoxamine monotherapy continued for 6 weeks with placebo or risperidone. Five patients responded to risperidone, and two responded to placebo. In a 9-week crossover study, Li and colleagues [47] compared the benefits of 2-week adjunctive treatments with risperidone, haloperidol, and placebo in 12 patients. Although results are difficult to interpret because of study design and small samples, the authors suggest that risperidone may improve obsessions and depressed mood compared with placebo, whereas haloperidol improved both obsessions and compulsions. All 12 patients completed the 2-week risperidone treatment, but 5 of the 12 terminated haloperidol treatment early because of intolerable side effects.

Olanzapine. Shapira and colleagues [48] added olanzapine, 5 to 10 mg, to patients who did not respond to an 8-week open-label fluoxetine trial. Both the fluoxetine-plus-olanzapine and fluoxetine-plus-placebo groups improved significantly over 6 weeks. This study does not indicate an additional advantage of adding olanzapine for 6 weeks in OCD patients and who have not had a satisfactory response to fluoxetine for 8 weeks compared with an extended fluoxetine monotherapy trial. Bystritsky and colleagues [49] examined the efficacy of adding olanzapine to SRIs in 26 patients who had treatment-refractory OCD. Six of 13 subjects in the olanzapine group showed a 25% or greater improvement in Y-BOCS score, compared with none in the placebo group.

Quetiapine. Atmaca and colleagues [50] included 28 patients in an 8-week placebo-controlled single-blind trial. Nine of 14 patients in the quetiapine-addition group improved with a mean 60% decrease on the Y-BOCS score, whereas none improved in the placebo group. Denys and colleagues [51] evaluated the efficacy of the addition of quetiapine to an SRI for patients who had not responded to courses of treatment with at least two different SRIs. Eight of 20 patients in the quetiapine group and 2 of 20 patients in the placebo group were responders. The most common side effects in the quetiapine group were somnolence, dry mouth, weight gain, and dizziness. In the study by Carey and colleagues [52], quetiapine did not demonstrate a significant benefit over placebo at the end of the 6-week treatment period and failed to separate from placebo in the subgroup of subjects (n = 10) who had comorbid tics. In the study by Fineberg and colleagues [53], 21 patients who had OCD resistant to SRI treatment were randomly assigned to 16 weeks of augmentation with either quetiapine or placebo. Three patients treated with quetiapine met criteria for clinical response, compared with one patient who was treated with placebo. There were no statistically significant differences between the groups on any of the outcome scores.

In general, risperidone, olanzapine, and quetiapine may be effective in addition to SRIs for patients who have treatment-refractory OCD, although one negative olanzapine addition study [48] and two negative quetiapine addition studies [51,52] have been published. A responder rate of 30% may be expected within 4 to 6 weeks. The best results are obtained with patients who are resistant to at least a 12-week SRI trial at maximum dose and who have comorbid tic disorders. Side effects include sedation, increased appetite, and akathesia. A small study by Maina and colleagues [54] showed that patients who respond to the addition of antipsychotics relapse when the antipsychotics are withdrawn.

Placebo-controlled addition studies with other drugs

Twenty-three patients who had not responded to two to six trials of SRIs were randomly assigned to 2-week blocks of once-weekly addition of morphine (15–45 mg), lorazepam (0.5–2 mg), or placebo [55]. In the morphine group, seven patients responded with decreases in the Y-BOCS score of 25% or more. Four patients in the lorazepam group responded. No patients in the placebo group responded. The effect of morphine may be attributed to morphine μ-opioid receptor blockade. Because some studies show a beneficial effect with omega-3 fatty acids in major affective disorders, it was hypothesized that addition of eicosapentaenoic acid might be effective in OCD [56]. Adjunctive eicosapentaenoic acid for 6 weeks showed no clinical meaningful effect in 11 patients who had OCD. Pallanti and colleagues [57] hypothesized that addition of mirtazapine might induce an earlier and higher response based on the assumption that increased 5-HT neurotransmission with mirtazapine does not require a time-dependent desensitization of 5-HT receptors but runs through indirect α_2-adrenoceptor antagonism. Mirtazapine did not enhance treatment response but was associated with an earlier onset of response. Pindolol addition to paroxetine, 60 mg/d, was effective for patients who had OCD and who had been treated unsuccessfully with at least two SRIs [58]. The authors explained the enhancement by pindolol's presynaptic 5-HT_{1A} and 5-HT_{1B} activity: Antagonism of 5-HT_{1A} and 5-HT_{1B} receptors may potentiate the effect of SRIs by increasing the 5-HT release from the nerve terminals. The results of this study, however, contradict the outcome of an earlier negative placebo-controlled trial of the addition of pindolol to fluvoxamine [59]. Crockett and colleagues [60] investigated whether clonazepam addition might accelerate and increase response in patients who are treated with sertraline. No significant difference was detected at end point between sertraline-treated patients and patients treated with sertraline plus clonazepam. The lack of effectiveness of clonazepam in OCD is consistent with a negative placebo-controlled trial in 27 patients who had OCD by Hollander and colleagues [61] (Table 6).

Open addition studies for therapy-refractory obsessive-compulsive disorder

Hollander and colleagues [62] included 39 patients of whom 29 were resistant to prior SRI treatment trials, in an open, naturalistic 18-month trial of venlafaxine, mean dose 232.2 mg/d (range, 37.5–375 mg/d). Although no Y-BOCS scores were taken, nearly 70% were rated as responders with final CGI scores of "much improved" or "very much improved." Fourteen of 18 patients who were unresponsive to an adequate dosage of SRIs for at least 6 months responded to citalopram (up to 40 mg/d) during a 4-month

Table 6
Placebo-controlled addition studies with other drugs for patients who have therapy-refractory OCD

Author	Drug	N	Weeks	Dose (mg/day)	Baseline*	End Point*	Change*
Koran [55]	oral morphine	23	2	15–45	28.4	24.1	4.3
	placebo	23	2		28.4	26.8	1.6
Fux [56]	epa	11	6	2 g	28.4	18.5	9.9
	placebo	11	6		28.4	17.6	10.8
Pallanti [57]	mirtazapine	21	12	15–30	32.6	12.9	19.7
	placebo	28	12		30.9	13.6	17.3
Dannon [58]	pindolol	8	6	7.5	28.8	21.4	7.4
	placebo	6	6		31.2	28.8	2.4
Crockett [60]	clonazepam	20	12	NA	NA	NA	NA
	placebo	17	12				

* Absolute Y-BOCS scores

trial [63]. In an open trial, Metin and colleagues [64] evaluated the efficacy of 200 to 600 mg/d of amisulpiride, a selective dopamine $D_{2/3}$ antagonist, in augmentation of ongoing SRI treatment in 20 patients who had treatment-resistant OCD. They observed a significant improvement in 95% of patients, with a mean reduction in Y-BOCS score of 14.2 points. Addition of lamotrigine (up to 100 mg/d) was ineffective for eight patients who had therapy-refractory OCD [65]. Because effective treatment of OCD with SRIs has been observed to lead to a reduction in glutaminergic tone in the cortical striatal network, Coric and colleagues [66] hypothesized that riluzole, a glutamate-modulating agent, might be effective in OCD. Of 13 patients, 7 demonstrated a reduction of more than 35% in Y-BOCS scores, and 5 were categorized as treatment responders. The authors hypothesize that riluzole may reduce synaptic glutamate by attenuating elevations in extrasynaptic glutamate levels that may arise because of impaired glial glutamate uptake. Topiramate (253.1 mg/d) was added to the treatment of 16 patients who had not responded to SRI monotherapy or SRI combination therapy for a minimum of 14 weeks [67]. Eleven of the 16 patients responded with a CGI-I score of "much improved" or "very much improved" (Table 7).

Increasing doses

Although the same drugs are used, the treatment of OCD differs fundamentally from the treatment of depression in that clinical response in OCD may be delayed for 8 to 12 weeks, and higher doses are needed. Controlled, fixed-dose studies clearly demonstrate superior efficacy with higher doses for fluoxetine, paroxetine, sertraline, and citalopram [68]. Remarkably, neither fluvoxamine nor clomipramine, the most extensively studied drug for OCD, has been examined in a controlled, fixed-dose design.

A recent study investigated whether patients who have not responded to standard therapeutic doses may respond to much higher doses. Ninan and colleagues [69] evaluated the efficacy of high doses of sertraline (400 mg/d) in 66 patients who had not responded to 16 weeks of sertraline treatment (200 mg/d). Thirty patients were assigned to receive 250 to 400 mg/d, and 36 continued with 200 mg/d for an additional 12 weeks. At end point, 40% of

Table 7
Open addition studies for patients who have therapy-refractory OCD

Author	Drug	N	Weeks	Dose (mg/day)	Baseline*	End Point*	Change*
Hollander [62]	venlafaxine	39			NA	NA	NA
Marazziti [63]	citalopram	18	16	40	NA	NA	NA
Metin [64]	amisulpiride	20	12	325	26.7	12.5	14.2
Kumar [65]	lamotrigine	8	4	100	24.0	18.9	5.1
Coric [66]	riluzole	13	12	100	30.7	17.7	13.0
Van Ameringen [67]	topiramate	16	6–18	253	NA	NA	NA

* Absolute Y-BOCS scores

patients receiving the highest dose responded, with a mean decrease in Y-BOCS score of 5.5 points; 33% of the patients receiving the regular dose had a mean decrease in Y-BOCS scale of 3.3 points. High doses of sertraline were generally well tolerated, and rates of adverse events were similar to those seen with regular doses. This study suggests that continued treatment with either regular or high doses of sertraline may result in higher responder rates and that patients who initially do not respond eventually may achieve a clinically meaningful response. Higher doses of sertraline may result in a faster and somewhat greater improvement.

Although clinical experience has shown that a dose–response relationship exists for some SRIs, empiric evidence from plasma levels does not support this widespread notion. No correlation was found between clinical outcome and plasma levels of clomipramine, sertraline, fluoxetine, and citalopram [70–73].

Switching drugs

Failure of response to one SRI does not necessarily preclude response to another. Although the likelihood of response diminishes with every trial, each new SRI may be effective. Switching drugs is perhaps the most common but least investigated treatment option in case of nonresponse. A few studies have retrospectively examined the chances of responding with a switch to another SRI. In a small, open study, 28 patients who had not responded to at least two previous SRI trials were randomly assigned to venlafaxine, 225 to 350 mg/d, or clomipramine, 125 to 225 mg/d, or citalopram, 40 to 60 mg/d, for 12 weeks [74]. Three of eight patients responded to venlafaxine, 3 of 11 responded to clomipramine, and one of seven responded to citalopram. In one prospective, double-blind, crossover trial, 43 patients who had not responded to paroxetine, 60 mg/d, or venlafaxine, 300 mg/d, were switched to 12 additional weeks of the alternate antidepressant after a 4-week tapering phase [75]. At the end of 12 weeks, responder rates were 56% for paroxetine (15 of 27) and 19% for venlafaxine (3 of 16). A last-observation-carried-forward analysis demonstrated a mean decrease on the Y-BOCS score of 1.8 in the venlafaxine group and 6.5 in the paroxetine group. To conclude, 42% of the nonresponders benefited from a crossover to the other antidepressant, and paroxetine clearly was more efficacious than venlafaxine in the treatment of patients who had not responded to a previous SRI trial.

Intravenous trials

Clomipramine and citalopram are the only SRIs that are currently available in an intravenous form. Some data suggest that intravenously administered drugs have a more rapid onset of response and higher improvement rates in OCD. In two placebo-controlled studies, intravenous clomipramine has been shown to be more effective than placebo for patients who had not responded to oral clomipramine [76,77]. In a 3-week open-label trial of intravenous citalopram administered daily for 21 days, 27 of 39 patients who had not responded to trials of at least two adequate oral SRIs showed significant improvement [78].

Pharmacotherapy with behavior therapy

The combination of pharmacotherapy and behavioral therapy is the optimal treatment for OCD. Although conclusions remain tentative because of the paucity of clinical trials combining pharmacotherapy and psychotherapy, effect sizes in a recent meta-analysis of combined therapies are higher than for pharmacotherapy or psychotherapy alone [22]. Foa and colleagues [79], on the other hand, failed to find a clear advantage for combined treatment over behavioral therapy in four trials. Combined treatment may be especially suitable for patients who have comorbid depression. During the past 5 years, a growing body of research has examined combination therapies. Three studies investigated the efficacy of short-term combined treatment (12 weeks) compared with either pharmacotherapy or behavior therapy alone. Five follow-up studies examined maintenance of different treatments over time (2–7 years). One study questioned the benefit of addition of behavioral therapy for patients who had not responded to pharmacotherapy, and another investigated the benefit of addition of behavioral therapy for patients who had responded to drug therapy. Behavioral therapy, which encompassing exposure and response prevention therapies, cognitive behavior therapy (CBT), and cognitive therapy, is difficult to compare because of specific procedural variants.

Acute treatment of pharmacotherapy versus pharmacotherapy plus behavior therapy

In an elegant placebo-controlled study, Foa and colleagues [80] tested the efficacy of placebo, clomipramine, behavioral therapy, and the combination. Interventions included intensive exposure and ritual prevention for 4 weeks followed by eight weekly maintenance sessions or clomipramine administered for 12 weeks, with a maximum dose of 250 mg/d. At week 12, the effects of all active treatments were superior to placebo. The effect of behavioral therapy did not differ from that of behavioral therapy plus clomipramine, and both were superior to clomipramine only. Responder rates were 10% for placebo, 48% for clomipramine, 86% for behavioral therapy, and 79% for behavioral therapy plus clomipramine. The authors conclude that intensive exposure and ritual prevention may be superior to clomipramine and, by implication, to monotherapy with the other SRIs.

Nakatani and colleagues [81] randomly assigned patients to one of three treatment conditions: behavioral therapy (behavior therapy with or without pill placebo), FLV (autogenic training [a psychological placebo for OCD] with or without fluvoxamine), or a control group (autogenic training with or without pill placebo) for 12 weeks. Patients in the behavioral therapy and FLV groups showed significantly more improvement than those in the control group. Patients who had lower baseline total Y-BOCS scores, past history of a major depressive episode, and absence of cleaning compulsion improved more with fluvoxamine.

Simpson and colleagues [82] followed 46 patients who had OCD and who responded to behavioral therapy (n = 18), clomipramine (n = 15), behavioral therapy plus clomipramine (n = 15), and placebo (n = 2) for 12 weeks after treatment discontinuation. As hypothesized, the relapse rate was considerably lower in those who responded to behavioral therapy and to behavioral therapy plus clomipramine responders than in those who responded to clomipramine (4 of 33 versus 5 of 11), and their time to relapse also was significantly longer (Table 8).

Long-term outcome of pharmacotherapy versus pharmacotherapy and behavior therapy

Hembree and colleagues [83] investigated the long-term outcome (17 months) of 62 patients who had OCD and who were treated with behavioral therapy alone, fluvoxamine (291 mg/day) or clomipramine (193 mg/d) alone, or their combination [83]. At follow-up, no differences in the severity of OCD symptoms were found among the three treatment groups. The findings indicate that OCD patients do show long-term improvement following behavioral therapy and medication treatment.

Rufer and colleagues [84] followed 30 patients for 6 to 8 years after treatment with CBT in combination with either fluvoxamine or placebo in a randomized design. No significant differences between treatment groups were found. Rehospitalization, which occurred in 11 patients (37%), was associated with more severe depressive symptoms at baseline and living without a partner. The short-term treatment outcome had no predictive value for the long-term course.

Table 8
Acute treatment of pharmacotherapy versus pharmacotherapy with behavior therapy

Author	Design	N	Weeks	Baseline*	End Point*	Change*
Foa [80]	behavioral therapy	29	12	24.6	11.0	13.6
	clomipramine	36	12	26.3	18.2	8.1
	clomipramine + behavioral therapy	31	12	25.4	10.5	14.9
	placebo	20	12	25.0	22.2	2.8
Nakatani [81]	behavioral therapy + pill placebo	10	24	29.9	12.9	17
	fluvoxamine + therapy placebo	10	24	28.4	20.2	8.2
	therapy placebo + pill placebo	8	24	30.5	28.4	2.1
Simpson [82]	behavioral therapy	18	24	23.1	9.33	13.7
	clomipramine + behavioral therapy	15	24	24.9	10.4	14.5
	clomipramine	15	24	24.5	17.0	7.5
	placebo	2	24	25.5	14.5	11.0

* Absolute Y-BOCS scores

Biondi and colleagues [85] studied the long-term effectiveness of behavioral therapy plus pharmacotherapy compared with pharmacotherapy alone in 20 patients. Eight of 10 patients receiving pharmacotherapy alone relapsed, compared with 1 of 10 receiving combined treatment. The estimated mean relapse-free interval was 25 months for pharmacotherapy and 132 months for the combined treatment. The probability of maintaining improvement after successful treatment was much higher in patients receiving combined treatment than in patients receiving pharmacotherapy alone.

Alonso and colleagues [86] examined the long-term course of 60 patients who were followed for 1 to 5 years. A substantial number of patients who had OCD showed persistent disabling symptoms at the long-term follow-up in spite of combined pharmacologic and behavioral treatment. Major benefits from behavioral therapy seemed to be the improvement of ritualistic behaviors. Sexual/religious obsessions predicted poorer long-term outcome, whereas short-term response to SRI treatment failed to achieve predictive value in the long-term course of OCD.

Van Oppen and colleagues [87] examined the long-term effectiveness (5 years) of cognitive therapy (n = 32), exposure in vivo with response prevention (n = 31), and CBT in combination with fluvoxamine (n = 39). At 5-year follow-up, the prevalence of OCD had decreased by more than 50% in all three treatment conditions. The long-term outcome did not differ between the three treatment conditions. About half of the patients initially treated with fluvoxamine continued antidepressant use.

In sum, most of these studies suggest that the addition of pharmacotherapy to behavioral therapy does not enhance the long-term effectiveness of behavioral therapy. Continued pharmacotherapy or behavioral therapy is needed to maintain long-term treatment gains.

Does the addition of behavior therapy benefit patients who do not respond to pharmacotherapy?

Kampman and colleagues [88] examined the effect of supplemental behavioral therapy to continued fluoxetine treatment in patients who had not responded to fluoxetine treatment. Fourteen of 56 patients who had not responded to 12 weeks of fluoxetine, 60 mg/d, subsequently received 12 sessions of CBT in addition to the continued fluoxetine treatment. The mean Y-BOCS score dropped by 9.0 points with supplemental CBT, suggesting that patients who do not respond to pharmacotherapy still may benefit CBT.

Does the addition of behavior therapy benefit patients who respond to pharmacotherapy?

Tenney and colleagues [89] tested whether addition of behavioral therapy would augment treatment outcome in responders to pharmacotherapy. Ninety-six patients who had responded to 3 months of drug treatment (venlafaxine or paroxetine) were randomly assigned to receive the addition of behavioral therapy or to continue with drug treatment alone [89]. Patients who received the addition of behavioral therapy showed a greater improvement in OCD, with a decrease in Y-BOCS score of 3.9 points, whereas the symptoms of patients who continued drug treatment alone increased on the Y-BOCS score by 3.9 points. These results indicate that the addition of behavior therapy is beneficial for patients who already have responded to drug treatment.

Prediction of response

Although pharmacotherapy is effective in treating OCD, 20% to 40% of patients do not respond. In view of the delayed onset and the side effects associated with pharmacotherapy, it is important to identify factors that may predict effective pharmacotherapy. Prediction of treatment response might be based on demographic and clinical variables, neurochemical and electrophysiologic parameters, imaging studies, and genetic markers.

Demographic and clinical variables

In the past, numerous studies reported on the predictive value of demographic and clinical variables in response to SSRIs, but conclusions are equivocal and often contradicting [90]. Recent studies suggested that a symptom-based dimensional approach may prove to be valuable in identifying significant predictors of treatment response [91]. For instance, some studies have shown that patients who have hoarding symptoms and patients who have sexual or religious and somatic obsessions respond less favorably to SRIs [91]. A common theme in these OCD symptom subtypes is their pronounced ego-syntonic nature with lack of insight, and a poorer motivation for treatment. Neziroglu and colleagues [92] reported a poorer outcome in the presence of overvalued ideation, and Ravi and colleagues [93] found poor insight (high baseline Brown Assessment of Beliefs Scale scores) to be highly predictive of poor treatment response. Denys and colleagues [94] developed an easily applicable prediction method based on the joint predictive value of several clinical characteristics that can be evaluated at the beginning of the pharmacologic treatment. The absence of previous pharmacotherapy, moderate baseline severity of OCD symptoms (Y-BOCS score < 23), and low Hamilton Depression scale scores (6–15) were prognostic determinants of response to pharmacotherapy.

Neurochemical and neurophysiologic markers

Since the origin of the serotonin hypothesis in OCD, there has been a search for direct links between 5-HT concentrations and treatment response with SRIs. In a small sample (n = 19), Delorme and colleagues [95] recently confirmed a positive relationship between pretreatment whole-blood 5-HT concentrations and good response to SRIs. In a sample of 44 patients who had OCD resistant to oral clomipramine, Mathew and colleagues [96] found that neuroendocrine measures such as plasma levels of prolactin, growth hormone, and cortisol may distinguish patients who respond to intravenous clomipramine treatment from those who do not. Low plasma levels of prolactin on day 1 on treatment with intravenous clomipramine and low cortisol levels overall were significantly associated with clinical response at day 14, and an overall increase in growth hormone secretion on the day-14 testing was associated with positive response. Earlier reports have shown that baseline quantitative electroencephalography, such as increased alpha and beta activity, may predict better treatment outcome with SRIs, whereas patients who do not respond show decreased delta and theta activity. Recently, in a sample of 20 patients, Hansen and colleagues [97] showed that responders had a strong baseline alpha activity that was normalized after paroxetine treatment.

Pharmacotherapy and neuroimaging

Imaging studies have been only moderately successful in identifying brain activity associated with clinical improvement. Both lower and higher activity in prefrontal cortex and basal ganglia have been associated with a more favorable response to medication. A possible explanation for the diverse findings may be that in OCD regional cerebral activity in basal ganglia and prefrontal cortex reflects the brain dysfunction as well as attempts to compensate for this dysfunction.

In nine patients who had contamination-related OCD, Rauch and colleagues [98] found that lower pretreatment PET measures of rCBF within the orbitofrontal cortex and higher rCBF levels within the posterior cingulate cortex predicted symptom improvement after a 12- week open trial of fluvoxamine [98]. The inverse relation between pretreatment rCBF in the orbitofrontal cortex and symptom improvement is remarkably consistent with results from three previous studies using clomipramine, fluoxetine, and paroxetine [99]. In contrast, Hoehn-Saric and colleagues [26], in a SPECT study comparing rCBF in responders (n = 11) versus patients who had not responded (n = 5) to a 12-week trial of sertraline (up to 200 mg/d), found that higher prefrontal and subcortical activity was associated with better response to drug treatment. Clinical change, but not the administration of medication as such, was associated with a decrease of prefrontal rCBF. Similarly, Carey and colleagues [100] found higher baseline perfusion levels in the left medial prefrontal region in responders using SPECT before and after a 12-week inositol treatment.

Saxena and colleagues [101] investigated brain glucose metabolism in 20 subjects who had OCD using [18F]-fluorodeoxyglucose positron-emission tomography (FDG-PET) scans before and after 8 to 12 weeks of treatment with paroxetine, 40 mg/d. In patients who responded to paroxetine, glucose metabolism decreased significantly in the right anterolateral occipitofrontal circumference and right caudate nucleus. Lower pretreatment metabolism in both the left and right occipitofrontal circumference predicted greater reduction in OCD severity with treatment [101]. In a subsequent study, which has been published twice, Saxena and colleagues [102,103] compared cerebral glucose metabolism using FDG-PET scans in 27 patients who had OCD alone, 27 who had MDD alone, and 17 who had concurrent OCD and MDD, all of whom were treated with paroxetine, 30 to 60 mg/d for 8 to 12 weeks. Subjects who had OCD alone showed significant metabolic decreases in the right caudate nucleus, right ventrolateral prefrontal cortex, bilateral orbitofrontal cortex, and thalamus. Both the MDD and concurrent OCD plus MDD groups showed metabolic decreases in the left ventrolateral prefrontal cortex and increases in the right striatum. Treatment response was associated with a decrease in striatal metabolism in nondepressed patients who had OCD but with an increase in striatal activity in patients who had OCD plus MDD. The authors conclude that, although both OCD and MDD respond to SRIs, the two syndromes have different neurobiologic substrates for response. Elevated activity in the right caudate may be a marker of responsiveness to anti-obsessional treatment, whereas lower right amygdala activity and higher midline prefrontal activity may be required for depressive symptoms to respond to treatment. The authors suggest that higher glucose metabolism reflects a greater release of glutamate in the caudate following paroxetine treatment, which would confirm an earlier finding reported by Rosenberg and colleagues [104]. In a preliminary study, Hurley and colleagues [99] report higher pretreatment rCMR glutamate in the right orbitofrontal cortex and bilateral thalamus but lower pretreatment rCMR glutamate in left parietal and bilateral dorsolateral prefrontal cortices in patients who have treatment-refractory OCD responding to adjunctive risperidone. An important implication of this finding is that patients who respond to the addition of atypical antipsychotics may have different and opposite neurochemical underpinnings than responders to SRIs [99].

Genetic markers

Three pharmacogenetic studies investigated the role of the promoter region of the serotonin transporter gene (*5-HTTLPR*) and treatment response in OCD. McDougle and colleagues [105] found a trend for an association of the L-allele with poorer response to SRIs (clomipramine, fluvoxamine, fluoxetine, sertraline, and paroxetine) in a sample of 33 patients. Billet and colleagues [106] examined 72 patients retrospectively after a 10-week trial with SRIs and found no association. Di Bella and colleagues [107] failed to find a relation between response and *5-HTTLPR* genotypes in a sample of 99 patients after 12 weeks of standardized fluvoxamine treatment.

Summary of pharmacotherapy of pharmacotherapy
for obsessive-compulsive disorder

The basics of pharmacotherapy of OCD have not changed substantially since 2000. First-line pharmacologic treatment of OCD still consists of drugs with potent serotonin-reuptake inhibition properties such as clomipramine, fluvoxamine, paroxetine, sertraline, fluoxetine, and citalopram. Clomipramine might be slightly more effective than the SSRIs, which are equally effective. Because of side effects, toxicity, and potential drug interactions, SSRIs usually are the first treatment of choice. The daily dose usually needs to be higher than in depression (ie, clomipramine, 250–300 mg; fluvoxamine, 200–300 mg; paroxetine, 40–60 mg; sertraline, 225 mg; citalopram, 40–60 mg, and fluoxetine 60–80 mg). Response is slow and may not occur for several weeks; a treatment period of at least 12 weeks is required to assess response. Concomitant depression is not necessary for improvement of OCD symptoms. Compared with depression, response to pharmacotherapy in OCD is moderate, with a 25% to 30% decrease in symptoms. The optimal time to maintain an individual who has responded to pharmacotherapy on medication is unclear, but after a satisfactory response patients should be maintained on anti-obsessional medication for 12 to 18 months before attempting to discontinue medication.

In case of nonresponse, treatment options consist of adding another drug, increasing the dose, switching drugs, or changing the mode of delivery. Risperidone, olanzapine, and quetiapine may be effective additions to SRIs for patients who have treatment-refractory OCD. A responder rate of 30% may be expected within 4 to 6 weeks. The best results are obtained with patients who are resistant to at least a 12-week trial of an SRI at maximum dose and who have comorbid tic disorders.

The combination of pharmacotherapy and behavioral therapy is still regarded as the optimal treatment for OCD. Addition of behavior therapy may be beneficial for responders as well as for patients who do not respond to drug treatment. Maintaining long-term treatment gains requires continued pharmacotherapy or behavioral therapy, but the addition of pharmacotherapy to behavioral therapy does not enhance the long-term effectiveness of behavioral therapy.

There is currently little consistency regarding clinical and demographic predictors to pharmacotherapy. Duration, severity, and comorbidity generally seem to identify patients who are at risk for nonresponse to treatment. Imaging studies may help identify predictors of treatment but are of limited use for the practicing clinician. There seems to be some agreement that lower pretreatment PET measurements of rCBF within the orbitofrontal cortex and higher activity in the caudate predict treatment response.

Obsessive-compulsive spectrum disorders

Obsessive-compulsive spectrum disorders encompass a broad range of compulsive and impulsive disorders that may be viewed along a continuum with overestimation of harm on the compulsive end and underestimation of harm on the impulsive end [108]. The common thread linking compulsive and impulsive behaviors is a shared clinical trait, which is, in essence, the inability to control one's own behavior. Obsessive-compulsive spectrum disorders often occur jointly and may share a common genetic background. Although not universally accepted, the responsiveness of obsessive-compulsive spectrum disorders to SRIs has led to the suggestion of a common serotonin-related dysfunction in these disorders [109,110].

At present, the treatment of obsessive-compulsive spectrum disorders has received little attention. There are no meta-analyses or reviews available on the pharmacotherapy of all obsessive-compulsive spectrum disorders (although there are reviews of individual disorders such as body dysmorphic disorder and pathologic gambling), and placebo-controlled trials are rare. This section deals with pharmacotherapy of skin picking, nail baiting, compulsive buying disorder, and compulsive non-paraphilic sexual disorders. Pharmacotherapy of Tourette's syndrome, body dysmorphic disorder, hypochondria, and trichotillomania is discussed in other articles in this issue.

Skin picking

Skin picking or neurotic excoriation is defined as the habitual picking of skin lesions or the excessive scratching, picking, or squeezing of otherwise healthy skin, often with numerous scars as result. Dermatologic treatment with antihistamines and corticosteroids is generally ineffective, but some case studies, open trials, and small double-blind studies have demonstrated the efficacy of SRIs [111]. Fluoxetine proved effective in a placebo-controlled trial in which 21 adults who had chronic pathologic skin picking received 10 weeks of fluoxetine with a flexible dosing schedule up to 80 mg/d [112]. In a similar study, 8 of 15 patients who responded to an open-label, 6-week trial of fluoxetine were subsequently randomly assigned to 6 weeks of double-blind fluoxetine or placebo. Four fluoxetine-treated patients maintained clinically significant improvement, whereas four placebo-treated patients returned to their baseline symptom level [113,114]. A preliminary 12-week open trial showed efficacy of fluvoxamine in 14 patients [115]. Recently, olanzapine (5–7.5 mg/d) has been shown to be effective in monotherapy as well as in addition to fluoxetine for a treatment-refractory case [116,117]. Other pharmacological treatments that have been successful in case reports are paroxetine, doxepin, clomipramine, naltrexone, inositol, and pimozide [116,118]. In 15 patients who had Prader-Willi syndrome with comorbid skin picking behavior, a double-blind trial of fenfluramine was ineffective [119]. Two patients who had Prader-Willi syndrome who displayed repetitive, self-mutilating skin picking were treated successfully with fluoxetine, and topiramate attenuated skin picking in an 8-week open-label trial in three patients who had Prader-Willi syndrome [120,121].

Nail biting

Nail biting or onychophagia involves habitual and excessive biting of nails or clipping the cuticles. At present, one controlled drug trial and one case report for nail biting have been published. Twenty-five adult subjects who had severe morbid nail biting and no history of OCD were enrolled in a 10-week double-blind crossover trial of clomipramine and desipramine. For the 14 subjects who completed the study, clomipramine (120 mg/d) was superior to desipramine (135 mg/d) [122]. Bupropion was effective in one case report [123].

Compulsive buying disorder

Compulsive buying disorder is the maladaptive preoccupation with buying/shopping, or excessive buying/shopping that does not occur exclusively during periods of hypomania or mania. Bullock and colleagues recently reviewed pharmacotherapy of compulsive buying [124]. McElroy and colleagues [125] were the first to report benefit from bupropion, nortriptyline, and fluoxetine in three cases of compulsive buying disorder with comorbid depression and anxiety. In an open study by Black and colleagues [126] compulsive buying behavior diminished in nine patients treated with fluvoxamine, 200 mg/d, whereas the comorbid major depression remained unchanged, suggesting that improvement was independent of the treatment of mood symptoms [126]. Two double-blind, placebo-controlled trials failed to show a significant difference between fluvoxamine and placebo [127,128]. Patients with compulsive buying exhibited high placebo rates, which were explained by the use of a self-report shopping diary that might itself be therapeutic. Koran and colleagues [129] reported a positive response in 17 of 24 patients during a 12-week open-label trial of citalopram (20–60 mg/d). The same group conducted a 7-week open-label trial of citalopram followed by a 9-week double-blind, placebo-controlled trial. In the placebo-controlled trial, none of the seven patients randomly assigned to the citalopram group relapsed, whereas five of eight placebo-treated patients relapsed [130]. Other drugs that have been successful in case reports include clomipramine and naltrexone [130].

Compulsive sexual disorder

Compulsive sexual behavior or sexual addiction involves conventional sexual behaviors (eg, compulsive searching for multiple partners, compulsive masturbation, compulsive love relationships, and compulsive sexuality in a relationship) that are recurrent, distressing, and interfere in daily functioning. Although no controlled trials are available, a number of case series support pharmacologic interventions. In a case report sexual obsessions diminished with a 125-mg/d dosage of clomipramine [131]. Three of a series of five patients who engaged in compulsive masturbation and who had comorbid OCD improved when treated with fluoxetine, 20 to 80 mg/d [132]. In a 12-week open study, fluoxetine titrated to 60 mg/d selectively reduced compulsive sexual behavior in 7 of 20 men who had comorbid mild-to-severe depressive symptoms [133]. The same authors observed response with sertraline (mean dose, 100 mg/d) for 18 weeks in 11 patients [134]. Two of five patients who did not respond to sertraline responded to fluoxetine, 60 mg/d. Six of 14 subjects who had compulsive sexual behavior treated with nefazodone, 200 mg/d, reported good control of sexual obsessions and compulsions, and 5 reported a remission of sexual obsessions and compulsions [135]. One trial with donepezil led to significant amelioration of compulsive hypersexual behavior without adverse motor effects in Parkinson disease [136].

Summary of pharmacotherapy of obsessive-compulsive spectrum disorders

Given the current limited evidence of drug treatment, no clear conclusions can be drawn regarding efficacy in the obsessive-compulsive spectrum disorders described here. Most pharmacologic studies comprise a mix of case reports, retrospective case series, or open-label studies. Placebo-controlled trials are lacking, and often sizes of study samples are too small. In many cases, high comorbidity rates hamper the precise evaluation of drug effects. Many early studies fail to describe clearly the characteristics of the patients, and outcome measures are difficult to interpret because standardized validated scales are lacking. At present, SSRIs and naltrexone are the best treatment options for obsessive-compulsive spectrum disorders. Some impulse-prone patients, however, might react with the emergence of impulsivity during SRI-treatment and eventually might develop obsessive-compulsive spectrum disorders [137,138]. Thus, although promising, there is still only preliminary evidence that pharmacotherapy is effective in obsessive-compulsive spectrum disorders.

References

[1] Rack M, Chir D. Experience with intravenous clomipramine. In: Obsessional states and their treatment with Anafranil. Geigy, 1970, p. 10–13.
[2] Denys D, van Megen H, Westenberg H. The adequacy of pharmacotherapy in outpatients with obsessive-compulsive disorder. Int Clin Psychopharmacol 2002;17(3):109–14.
[3] Fineberg NA, Gale TM. Evidence-based pharmacotherapy of obsessive-compulsive disorder. Int J Neuropsychopharmacol 2005;8(1):107–29.
[4] Kaplan A, Hollander E. A review of pharmacologic treatments for obsessive-compulsive disorder. Psychiatr Serv 2003;54(8):1111–8.
[5] Hollander E, Kaplan A, Allen A, et al. Pharmacotherapy for obsessive-compulsive disorder. Psychiatr Clin North Am 2000;23(3):643–56.
[6] Jenike MA, Baer L, Minichiello WE. Obsessive-compulsive disordersPractical management. 3rd edition. St. Louis (MO): Mosby; 1998.
[7] Goodman WK, Price LH, Rasmussen SA, et al. The Yale-Brown Obsessive Compulsive Scale. I. Development, use, and reliability. Arch Gen Psychiatry 1989;46(11):1006–11.
[8] Goodman WK, Price LH, Rasmussen SA, et al. The Yale-Brown Obsessive Compulsive Scale. II. Validity. Arch Gen Psychiatry 1989;46(11):1012–6.
[9] Tolin DF, Abramowitz JS, Diefenbach GJ. Defining response in clinical trials for obsessive-compulsive disorder: a signal detection analysis of the Yale-Brown Obsessive Compulsive Scale. J Clin Psychiatry 2005;66(12):1549–57.

[10] Ackerman DL, Greenland S. Multivariate meta-analysis of controlled drug studies for obsessive-compulsive disorder. J Clin Psychopharmacol 2002;22(3):309–17.

[11] Dell'osso B, Allen A, Hollander E. Fluvoxamine: a selective serotonin re-uptake inhibitor for the treatment of obsessive-compulsive disorder. Expert Opin Pharmacother 2005;6(15): 2727–40.

[12] Hollander E, Koran LM, Goodman WK, et al. A double-blind, placebo-controlled study of the efficacy and safety of controlled-release fluvoxamine in patients with obsessive-compulsive disorder. J Clin Psychiatry 2003;64(6):640–7.

[13] Montgomery SA, McIntyre A, Osterheider M, et al. A double-blind, placebo-controlled study of fluoxetine in patients with DSM-III-R obsessive-compulsive disorder. The Lilly European OCD Study Group. Eur Neuropsychopharmacol 1993;3(2):143–52.

[14] Bogetto F, Albert U, Maina G. Sertraline treatment of obsessive-compulsive disorder: efficacy and tolerability of a rapid titration regimen. Eur Neuropsychopharmacol 2002;12(3): 181–6.

[15] Zohar J, Judge R. Paroxetine versus clomipramine in the treatment of obsessive-compulsive disorder. OCD Paroxetine Study Investigators. Br J Psychiatry 1996;169(4):468–74.

[16] Ninan PT. Obsessive-compulsive disorder: implications of the efficacy of an SSRI, paroxetine. Psychopharmacol Bull 2003;37(Suppl 1):89–96.

[17] Kamijima K, Murasaki M, Asai M, et al. Paroxetine in the treatment of obsessive-compulsive disorder: randomized, double-blind, placebo-controlled study in Japanese patients. Psychiatry Clin Neurosci 2004;58(4):427–33.

[18] Hollander E, Allen A, Steiner M, et al. Acute and long-term treatment and prevention of relapse of obsessive-compulsive disorder with paroxetine. J Clin Psychiatry 2003;64(9): 1113–21.

[19] Montgomery SA, Kasper S, Stein DJ, et al. Citalopram 20 mg, 40 mg and 60 mg are all effective and well tolerated compared with placebo in obsessive-compulsive disorder. Int Clin Psychopharmacol 2001;16(2):75–86.

[20] Stein DJ, Montgomery SA, Kasper S, et al. Predictors of response to pharmacotherapy with citalopram in obsessive-compulsive disorder. Int Clin Psychopharmacol 2001;16(6):357–61.

[21] Bareggi SR, Bianchi L, Cavallaro R, et al. Citalopram concentrations and response in obsessive-compulsive disorder. Preliminary results. CNS Drugs 2004;18(5):329–35.

[22] Eddy KT, Dutra L, Bradley R, Westen D. A multidimensional meta-analysis of psychotherapy and pharmacotherapy for obsessive-compulsive disorder. Clin Psychol Rev 2004; 24(8):1011–30.

[23] Mundo E, Rouillon F, Figuera ML, et al. Fluvoxamine in obsessive-compulsive disorder: similar efficacy but superior tolerability in comparison with clomipramine. Hum Psychopharmacol 2001;16(6):461–8.

[24] Bergeron R, Ravindran AV, Chaput Y, et al. Sertraline and fluoxetine treatment of obsessive-compulsive disorder: results of a double-blind, 6-month treatment study. J Clin Psychopharmacol 2002;22(2):148–54.

[25] Hoehn-Saric R, Ninan P, Black DW, et al. Multicenter double-blind comparison of sertraline and desipramine for concurrent obsessive-compulsive and major depressive disorders. Arch Gen Psychiatry 2000;57(1):76–82.

[26] Hoehn-Saric R, Schlaepfer TE, Greenberg BD, et al. Cerebral blood flow in obsessive-compulsive patients with major depression: effect of treatment with sertraline or desipramine on treatment responders and non-responders. Psychiatry Res 2001;108(2):89–100.

[27] Phelps NJ, Cates ME. The role of venlafaxine in the treatment of obsessive-compulsive disorder. Ann Pharmacother 2005;39(1):136–40.

[28] Yaryura-Tobias JA, Neziroglu FA. Venlafaxine in obsessive-compulsive disorder [letter; comment]. Arch Gen Psychiatry 1996;53(7):653–4.

[29] Albert U, Aguglia E, Maina G, et al. Venlafaxine versus clomipramine in the treatment of obsessive-compulsive disorder: a preliminary single-blind, 12-week, controlled study. J Clin Psychiatry 2002;63(11):1004–9.

[30] Denys D, Van Der WN, van Megen HJ, et al. A double blind comparison of venlafaxine and paroxetine in obsessive-compulsive disorder. J Clin Psychopharmacol 2003;23(6):568–75.

[31] Koran LM, Hackett E, Rubin A, et al. Efficacy of sertraline in the long-term treatment of obsessive-compulsive disorder. Am J Psychiatry 2002;159(1):88–95.

[32] Romano S, Goodman W, Tamura R, et al. Long-term treatment of obsessive-compulsive disorder after an acute response: a comparison of fluoxetine versus placebo. J Clin Psychopharmacol 2001;21(1):46–52.

[33] March JS. Treatment of obsessive-compulsive disorder. The Expert Consensus Panel for Obsessive-compulsive Disorder. J Clin Psychiatry 1997;58(Suppl 4):2–72.

[34] Greist JH, Bandelow B, Hollander E, et al. WCA recommendations for the long-term treatment of obsessive-compulsive disorder in adults. CNS Spectr 2003;8(Suppl 1):7–16.

[35] Connor KM, Payne VM, Gadde KM, et al. The use of aripiprazole in obsessive-compulsive disorder: preliminary observations in 8 patients. J Clin Psychiatry 2005;66(1):49–51.

[36] Koran LM, Gamel NN, Choung HW, et al. Mirtazapine for obsessive-compulsive disorder: an open trial followed by double-blind discontinuation. J Clin Psychiatry 2005;66(4): 515–20.

[37] Hewlett WA, Schmid SP, Salomon RM. Pilot trial of ondansetron in the treatment of 8 patients with obsessive-compulsive disorder. J Clin Psychiatry 2003;64(9):1025–30.

[38] Vulink NC, Denys D, Westenberg HG. Bupropion for patients with obsessive-compulsive disorder: an open-label, fixed-dose study. J Clin Psychiatry 2005;66(2):228–30.

[39] Pasquini M, Garavini A, Biondi M. Nicotine augmentation for refractory obsessive-compulsive disorder. A case report. Prog Neuropsychopharmacol Biol Psychiatry 2005;29(1): 157–9.

[40] Taylor LH, Kobak KA. An open-label trial of St. John's Wort (*Hypericum perforatum*) in obsessive-compulsive disorder. J Clin Psychiatry 2000;61(8):575–8.

[41] Pallanti S, Hollander E, Bienstock C, et al. Treatment non-response in OCD: methodological issues and operational definitions. Int J Neuropsychopharmacol 2002;5(2):181–91.

[42] Sareen J, Kirshner A, Lander M, et al. Do antipsychotics ameliorate or exacerbate obsessive compulsive disorder symptoms? A systematic review. J Affect Disord 2004;82(2): 167–74.

[43] Keuneman RJ, Pokos V, Weerasundera R, et al. Antipsychotic treatment in obsessive-compulsive disorder: a literature review. Aust N Z J Psychiatry 2005;39(5):336–43.

[44] McDougle CJ, Epperson CN, Pelton GH, et al. A double-blind, placebo-controlled study of risperidone addition in serotonin reuptake inhibitor-refractory obsessive-compulsive disorder. Arch Gen Psychiatry 2000;57(8):794–801.

[45] Hollander E, Baldini RN, Sood E, et al. Risperidone augmentation in treatment-resistant obsessive-compulsive disorder: a double-blind, placebo-controlled study. Int J Neuropsychopharmacol 2003;6(4):397–401.

[46] Erzegovesi S, Guglielmo E, Siliprandi F, et al. Low-dose risperidone augmentation of fluvoxamine treatment in obsessive-compulsive disorder: a double-blind, placebo-controlled study. Eur Neuropsychopharmacol 2005;15(1):69–74.

[47] Li X, May RS, Tolbert LC, et al. Risperidone and haloperidol augmentation of serotonin reuptake inhibitors in refractory obsessive-compulsive disorder: a crossover study. J Clin Psychiatry 2005;66(6):736–43.

[48] Shapira NA, Ward HE, Mandoki M, et al. A double-blind, placebo-controlled trial of olanzapine addition in fluoxetine-refractory obsessive-compulsive disorder. Biol Psychiatry 2004;55(5):553–5.

[49] Bystritsky A, Ackerman DL, Rosen RM, et al. Augmentation of serotonin reuptake inhibitors in refractory obsessive-compulsive disorder using adjunctive olanzapine: a placebo-controlled trial. J Clin Psychiatry 2004;65(4):565–8.

[50] Atmaca M, Kuloglu M, Tezcan E, et al. Quetiapine augmentation in patients with treatment resistant obsessive-compulsive disorder: a single-blind, placebo-controlled study. Int Clin Psychopharmacol 2002;17(3):115–9.

[51] Denys D, De Geus F, van Megen HJ, et al. A double-blind, randomized, placebo-controlled trial of quetiapine addition in patients with obsessive-compulsive disorder refractory to serotonin reuptake inhibitors. J Clin Psychiatry 2004;65(8):1040–8.

[52] Carey PD, Vythilingum B, Seedat S, et al. Quetiapine augmentation of SRIs in treatment refractory obsessive-compulsive disorder: a double-blind, randomised, placebo-controlled study [ISRCTN83050762]. BMC Psychiatry 2005;5(1):5.

[53] Fineberg NA, Sivakumaran T, Roberts A, et al. Adding quetiapine to SRI in treatment-resistant obsessive-compulsive disorder: a randomized controlled treatment study. Int Clin Psychopharmacol 2005;20(4):223–6.

[54] Maina G, Albert U, Ziero S, et al. Antipsychotic augmentation for treatment resistant obsessive-compulsive disorder: what if antipsychotic is discontinued? Int Clin Psychopharmacol 2003;18(1):23–8.

[55] Koran LM, Aboujaoude E, Bullock KD, et al. Double-blind treatment with oral morphine in treatment-resistant obsessive-compulsive disorder. J Clin Psychiatry 2005; 66(3):353–9.

[56] Fux M, Benjamin J, Nemets B. A placebo-controlled cross-over trial of adjunctive EPA in OCD. J Psychiatr Res 2004;38(3):323–5.

[57] Pallanti S, Quercioli L, Bruscoli M. Response acceleration with mirtazapine augmentation of citalopram in obsessive-compulsive disorder patients without comorbid depression: a pilot study. J Clin Psychiatry 2004;65(10):1394–9.

[58] Dannon PN, Sasson Y, Hirschmann S, et al. Pindolol augmentation in treatment-resistant obsessive compulsive disorder: a double-blind placebo controlled trial. Eur Neuropsychopharmacol 2000;10(3):165–9.

[59] Mundo E, Guglielmo E, Bellodi L. Effect of adjuvant pindolol on the antiobsessional response to fluvoxamine: a double-blind, placebo-controlled study. Int Clin Psychopharmacol 1998;13(5):219–24.

[60] Crockett BA, Churchill E, Davidson JR. A double-blind combination study of clonazepam with sertraline in obsessive-compulsive disorder. Ann Clin Psychiatry 2004;16(3): 127–32.

[61] Hollander E, Kaplan A, Stahl SM. A double-blind, placebo-controlled trial of clonazepam in obsessive-compulsive disorder. World J Biol Psychiatry 2003;4(1):30–4.

[62] Hollander E, Friedberg J, Wasserman S, et al. Venlafaxine in treatment-resistant obsessive-compulsive disorder. J Clin Psychiatry 2003;64(5):546–50.

[63] Marazziti D, Dell'Osso L, Gemignani A, et al. Citalopram in refractory obsessive-compulsive disorder: an open study. Int Clin Psychopharmacol 2001;16(4):215–9.

[64] Metin O, Yazici K, Tot S, et al. Amisulpiride augmentation in treatment resistant obsessive-compulsive disorder: an open trial. Hum Psychopharmacol 2003;18(6):463–7.

[65] Kumar TC, Khanna S. Lamotrigine augmentation of serotonin re-uptake inhibitors in obsessive-compulsive disorder. Aust N Z J Psychiatry 2000;34(3):527–8.

[66] Coric V, Milanovic S, Wasylink S, et al. Beneficial effects of the antiglutamatergic agent riluzole in a patient diagnosed with obsessive-compulsive disorder and major depressive disorder. Psychopharmacology (Berl) 2003;167(2):219–20.

[67] Van Ameringen M, Mancini C, Patterson B, et al. Topiramate augmentation in treatment-resistant obsessive-compulsive disorder: a retrospective, open-label case series. Depress Anxiety 2005.

[68] Fineberg NA, Gale TM. Evidence-based pharmacotherapy of obsessive-compulsive disorder. Int J Neuropsychopharmacol 2005;8(1):107–29.

[69] Ninan PT, Koran LM, Kiev A, et al. High-dose sertraline strategy for nonresponders to acute treatment for obsessive-compulsive disorder: a multicenter double-blind trial. J Clin Psychiatry 2006;67(1):15–22.

[70] Kasvikis Y, Marks IM. Clomipramine in obsessive-compulsive ritualisers treated with exposure therapy: relations between dose, plasma levels, outcome and side effects. Psychopharmacology (Berl) 1988;95(1):113–8.

[71] Greist JH, Jefferson JW, Kobak KA, et al. A 1 year double-blind placebo-controlled fixed dose study of sertraline in the treatment of obsessive-compulsive disorder. Int Clin Psychopharmacol 1995;10(2):57–65.

[72] Koran LM, Cain JW, Dominguez RA, et al. Are fluoxetine plasma levels related to outcome in obsessive-compulsive disorder? Am J Psychiatry 1996;153(11):1450–4.

[73] Bareggi SR, Bianchi L, Cavallaro R, et al. Citalopram concentrations and response in obsessive-compulsive disorder. Preliminary results. CNS Drugs 2004;18(5):329–35.

[74] Hollander E, Bienstock CA, Koran LM, et al. Refractory obsessive-compulsive disorder: state-of-the-art treatment. J Clin Psychiatry 2002;63(Suppl 6):20–9.

[75] Denys D, van Megen HJ, Van Der WN, et al. A double-blind switch study of paroxetine and venlafaxine in obsessive-compulsive disorder. J Clin Psychiatry 2004;65(1):37–43.

[76] Fallon BA, Liebowitz MR, Campeas R, et al. Intravenous clomipramine for obsessive-compulsive disorder refractory to oral clomipramine: a placebo-controlled study. Arch Gen Psychiatry 1998;55(10):918–24.

[77] Koran LM, Sallee FR, Pallanti S. Rapid benefit of intravenous pulse loading of clomipramine in obsessive-compulsive disorder. Am J Psychiatry 1997;154(3):396–401.

[78] Pallanti S, Quercioli L, Koran LM. Citalopram intravenous infusion in resistant obsessive-compulsive disorder: an open trial. J Clin Psychiatry 2002;63(9):796–801.

[79] Foa EB, Franklin ME, Moser J. Context in the clinic: how well do cognitive-behavioral therapies and medications work in combination? Biol Psychiatry 2002;52(10): 987–97.

[80] Foa EB, Liebowitz MR, Kozak MJ, et al. Randomized, placebo-controlled trial of exposure and ritual prevention, clomipramine, and their combination in the treatment of obsessive-compulsive disorder. Am J Psychiatry 2005;162(1):151–61.

[81] Nakatani E, Nakagawa A, Nakao T, et al. A randomized controlled trial of Japanese patients with obsessive-compulsive disorder—effectiveness of behavior therapy and fluvoxamine. Psychother Psychosom 2005;74(5):269–76.

[82] Simpson HB, Liebowitz MR, Foa EB, et al. Post-treatment effects of exposure therapy and clomipramine in obsessive-compulsive disorder. Depress Anxiety 2004;19(4):225–33.

[83] Hembree EA, Riggs DS, Kozak MJ, et al. Long-term efficacy of exposure and ritual prevention therapy and serotonergic medications for obsessive-compulsive disorder. CNS Spectr 2003;8(5):363–71, 381.

[84] Rufer M, Hand I, Alsleben H, et al. Long-term course and outcome of obsessive-compulsive patients after cognitive-behavioral therapy in combination with either fluvoxamine or placebo: a 7-year follow-up of a randomized double-blind trial. Eur Arch Psychiatry Clin Neurosci 2005;255(2):121–8.

[85] Biondi M, Picardi A. Increased maintenance of obsessive-compulsive disorder remission after integrated serotonergic treatment and cognitive psychotherapy compared with medication alone. Psychother Psychosom 2005;74(2):123–8.

[86] Alonso P, Menchon JM, Pifarre J, et al. Long-term follow-up and predictors of clinical outcome in obsessive-compulsive patients treated with serotonin reuptake inhibitors and behavioral therapy. J Clin Psychiatry 2001;62(7):535–40.

[87] van Oppen P, Van Balkom AJ, de Haan E, et al. Cognitive therapy and exposure in vivo alone and in combination with fluvoxamine in obsessive-compulsive disorder: a 5-year follow-up. J Clin Psychiatry 2005;66(11):1415–22.

[88] Kampman M, Keijsers GP, Hoogduin CA, et al. Addition of cognitive-behaviour therapy for obsessive-compulsive disorder patients non-responding to fluoxetine. Acta Psychiatr Scand 2002;106(4):314–9.

[89] Tenny NH, van Megen HJ, Denys DA, et al. Behavior therapy augments response of patients with obsessive-compulsive disorder responding to drug treatment. J Clin Psychiatry 2005;66(9):1169–75.

[90] Denys D, Burger H, van Megen H, et al. A score for predicting response to pharmacotherapy in obsessive-compulsive disorder. Int Clin Psychopharmacol 2003;18(6):315–22.

[91] Mataix-Cols D, Rauch SL, Manzo PA, et al. Use of factor-analyzed symptom dimensions to predict outcome with serotonin reuptake inhibitors and placebo in the treatment of obsessive-compulsive disorder. Am J Psychiatry 1999;156(9):1409–16.

[92] Neziroglu F, Stevens KP, McKay D, et al. Predictive validity of the overvalued ideas scale: outcome in obsessive-compulsive and body dysmorphic disorders. Behav Res Ther 2001; 39(6):745–56.

[93] Ravi KV, Samar R, Janardhan Reddy YC, et al. Clinical characteristics and treatment response in poor and good insight obsessive-compulsive disorder. Eur Psychiatry 2004;19(4): 202–8.

[94] Denys D, Burger H, van Megen H, et al. A score for predicting response to pharmacotherapy in obsessive-compulsive disorder. Int Clin Psychopharmacol 2003;18(6):315–22.

[95] Delorme R, Betancur C, Callebert J, et al. Platelet serotonergic markers as endophenotypes for obsessive-compulsive disorder. Neuropsychopharmacology 2005;30(8):1539–47.

[96] Mathew SJ, Coplan JD, Perko KA, et al. Neuroendocrine predictors of response to intravenous clomipramine therapy for refractory obsessive-compulsive disorder. Depress Anxiety 2001;14(4):199–208.

[97] Hansen ES, Prichep LS, Bolwig TG, et al. Quantitative electroencephalography in OCD patients treated with paroxetine. Clin Electroencephalogr 2003;34(2):70–4.

[98] Rauch SL, Shin LM, Dougherty DD, et al. Predictors of fluvoxamine response in contamination-related obsessive compulsive disorder: a PET symptom provocation study. Neuropsychopharmacology 2002;27(5):782–91.

[99] Hurley RA, Saxena S, Rauch SL, et al. Predicting treatment response in obsessive-compulsive disorder. J Neuropsychiatry Clin Neurosci 2002;14(3):249–53.

[100] Carey PD, Warwick J, Harvey BH, et al. Single photon emission computed tomography (SPECT) in obsessive-compulsive disorder before and after treatment with inositol. Metab Brain Dis 2004;19(1–2):125–34.

[101] Saxena S, Brody AL, Maidment KM, et al. Localized orbitofrontal and subcortical metabolic changes and predictors of response to paroxetine treatment in obsessive-compulsive disorder. Neuropsychopharmacology 1999;21(6):683–93.

[102] Saxena S, Brody AL, Ho ML, et al. Differential cerebral metabolic changes with paroxetine treatment of obsessive-compulsive disorder vs major depression. Arch Gen Psychiatry 2002;59(3):250–61.

[103] Saxena S, Brody AL, Ho ML, et al. Differential brain metabolic predictors of response to paroxetine in obsessive-compulsive disorder versus major depression. Am J Psychiatry 2003;160(3):522–32.

[104] Rosenberg DR, MacMaster FP, Keshavan MS, et al. Decrease in caudate glutamatergic concentrations in pediatric obsessive-compulsive disorder patients taking paroxetine. J Am Acad Child Adolesc Psychiatry 2000;39(9):1096–103.

[105] McDougle CJ, Epperson CN, Price LH, et al. Evidence for linkage disequilibrium between serotonin transporter protein gene (SLC6A4) and obsessive compulsive disorder. Mol Psychiatry 1998;3(3):270–3.

[106] Billett EA, Richter MA, King N, et al. Obsessive compulsive disorder, response to serotonin reuptake inhibitors and the serotonin transporter gene. Mol Psychiatry 1997;2(5):403–6.

[107] Di Bella D, Erzegovesi S, Cavallini MC, et al. Obsessive-compulsive disorder, 5-HTTLPR polymorphism and treatment response. Pharmacogenomics J 2002;2(3):176–81.

[108] Hollander E, Kwon JH, Stein DJ, et al. Obsessive-compulsive and spectrum disorders: overview and quality of life issues. J Clin Psychiatry 1996;57(Suppl 8):3–6.

[109] Rasmussen SA. Obsessive compulsive spectrum disorders [see comments]. J Clin Psychiatry 1994;55(3):89–91.

[110] Stein DJ. Neurobiology of the obsessive-compulsive spectrum disorders. Biol Psychiatry 2000;47(4):296–304.

[111] Gupta MA, Gupta AK, Haberman HF. Neurotic excoriations: a review and some new perspectives. Compr Psychiatry 1986;27(4):381–6.

[112] Simeon D, Stein DJ, Gross S, et al. A double-blind trial of fluoxetine in pathologic skin picking. J Clin Psychiatry 1997;58(8):341–7.

[113] Bloch MR, Elliott M, Thompson H, et al. Fluoxetine in pathologic skin-picking: open-label and double-blind results. Psychosomatics 2001;42(4):314–9.

[114] Ravindran AV, Lapierre YD, Anisman H. Obsessive-compulsive spectrum disorders: effective treatment with paroxetine. Can J Psychiatry 1999;44(8):805–7.

[115] Arnold LM, Mutasim DF, Dwight MM, et al. An open clinical trial of fluvoxamine treatment of psychogenic excoriation. J Clin Psychopharmacol 1999;19(1):15–8.

[116] Blanch J, Grimalt F, Massana G, et al. Efficacy of olanzapine in the treatment of psychogenic excoriation. Br J Dermatol 2004;151(3):714–6.

[117] Christensen RC. Olanzapine augmentation of fluoxetine in the treatment of pathological skin picking. Can J Psychiatry 2004;49(11):788–9.

[118] Seedat S, Stein DJ, Harvey BH. Inositol in the treatment of trichotillomania and compulsive skin picking. J Clin Psychiatry 2001;62(1):60–1.

[119] Selikowitz M, Sunman J, Pendergast A, et al. Fenfluramine in Prader-Willi syndrome: a double blind, placebo controlled trial. Arch Dis Child 1990;65(1):112–4.

[120] Warnock JK, Kestenbaum T. Pharmacologic treatment of severe skin-picking behaviors in Prader-Willi syndrome. Two case reports. Arch Dermatol 1992;128(12):1623–5.

[121] Schepis C, Failla P, Siragusa M, et al. Failure of fluoxetine to modify the skin-picking behaviour of Prader-Willi syndrome. Australas J Dermatol 1998;39(1):57–8.

[122] Leonard HL, Lenane MC, Swedo SE, et al. A double-blind comparison of clomipramine and desipramine treatment of severe onychophagia (nail biting). Arch Gen Psychiatry 1991;48(9):821–7.

[123] Wadden P, Pawliuk G. Cessation of nail-biting and bupropion. Can J Psychiatry 1999; 44(7):709–10.

[124] Bullock K, Koran L. Psychopharmacology of compulsive buying. Drugs Today (Barc) 2003;39(9):695–700.

[125] McElroy SL, Keck PE Jr, Pope HG Jr, et al. Compulsive buying: a report of 20 cases. J Clin Psychiatry 1994;55(6):242–8.

[126] Black DW, Monahan P, Gabel J. Fluvoxamine in the treatment of compulsive buying. J Clin Psychiatry 1997;58(4):159–63.

[127] Ninan PT, McElroy SL, Kane CP, et al. Placebo-controlled study of fluvoxamine in the treatment of patients with compulsive buying. J Clin Psychopharmacol 2000;20(3): 362–6.

[128] Black DW, Gabel J, Hansen J, et al. A double-blind comparison of fluvoxamine versus placebo in the treatment of compulsive buying disorder. Ann Clin Psychiatry 2000;12(4): 205–11.

[129] Koran LM, Bullock KD, Hartston HJ, et al. Citalopram treatment of compulsive shopping: an open-label study. J Clin Psychiatry 2002;63(8):704–8.

[130] Bullock K, Koran L. Psychopharmacology of compulsive buying. Drugs Today (Barc) 2003;39(9):695–700.

[131] Rubey R, Brady KT, Norris GT. Clomipramine treatment of sexual preoccupation. J Clin Psychopharmacol 1993;13(2):158–9.

[132] Stein DJ, Hollander E, Anthony DT, et al. Serotonergic medications for sexual obsessions, sexual addictions, and paraphilias. J Clin Psychiatry 1992;53(8):267–71.

[133] Kafka MP, Prentky R. Fluoxetine treatment of nonparaphilic sexual addictions and paraphilias in men. J Clin Psychiatry 1992;53(10):351–8.

[134] Kafka MP. Sertraline pharmacotherapy for paraphilias and paraphilia-related disorders: an open trial. Ann Clin Psychiatry 1994;6(3):189–95.

[135] Coleman E, Gratzer T, Nesvacil L, et al. Nefazodone and the treatment of nonparaphilic compulsive sexual behavior: a retrospective study. J Clin Psychiatry 2000;61(4):282–4.

[136] Ivanco LS, Bohnen NI. Effects of donepezil on compulsive hypersexual behavior in Parkinson disease: a single case study. Am J Ther 2005;12(5):467–8.

[137] Kindler S, Dannon PN, Iancu I, et al. Emergence of kleptomania during treatment for depression with serotonin selective reuptake inhibitors. Clin Neuropharmacol 1997;20(2): 126–9.

[138] Denys D, van Megen HJ, Westenberg HG. Emerging skin-picking behaviour after serotonin reuptake inhibitor-treatment in patients with obsessive-compulsive disorder: possible mechanisms and implications for clinical care. J Psychopharmacol 2003;17(1):127–9.

ELSEVIER
SAUNDERS

PSYCHIATRIC
CLINICS
OF NORTH AMERICA

Psychiatr Clin N Am 29 (2006) 585–604

Psychotherapy of Obsessive-Compulsive Disorder and Spectrum: Established Facts and Advances, 1995–2005

Fugen Neziroglu, PhD, ABBP, ABPP*,
Jill Henricksen, MA, Jose A. Yaryura-Tobias, MD

*Bio-Behavioral Institute,
935 Northern Boulevard, Great Neck, NY 11021, USA*

Learning theory model

Current psychologic approaches to obsessive-compulsive disorder (OCD) are not much different from those of the early 1980s except for the addition of cognitive therapy. Behavior therapy, specifically ERP, dominated treatment and research from the late 1970s to the mid-1990s.

Behavioral treatment has its roots in learning theory. Mowrer [1] described a two-factor model of fear and avoidance behavior in anxiety disorders. He suggested that fear is acquired through classical conditioning and maintained by operant conditioning. Dollard and Miller [2] later applied this theory to the acquisition of OCD. Through classical conditioning a neutral stimulus that is paired with an unconditional stimulus acquires the same properties as the unconditional stimulus and thus elicits anxiety. The second stage consists of negative reinforcement, in which new responses are learned to decrease the anxiety in the presence of the conditioned (neutral) stimulus. These learned responses are termed avoidance or escape responses. They remove anxiety and therefore are negatively reinforcing. A checker may associate an electrical appliance (conditioned stimulus) with death (unconditional stimulus, ie, danger of fire) and thus feel anxiety (unconditional response and conditioned response) in the presence of a stove. The checking behavior is negatively reinforced because it removes anxiety.

---

* Corresponding author.
E-mail address: Neziroglu@aol.com (F. Neziroglu).

Development of exposure and response prevention

In 1966, Meyer [3] was the first to expose two patients who had OCD to anxiety-evoking stimuli and with constant staff supervision prevented them from engaging in compulsions. One patient had a hand washing/cleaning ritual, and another had an obsession of eternal damnation after performing certain acts such as imagining have intercourse with the Holy Ghost, cleaning a smoking pipe, swearing, eating sausages, and walking straight. Both patients remained improved at the end of 2 years follow-up. These procedures of ERP were derived from animal experiments. Fixated or stereotyped behaviors in animals, which are analogous to human compulsive behaviors, are difficult to remove. Maier [4] found that the guidance technique could be successful. The method consists of preventing a rat from carrying out a fixed response by guiding it manually toward the previously avoided situation. Baum [5], in a similar manner, taught rats avoidance behaviors and then prevented their response. The avoidance behavior was extinguished. When Meyer [3] adapted this technique to humans, ERP became the first effective psychologic treatment model for OCD.

Efficacy rates of responders and nonresponders

Once Meyer [3] developed the early forms of ERP treatment for OCD, many researchers began to test its efficacy. In the 1970s and 1980s a series of investigations proved the efficacy of ERP (for a review of the early literature, see Foa and Kozak [6]). Despite the reported efficacy (75% patients experiencing clinical improvement), those who improve have an average reduction of symptoms of only 48% [7–11]. Because this is a modal response rate, it includes both low and high responders; therefore, it may be assumed that symptom reduction was greater for high responders. Nonetheless, it is not an impressive response rate, and patients are still left with many symptoms. If reports included the individuals who refused treatment or dropped out, the response rate would be even lower. Most studies do not report on intent-to-treat analysis (individuals who entered a study but do not complete it). In addition, most studies accept a 30% reduction in symptoms as improvement [12]. Where does this treatment leave patients in their naturalistic environment and their quality of life? Most patients at the end of a study still met criteria for entrance into another study if the common criterion of a score higher than 16 on the Yale-Brown Obsessive-Compulsive Scale (Y-BOCS) is used.

Within the disorders on the obsessive-compulsive spectrum, engaging patients in treatment is the first priority. Most patients are not ready for change, probably because of their higher levels of overvalued ideation (OVI). Because of the small number of studies, the percentage of patients who are treatment refractory cannot be ascertained, and of course it is necessary to study each disorder separately. Although patients do demonstrate improvement (eg, in body dysmorphic disorder), more studies are needed to determine what percentages of patientes improve, recover, or are refractory.

This article reviews what already has been established within cognitive behavior therapy (CBT) and then evaluates the advances, if any, that have been made during the last decade. Some of the questions the authors set out to explore are

Has knowledge increased, and have new and more effective approaches been discovered?
Have rates of treatment resistance and refractory rates been reduced?
Have the limitations of the previous research been addressed?

Facts established before 1995

Exposure versus response prevention

Combined ERP is the most commonly applied treatment technique for OCD. Typically, exposure and response prevention are implemented concurrently. Previous studies determined the unique contribution of each component. Foa and colleagues [13] assigned patients who had washing rituals to three separate treatment conditions: exposure only, ritual prevention only, and combined ERP. Participants received intensive treatment consisting of 2-hour sessions for 15 days over the course of 3 weeks. Foa and colleagues [13] reported symptom reductions across all treatment groups at posttreatment evaluation and follow-up, but the combined-treatment group was superior to the single-component groups on almost all measures. At posttreatment evaluation, Foa and colleagues [13] reported a 36% reduction of obsessions for the exposure group, a 28% reduction for the response prevention, and a 63% reduction for the combined ERP group. On ratings of ritual severity at posttreatment, Foa and colleagues [13] reported a 50% reduction for the exposure group, a 45% reduction for response prevention, and a 63% reduction for the combined ERP group. Foa and colleagues' [13] finding demonstrated that the combined ERP is the most effective treatment method and also suggested how the different components of the treatment work to reduce symptoms in OCD. They noted that patients who received exposure alone reported lower anxiety when confronted with their fear contaminants than did patients who received response prevention alone. Patients who received response prevention alone reported a greater decrease in the urge to engage in compulsions than did the exposure-alone group.

In vivo versus imaginal exposure

Overall, there is agreement that the additional of imaginal exposure has added benefits for patients who are obsessive compulsive. Foa and colleagues [14] report that imaginal exposure has important clinical utility, especially for patients who are obsessive compulsive and whose obsessional fears focus on disastrous consequences. Additionally, imaginal exposure plays an essential role when in vivo exposures are not readily available. Imaginal exposure also may be helpful with patients who have a tendency to engage in extensive mental rituals during in vivo exposures. For instance, during in vivo exposure exercises certain patients may attempt to neutralize or undo the exposure mentally while facing the feared stimuli. Imaginal exposure may minimize cognitive avoidance strategies [14]. Last, imaginal exposure provides additional clinical utility because it frequently can be assigned for homework. In fact, the exposure scenes can be recorded in session, and patients can be asked to listen to the audiotapes between sessions.

Frequency of sessions

Throughout the 1980s many of the published studies of ERP were based on an intensive treatment program with therapist-guided exposures. Exposure sessions were conducted daily, and these intensive treatment programs were efficacious [15]. Today, therapists are faced with increased treatment costs and the demands of managed health care. Consequently, research has turned to other treatment options, such as CBT and psychopharmacology. Additionally, ERP techniques applied in clinics and in the outpatient setting may be more diluted than those initially used in treatment research. For example, sessions are often held once per week, and the patient is largely responsible for self-guided exposure exercises between sessions. Session time has decreased from the recommended session duration of 90 to 120 minutes. The results of the literature review by the Franklin and Foa [15] indicated that these modifications to ERP treatment guidelines have resulted in diminished treatment efficacy.

Inpatient versus outpatient treatment

Throughout the 1970s ERP was applied mostly in hospital settings, although some treated OCD on an outpatient basis [16–18] Yaryura-Tobias and Neziroglu [12,19] recommended that OCD is a disorder best treated in the patient's natural environment or at least in the outpatient setting. At times, hospitalization may be necessary, primarily for severely afflicted patients who do not have adequate support systems and resources. Severe comorbidity also may warrant short-term hospitalization.

Overvalued ideation

OVI frequently is referred to incorrectly as "poor insight." Although poor insight is one component of OVI, it is not the total essence of OVI. The most recent revision to the *Diagnostic and Statistical Manual of Mental*

Disorders [20] has added the identifier "with poor insight" for diagnoses of OCD. This addition is intended to denote persons who have OCD and who view their symptoms as reasonable. In the research literature on OCD, this condition has been termed "overvalued ideation" [21,22]. It is important to distinguish poor insight from overvalued ideas, because the two connote different psychologic phenomena. "Insight" is a term describing a gradation of personal awareness into one's disorder as giving rise to disorder-specific beliefs. The term "overvalued ideas," on the other hand, refers more to ideas or beliefs regarding the sensibility of the patient's pattern of thinking; it is affect driven, and the patient holds on to the belief without fluctuation in conviction. Different positions adopted regarding the relation between overvalued ideas and psychopathology have been stated. For example, Wernicke [23] determined that overvalued ideas were the source of attention disturbance and impaired judgment. Jaspers [24], on the other hand, believed that overvalued ideas were associated with righteousness or behaviors that had societal gain at personal cost. Kozak and Foa [22] more recently suggested overvalued ideas lie on a continuum between rational thoughts and delusions, with fluctuations along this continuum over time.

Preliminary research studies and clinical observations indicate that the presence of high OVI is a poor prognostic indicator. Patients who have OCD and who have high OVIs are less likely to resist compulsions and are more likely to believe in their obsessions. Although OVI have been linked theoretically to poorer treatment outcome [25,26] and has been identified in individual and small-group case analyses [27], assessment tools for quantifying OVI have been few and with undetermined psychometric properties. Most assessments of overvalued ideas have been single-item assessments (as in the Y–BOCS) [28], dichotomous ratings based on clinical criteria but without established psychometric properties [29], and a scale that assesses delusions in a variety of distinct disorders [30]. Either because the scales have not established reliability and validity or because they do not specifically measure OVI, the Overvalued Ideas Scale (OVIS) was developed [31].

The OVIS measures strength of belief, reasonableness of belief, lowest and highest strength of belief in the past week, accuracy of belief, extent of adherence by others, attribution of differing views by others, effectiveness of compulsions, insight, and strength of resistance. The OVIS has been shown to have acceptable test–retest and inter-rater reliability and acceptable convergent validity with measures of OCD and psychotic experiences. Research by Neziroglu and colleagues [32] found that the OVIS has better predictive validity than a single-item assessment of OVI (item 11 from the Y–BOCS) in a sample of patients diagnosed as having OCD. In addition, Neziroglu and colleagues [32] found that patients who have OCD and who have a high level of OVI do not do as well with behavioral therapy as patients who have a low level of OVI.

Depression

OCD significantly impairs an individual's quality of life. OCD is a disorder that truly affects all spheres of life, including personal relationships, home, work, and school. Approximately one third of patients who have OCD have a comorbid diagnosis of depression [33]. In addition, many patients experience secondary depressive symptoms because of the severe and intense feelings of frustration resulting from the inability to control symptoms that dominate the patient's life. For patients whose depression is severe and is interfering with treatment for the OCD symptoms, psychologic treatment to address the depressive symptoms is often recommended. Depression affects a patient's compliance with and motivation for treatment. More specifically, when Ricciardi and McNally [34] compared patients who were obsessive compulsive and who had a mood disorder with patients who were obsessive compulsive but who did not experience a mood disorder, they found that depressive symptoms lead to an increase in the severity of obsessions but not to more severe compulsive symptoms. It is believed that depression impedes ERP treatment.

When to use pharmacotherapy combined with cognitive behavior therapy

There are several full reviews of combined treatment for OCD patients and controlled comparisons of ERP with medication [35–38]. In general, strong or selective serotonin reuptake inhibitors are used to treat OCD. The clinical efficacy of clomipramine, a strong serotonin reuptake inhibitor, led to the hypothesis of a faulty serotonin metabolism and subsequent measurements of serotonin levels in patients who have OCD [39,40]. Later more select serotonin reuptake blockers, such as fluoxetine, fluvoxamine, paroxetine, sertraline, and the strong inhibitor clomipramine, were developed. In general, best practices suggest that for mild forms of OCD in adult patients, ERP should be the first line of treatment attempted. If the patient's symptoms do not improve with ERP alone, or for patients who have more severe forms of OCD, the combined treatment of selective serotonin reuptake inhibitors and ERP is the recommended course of treatment [41]. Although additional controlled studies are warranted, it seems logical that, because comorbid disorders such as depression and anxiety respond well to medication, pretreating these disorders might improve ERP outcomes. In addition, Simpson and Liebowitz [37] report that combined treatments may also increase compliance with ERP. When Foa and colleagues [42] compared ERP with clomipramine, alone and in combination, however, they noted that intensive ERP may be superior to clomipramine alone and thus by implication superior to other serotonin reuptake inhibitors.

Preventing relapse

To maintain treatment gains, patients seem to benefit from a psychoeducational session toward the end of a treatment program. These sessions should teach patients to expect setbacks and to devise a plan to engage in ERP techniques when they experience a minor worsening of symptoms. A contract of expectations between the patient and therapist is also helpful to secure treatment gains. Hiss and colleagues [43] examined the value of relapse prevention. In a study comparing a relapse-prevention group with a control group, Hiss and colleagues [43] found that at 6-month follow-up 87% of the relapse-prevention patients and only 50% of the control patients had maintained improvements. In addition, McKay and colleagues [44] proposed a preliminary maintenance program. Their findings suggested that at the 6-month follow-up patients continued to improve and remained stable for obsessive-compulsive symptoms; however, patients continued to suffer from depression. Similarly, Breytman [45] reported that after an initial course of CBT and 3 weeks of baseline assessment, patients who received 20 sessions of maintenance intervention retained their treatment gains. Her maintenance program consisted of behavioral exercises, cognitive therapy, and discussion of issues related to relapse. In a final thought on the importance of relapse prevention, Marlatt and Gordon [46] suggested that when patients encounter minor setbacks and regain control of their symptoms, treatment gains are solidified by the increase in self-efficacy.

Cognitive therapy

In a series of studies starting in the late 1970s, Emmelkamp [47] began testing the efficacy of cognitive therapy. A study comparing the efficacy of adding self-instructional training as a form of cognitive therapy to ERP led to the conclusion that self-instructional training did not enhance ERP. In a head-to-head comparison, cognitive therapy and ERP were found to be equally effective [48]. In addition, both treatments led to a reduction of social anxiety; however, the cognitive-therapy group also had significant changes in depression. Similarly, another study noted no differences between cognitive therapy and ERP nor between cognitive therapy administered before ERP and ERP alone [49] In a study by Neziroglu and Neuman [50], rational emotive therapy, ERP, and thought stopping were compared in a purely obsessional population. ERP and rational emotive therapy were equally effective, but thought stopping was ineffective in decreasing obsessions. Although these studies tested the efficacy of cognitive therapy, it was Salkovskis [51] who put forth the cognitive model for OCD. Cognitive models were developed to deal with the high rate of patients who refused treatment and dropouts within ERP treatment. Despite its effectiveness, Riggs and Foa [52] report that 10% of persons who complete ERP therapy fail to respond and that 20% of patients relapse after treatment. Additionally, Salkovskis [53] reported that the theoretical conceptualization of behavioral theory limited its ability to differentiate OCD from other anxiety disorders.

The foundation for cognitive models of OCD stemmed largely from the work of Rachman and De Silva [54] who found that intrusive thoughts were reported by almost 90% of a nonclinical population. In their content, these intrusive thoughts were indistinguishable from obsessional thoughts. Because intrusive thoughts occur in a high percentage of individuals, researchers began to investigate which features distinguish obsessions from regularly occurring intrusive thoughts and the factors that lead to the development and maintenance of OCD in some individuals and not others.

The cognitive models assume that obsessions originate from normal intrusive thoughts, thus making an individual's interpretation of these thoughts the distinguishing factor that separates obsessions from normal intrusive thoughts. Salkovskis [51] referred to the interpretation or meaning that individuals who have OCD attach to an intrusive belief as "responsibility." According to Salkovskis [53], the notion of responsibility affects OCD in several ways. First it leads to increased discomfort, anxiety, and depression. Second, it allows greater access to the original thoughts and other related thoughts. Last, it leads to behavioral responses with the intent to neutralize or escape anxiety. These factors, singly and in combination, are believed to lead to the maintenance and worsening of anxiety along with intrusive thoughts.

The notion of responsibility differentiates the thought patterns of patients who hare OCD from those of individuals in the general population and also can separate OCD from other psychiatric disorders. The cognitive approach proposed by Salkovskis [51] was similar to other models in anxiety disorders; however, it considered the specific consequences attached to the specific belief. The notion of responsibility differentiates obsessional thinking in depression and other anxiety disorders from OCD. As stated by Salkovskis [53]:

> Appraisal of responsibility and consequent neutralizing can arise from a sensitivity to responsibility arising from a failure to control thoughts, from an increase in the level of perceived personal responsibility, and from an increased perception of the awfulness of being responsible for harm

The notion of responsibility is important in the maintenance of OCD because it accounts for both distress and the neutralizing behaviors. If the individual did not somehow feel a personal sense of harm to themselves or others, and only distress was present, the outcome would more likely be associated with depression or anxiety. Therefore, it is not the idea of danger and threat that is unique to OCD, but rather the motivation to carry out compulsions to neutralize or undo the perceived sense of harm.

Similarly, Rachman [55] proposed that obsessions are caused by catastrophic misinterpretations of the significance of one's thoughts, images, and impulses. Rachman [55] proposed that obsessions persist as long as these misinterpretations continue. Furthermore, it is believed that obsessions will diminish when the misinterpretations are weakened. Therefore, Rachman [55] also concluded that by decreasing the importance that patients attach to their obsessions, their compulsive behaviors also decrease.

In researching OCD primarily in patients who did not have overt compulsions, Freeston and colleagues [56] found several common features among this population. First, individuals interpret the presence of their obsessions as meaningfully important. Second, these individuals believe that their obsessions must reflect their true nature. Often these individuals possess a sense of moral thought–action fusion. In other words, having a particular image, thought, or impulse is the equivalent to acting upon it, thus making the patient a morally bad person. Last, some patients have likelihood thought–action fusion: the patient believes that the more one thinks about a particular thought, the greater is the likelihood that it actually will occur.

Cognitive therapy can be particularly useful clinically in several areas that are relevant in the maintenance of OCD. These areas were outlined originally by the Obsessive Compulsive Cognitions Working Group [57] and include an inflated sense of personal responsibility; attaching undue importance to thoughts; a need to control thoughts; an overestimation of treat; an intolerance of uncertainty; and perfectionism [58]. These areas can be targeted through cognitive therapy alone or within the context of behavioral experiments and ERP.

To support further the efficacy of cognitive therapy, van Oppen and colleagues [59] completed a controlled study comparing cognitive therapy with ERP. The cognitive therapy treatment focused on themes of danger and overestimation of personal responsibility. The ERP group consisted of self-controlled in vivo ERP. The findings of this study were pivotal in the treatment of OCD because it was the first randomized, controlled study using cognitive therapy. The researchers reported that cognitive therapy and ERP equally led to statistically significant improvements, with cognitive therapy showing more changes in faulty belief measurements. Franklin and Foa [15] emphasized that the ERP treatment used in the study by van Oppen and colleagues [59] was inadequate compared with the recommended treatment protocol for ERP. The ERP treatment group received one 45-minute session per week. Additionally, Franklin and Foa [15] pointed out that van Oppen and colleagues [59] were unclear about how much homework patients were asked to complete between sessions and that discussion of negative consequences was not permitted during the first six ERP sessions. Last, patients did not benefit from therapist-guided exposure exercises. Methodologic weaknesses in the ERP arm may weaken van Oppen colleagues' [59] findings that cognitive therapy is effective as ERP for the treatment of OCD.

Within the obsessive-compulsive literature, researchers still debate whether cognitive therapy is as effective as ERP and the additive benefits of adding cognitive therapy to an ERP treatment program. Results from Abramowitz and colleagues [60] concluded that, for the average patient who is obsessive compulsive, cognitive interventions either alone or combined with ERP are no more effective than ERP alone. Abramowitz and colleagues [60] suggest that the primary advantage of cognitive interventions is that they reduce the patient dropout rate. It is hoped that future research will focus on the type of treatment method that works best for certain subtypes of patients who have OCD. For example, some researchers are finding that patients who have hoarding compulsions may be more responsive to cognitive therapy [61]. In addition, cognitive therapy may emerge as a preferred form of treatment for patients who have high OVIs and comorbid depression. Franklin and Foa [15] suggest that future research should focus on identifying the point in a treatment program at which it is more beneficial to use cognitive therapy than ERP rather than continuing the debate as to which model of treatment is superior overall. For instance, are avoidance behaviors better addressed through ERP, and is an individual's overestimation of personal responsibility better addressed through cognitive therapy? Randomized, controlled studies in this area are likely to provide more clinical utility.

Advances between 1995 and 2005

To search PsychINFO for CBT studies published between 1995 and 2005, the authors used the keywords "obsessive compulsive disorder" and "cognitive behavior therapy." They were interested in investigating whether (1) any new information regarding CBT, behavior therapy, or cognitive therapy was reported and (2) whether the reported studies were generalizable to clinical practice. All information on CBT versus pharmacotherapy was excluded in the analyses. Eighteen articles were found that dealt with treatment outcome and were not single-case studies or meta-analyses.

In each article, the authors analyzed the following variables:

1. How many individuals participated
2. Whether the population studied was adults, children, or a group
3. How individuals were diagnosed
4. If the numbers screened, entered, dropped out, and completed were reported
5. If Axis I or II comorbidities were reported
6. If the specific therapy (eg, cognitive alone, ERP, behavior therapy, medication) was indicated
7. If recovery or improvement rate was reported
8. If effect size was presented
9. How improvement was assessed
10. Whether self- and interview ratings were used
11. Whether medication usage was mentioned
12. Whether there was a comparison group
13. Whether there was follow-up

Some of these factors are reported in Table 1.

Four of 18 studies were on a pediatric population [64,67,73,78]. Eight of the 18 studies (44%) reported on the number of individuals screened, but only a few indicated why individuals were not included in the study (eg, did not meet inclusion criteria, became homebound before treatment). Many studies (67%) indicated dropout rates; seven studies (39%) did not specify the reason for dropout, and five (28%) provided a reason. Thus it is still uncertain how many patients at screening may actually meet inclusion criteria but choose not to enter. Why do people not enter treatment? At least studies now seem to report dropout rates, but because the reasons for dropout are not systematically studied, it is unclear whether patients are truthful about why they drop out (Table 1). Could it be that unmotivated patients, patients not ready for treatment, and patients who have personality disorders or OVI provide environmental reasons for dropping out? In other words, would other patients with the same set of life circumstances have continued?

Twelve of the 18 studies (67%) reported Axis I comorbidities. Most comorbid conditions included phobias, anxiety, and major depressive disorder (MDD). Patients who had comorbid posttraumatic stress disorder (PTSD) and MDD did not do as well as those who were free of those comorbidities. Eight studies (44%) reported the presence of concomitant Axis II disorders, and three studies indicated the type of comorbidity. One study noted that personality disorders did not interfere with treatment [69].

Most studies reported on ERP variations, and others reported on the use of cognitive therapy and ERP. When CBT was specified, it usually meant cognitive therapy combined with ERP. All studies used the child or adult version of the Y–BOCS as the main indicator of improvement. Five of the studies (32%) reported effect size. Thirteen of the studies (72%) reported on the percentage of patients who improved at posttreatment evaluation, whereas others reported on statistical significance. (The term "recovery" referred to symptom reduction of 30% to 50%.) Fifteen of the studies (83%) indicated that medications were used but did not specify which medications, dosage levels, duration, or other details. Only three studies reported that medicated patients did equally well as nonmedicated patients [65,67,79]. Although some studies specified that medication was kept stable during the treatment, many did not indicate whether medication dosages were changed. For the most part, it is difficult to evaluate from these studies the role medication plays in treatment outcome. Also, it is unclear why some patients were receiving medication and others were not, the selection process was not explained.

Comparison groups were cognitive versus behavior therapy, wait-list control group, patients who did or did not have PTSD or depression, and intensive therapy versus weekly sessions. Results indicated that ERP and cognitive therapy were equally effective; that patients who had PTSD and MDD did not fare as well; and that patients who lack insight, have high OVI, are more severely ill, and are more impaired in functioning do better

Table 1
Cognitive behavioral treatment outcome studies published between 1995–2005

Author (date)	Screened	Entered	Dropped Out	Completed	Axis I	Axis II	Therapy Type	Improvement (% patients)	Medication	F/U
Abramowitz et al (2003) [62]	N/A	40	8 reason not specified	32	MDD, GAD, panic, ADD, Tourettes	schizotypal OCPD	ERP	85 with intensive therapy 55 in twice weekly therapy	SSRI (45%)	3 mo
Abramowitz et al (2000) [63]	N/A	48	15 at follow-up; reason not specified	48	MDD	yes; not specified	ERP	80 w/o MDD, 73 w/ MDD	SSRI	4–6 mo
Benazon et al (2002)[a] [64]	N/A	16	0	16	anxiety disorders	N/A	ERP	81	none	N/A
Cordioli et al (2003) [65]	65; 18 met exclusion criteria	47	2 because of anxiety and failure to attend evaluation	45	none	N/A	CBGT	treatment group: 69.6 control group: 4.2	none up to 3 months before treatment	3 mo
Cottraux et al (2001) [66]	85; 20 met exclusion criteria	65	37 reason not specified	28	none	N/A	CT + BT	CT: 19 patients BT: 20 patients	irregular use of anti-depressants by some	52 wk
Franklin et al (2000) [9]	N/A	110	10 reason not specified	100	MDD, bipolar, psychotic	yes; not specified	CBT + ERP	statistical significance	N/A	N/A

Franklin et al (1998)[a] [67]	N/A	14	0	14	motor tics, trichotillomania	N/A	ERP	86	CMI fluoxetine clonazepam	9 mo
Freeston et al (1997)[b] [68]	199	28	6 4 refused ERP 2 backed out	22	depression	N/A	CBT + ERP	67	anxiolytics, clomipramine, fluvoxamine, fluoxetine	6 mo
Fricke et al (2005)[b] [69]	70; 8 not primarily OCD; 7 N/A	55	0	55	MDD	many listed	ERP + CT	statistical significance provided	73% antidepressants during CBT; 64% at follow-up	6 mo
Gershuny et al (2002) [70]	N/A	15	0	15	MDD, PTSD, BDD, social phobia eating disorders	borderline	ERP	statistical significance provided	SSRIs benzodiazepines	N/A
Jones et al (1998) [71]	29 met criteria	23 agreed	2- reason not specified	21	N/A	N/A	CT + DIRT		fluoxetine, sertraline, other OCD meds for symptom reduction	3 mo
McLean et al (2001) [72]	93	76	17 2 changed medication 1 social/ impulse problems 1 refused treatment	63	MDD, GAD, social phobias	yes; not specified	CBT + ERP	CBT: 16 ERP: 38	48% psychotropics	3 mo

(continued on next page)

Table 1 (continued)

Author (date)	Screened	Entered	Dropped Out	Completed	Axis I	Axis II	Therapy Type	Improvement (% patients)	Medication	F/U
Piacentini et al (2002)[a] [73]	44	42	0	42	N/A	N/A	CBT + ERP	mean decrease of 45 on NIMH Global Score	52% SSRIs	N/A
Rosquist et al (2001) [74]	N/A	11	3: 1 pregnant 1 MD 1 diabetes	8	Tourettes, MDD, hoarding	yes; not specified	ERP ("home-based")	36	yes; not specified	N/A
Thienemann et al (2001)[a] [75]	N/A	18	1 counted in the final analysis, however; reason not specified	17	depression, social phobia, eating disorders, Tourettes	no	CBT	50	yes; not specified	N/A
Vogel et al (2004) [76]	54; 39 met inclusion material but 4 refused treatment	35	8 reason not specified	27	yes; not specified	yes; not specified	ERP + relaxation ERP + CT	ERP + relaxation: 53 ERP + CT: 56	SSRIs	12 mo

Wetzel et al (1999) [77]	N/A	85	0	85	none	N/A	high-density exposure + ERP	68.5	20% using anti-depressants 4.9% using tranquilizers	1 year
Wilhelm et al (2005) [78]	N/A	15	21 improved OC symptoms 1 moved to another state	13	none	N/A	ERP + CT	patients naive to ERP all improved	SSRIs	N/A

Abbreviations: ADD, attention deficit disorder; BDD, body dysphoric disorder; BT, behavioral therapy; CBGT, cognitive behavior group therapy; CBT, cognitive behavioral therapy; CMI, clomipramine; DIRT, danger ideation reduction therapy; ERP, exposure and response prevention; F/U, follow-up; GAD, generalized anxiety disorder; OCD, obsessive-compulsive disorder; OCPD, obsessive-compulsive personality disorder; MDD, major depressive disorder; N/A, not available; NIMH, National Institutes of Mental Health; PTSD, posttraumatic stress disorder; SSRI, selective serotonin reuptake inhibitor.

[a] Pediatric study.

[b] Adult study.

with more intensive treatment. Eleven studies (61%) reported on follow-up ranging from 3 months to 1 year.

The search led the authors to conclude that the newer studies have not addressed some of the limitations of older studies properly although there have been improvements in including patients who have comorbid conditions and in reporting on follow-up. Problems identified in the literature before 2000 were [36]

1. Poor reporting of screening and inclusion/exclusion criteria, which limit knowledge about generalizability
2. High exclusion rates, particularly for patients who have comorbid psychopathology
3. Exclusive focus in reviews on indices such as effect size and not on the percentage of patients whose symptoms actually remit with treatment
4. Limited data on long-term maintenance of treatment gains

Some of the previous problems have been addressed. There is less reliance on effect size, and generalizability to clinical practice has increased to some extent because comorbid Axis I disorders are included more systematically [80]. Axis II disorders, which usually provide the most difficult challenge to clinicians, are still not reported, however. Follow-up is limited to several months and is not really long term. More has been written about cognitive therapy, but when, where, and how cognitive therapy might enhance treatment results has not actually been tested. For example, it could be useful to test whether cognitive therapy might contribute to increasing motivation, decreasing poor insight and OVI (an area totally ignored in the literature), reducing dropout rates, or dealing with personality disorders before ERP, among other possible benefits. Most importantly, new methods to increase treatment efficacy have not been developed.

Summary

Dropout rates and refractory cases persist, for reasons that remain unexplained. There are few predictor variables and few innovative approaches to deal with them. New treatment approaches must be developed to improve treatment response even for the responders. Studies show that symptoms are reduced minimally (30%–50%). No new ways of dealing with treatment-refractory cases have been developed. Studies now include more comorbid cases, however, and their inclusion may account for some of the lack of progress in improvement rates. It needs to be seen whether patients who have one or more comorbid conditions do as well as patients who do not have comorbidity and whether the number or type of comorbid disorders accounts for treatment response. Perhaps better results would be seen with pure OCD cases. Certainly results now are more generalizable to clinical practice. Now it is important to look for alternative treatment approaches and to apply cognitive therapy to more specific problems. Cognitive therapy seems to be helpful with the disorders of the obsessive-compulsive spectrum. The attrition rate is lower when cognitive therapy is used in the treatment of hypochondriasis, and cognitive therapy also is helpful in reducing OVI , which is more severe in body dysmorphic disorder and hypochondriasis. The role of cognitive therapy in OVI needs further exploration.

References

[1] Mowrer H. On the dual nature of learning: a reinterpretation of "conditioning" and "problem solving." Harv Educ Rev 1947;17:102–48.

[2] Dollard J, Miller E. Personality and psychotherapy: an analysis in terms of learning, thinking, and culture. New York: McGraw-Hill; 1950.

[3] Meyer V. Modification of expectations in cases with obsessional rituals. Behav Res Ther 1966;4:273–80.

[4] Maier N. Frustration: the study of behavior without a goal. New York: McGraw- Hill; 1949.

[5] Baum M. Rapid extinction of an avoidance response following a period of response prevention in the avoidance apparatus. Psychol Rep 1966;18:55–64.

[6] Foa E, Kozak J. Psychological treatment for obsessive compulsive disorder. In: Mavissakalian MR, Prien RF, editors. Long-term treatments of anxiety disorders. Washington (DC): American Psychiatric Association; 1996. p. 285–309.

[7] Abel J. Exposure with response prevention and serotonergic antidepressants in the treatment of obsessive compulsive disorder: a review and implications for interdisciplinary treatment. Behav Res Ther 1993;3:463–78.

[8] Abramowitz J. Effectiveness of psychological and pharmacological treatment for obsessive compulsive disorder: a quantitative review. J Consult Clin Psychol 1997;65:44–52.

[9] Franklin M, Abramowitz J, Kozak M, et al. Effectiveness of exposure and ritual prevention for obsessive-compulsive disorder: randomized compared with nonrandomized samples. J Consult Clin Psychol 2000;68(4):594–602.

[10] Kozak M, Leibowitz M, Foa E. Cognitive behavior therapy and pharmacotherapy for obsessive compulsive disorder: the NIMH-sponsored collaborative study. In: Goodman WK, Rudorfer MV, Maser JD, editors. Obsessive compulsive disorder: contemporary issues in treatment. MaHwah (NJ): Lawrence Erlbaum; 2000. p. 501–32.

[11] Abramowitz J, Franklin M, Foa E. Information processing in obsessive compulsive disorder. In: Frost RO, Stektee G, editors. Cognitive approaches to obsessions and compulsions: theory, assessment, and treatment. Oxford (UK): Elsevier; 2002. p. 165–81.

[12] Yaryura-Tobias J, Neziroglu F. Obsessive compulsive disorder spectrum: pathogenesis, diagnosis and reatment. Washington (DC): American Psychiatric Association; 1997.

[13] Foa E, Steketee G, Grayson J, et al. Deliberate exposure and blocking of obsessive-compulsive rituals: immediate and long-term effects. Behav Ther 1984;15:450–72.

[14] Foa E, Franklin M, Kozak M. Psychosocial treatments for obsessive-compulsive disorder: literature review. In: Swinson RP, Antony MM, Rachman S, et al, editors. Obsessive-compulsive disorder: theory, research, and treatment. New York: Guilford; 1998. p. 258–76.

[15] Franklin M, Foa E. Cognitive-behavioral treatment for obsessive compulsive disorders. In: Nathan PE, Gorman JM, editors. A guide to treatments that work. New York: Oxford University Press; 1998. p. 339–57.

[16] Boersma K, Den Hengst S, Dekker J, et al. Exposure and response prevention in the natural environment: a comparison with obsessive-compulsive patients. Behav Res Ther 1976;14: 19–24.

[17] Neziroglu F. A combined behavioral-pharmacotherapy approach to obsessive-compulsive disorders. In: Obiols J, Ballus C, Gonzalez-Monclus E, et al, editors. Biological psychiatry today. Amsterdam: Elsevier; 1979. p. 591–6.

[18] Foa E, Steketee G. Obsessive-compulsives: conceptual issues and treatment interventions. In: Hersen M, Eisler RM, Miller PM, editors. Progress in behavior modification, vol. VII. New York: Academic Press; 1979.

[19] Yaryura-Tobias J, Neziroglu F. Obsessive-compulsive disorders: pathogenesis, diagnosis, treatment. New York: Marcel Dekker; 1983.

[20] American Psychiatric Association. Diagnostic and statistical manual of mental disorders, 4th edition. Washington (DC): American Psychiatric Association; 1994.

[21] Foa E. Failures in treating obsessive compulsives. Behav Res Ther 1979;17:169–76.

[22] Kozak M, Foa E. Obsessions, overvalued ideas and delusions in obsessive–compulsive disorder. Behav Res Ther 1994;32:343–53.

[23] Wernicke C. Grundrisse der Psychiatrie [Foundations of psychiatry]. Leipzig (Germany): Verlag; 1906. [in German].

[24] Jaspers K. General psychopathology. Buenos Aires (Argentina): Beta Publishers; 1913. [Subidet, RO, Trans.].

[25] Basoglu M, Lax T, Kasvikis Y, Marks I. Predictors of improvement in obsessive–compulsive disorder. J Anxiety Disord 1988;2:299–317.

[26] Lelliot P, Noshirvani H, Basoglu M. Obsessive compulsive beliefs and treatment outcome. Psychol Med 1988;18:697–702.

[27] Insel T, Akiskal H. Obsessive–compulsive disorder with psychotic features: a phenomenological analysis. Am J Psychiatry 1986;143:1527–33.

[28] Goodman W, Price H, Rasmussen S, et al. The Yale–Brown Obsessive–Compulsive Scale: I. Development, use, and reliability. Arch Gen Psychiatry 1989;46:1006–11.

[29] Foa E, Kozak M, Goodman W, et al. DSM-IV Field Trial: Obsessive–Compulsive Disorder. Am J Psychiatry 1995;152:90–6.

[30] Eisen J, Phillips K, Baer L, et al. The Brown Assessment of Beliefs Scale: reliability and validity. Am J Psychiatry 1998;155:102–8.

[31] Neziroglu F, McKay D, Yayura-Tobias J, et al. The overvalued ideas scale: development, reliability, and validity in obsessive-compulsive disorder. Behav Res Ther 1999;37:881–902.

[32] Neziroglu F, Stevens K, McKay D, et al. Predictive validity of the overvalued ideas scale: outcome in obsessive-compulsive and body dysmorphic disorders. Behav Rea Ther 2000; 38:1–12.

[33] Marks I. Behaviour therapy for obsessive-compulsive disorder: a decade of progress. Can J Psychiatry 1997;42:1021–7.

[34] Ricciardi JN, McNally RJ. Depressed mood is related to obsession but not compulsions in obsessive-compulsive disorder. J Anxiety Disord 1995;9:249–56.

[35] Van Balkom A, Van Dyck R. Combination treatments for obsessive-compulsive disorder. In: Swinson RP, Antony MM, Rachman S, et al, editors. Obsessive-compulsive disorder: theory, research, and treatment. New York: Guilford; 1998. p. 349–66.

[36] Eddy K, Dutra L, Bradley R, et al. A multidimensional meta-analysis of psychotherapy and pharmacotherapy for obsessive-compulsive disorder. Clin Psychol Rev 2004;24:1011–30.

[37] Simpson H, Liebowitz M. Combining pharmacotherapy and cognitive-behavioral therapy in the treatment of OCD. In: Abramowitz JS, Houts AC, editors. Concepts and controversies in obsessive-compulsive disorder. New York: Springer; 2005. p. 359–76.

[38] Franklin M. Combining serotonin medication with cognitive-behavior therapy: Is it necessary for all OCD patients? In: Abramowitz JS, Houts AC, editors. Concepts and controversies in obsessive-compulsive disorder. New York: Springer; 2005. p. 377–89.

[39] Yaryura-Tobias J. Obsessive compulsive disorder: a serotonergic hypothesis. Journal of Orthomolecular Psychiatry 1977;6:317–26.

[40] Yaryura-Tobias J, Bebirian R, Neziroglu F, et al. Obsessive compulsive disorders as a serotonin defect. Res Commun Psychol Psychiatr Behav 1977;2:279–86.

[41] March J, Frances A, Carpenter L, et al. Expert consensus treatment guidelines for obsessive-compulsive disorder: a guide for patients and families. J Clin Psychiatry 1997;58: 65–72.

[42] Foa E, Liebowitz M, Kozak M, et al. Randomized, placebo-controlled trial of exposure and ritual prevention, clomipramine, and their combination in the treatment of obsessive-compulsive disorder. Am J Psychiatry 2005;162:151–61.

[43] Hiss H, Foa EB, Kozak MJ. Relapse prevention program for treatment of obsessive-compulsive disorder. J Consult Clin Psychol 1994;62:801–8.

[44] McKay D, Todaro J, Neziroglu F, et al. Evaluation of a naturalistic maintenance program in the treatment of obsessive-compulsive disorder: a preliminary investigation. J Anxiety Disord 1996;10:211–7.

[45] Breytman A. Comparison of efficacy of maintenance intervention for obsessive compulsive disorder and body dysmorphic disorder [dissertation]. Hofstra University, Hempstead (NY): Hofstra University; 2002.

[46] Marlatt GA, Gordon JR. Relapse prevention. New York: Guilford; 1985.

[47] Emmelkamp P, Van der Helm M, Van Zanten B, et al. Contributions of self-instructional training to the effectiveness of exposure in vivo: a comparison with obsessive-compulsive patients. Behav Res Ther 1980;18:61–6.

[48] Emmelkamp P, Visser S, Hoekstra R. Cognitive therapy versus exposure in vivo in the treatment of obsessive-compulsives. Cognit Ther Res 1988;12:103–14.

[49] Emmelkamp P, Beens H. Cognitive therapy with obsessive compulsive disorder: a comparative evaluation. Behav Res Ther 1991;29:293–300.

[50] Neziroglu F, Neuman J. Three approaches to the treatment of obsessions. International Journal of Cognitive Therapy 1990;4:371–92.

[51] Salkovskis P. Obsessional-compulsive problems: a cognitive-behavioural analysis. Behav Res Ther 1985;25:571–83.

[52] Riggs D, Foa E. Obsessive compulsive disorder. In: Barlow DH, editor. Clinical handbook of psychological disorders: a step-by-step treatment manual. 2nd edition. New York: Guilford Press; 1993. p. 189–239.

[53] Salkovskis P. Psychological approaches to the understanding of obsessional problems. In: Swinson RP, Antony MM, Rachman S, et al, editors. Obsessive-compulsive disorder: theory, research, and treatment. New York: Guilford Press; 1998. p. 258–76.

[54] Rachman S, De Silva P. Abnormal and normal obsessions. Behav Res Ther 1978;16: 233–48.

[55] Rachman S. A cognitive theory of obsessions. Behav Res Ther 1997;35:793–802.

[56] Freeston M, Rheaume J, Ladouceur R. Correcting faulty appraisals of obsessional thoughts. Behav Res Ther 1996;34:433–46.

[57] Obsessive Compulsive Cognition Working Group. Cognitive assessment of obsessive-compulsive disorder. Behav Res Ther 1997;35:667–81.

[58] Fama J, Wilhelm S. Formal cognitive therapy: a new treatment for OCD. In: Abramowitz JS, Houts AC, editors. Concepts and controversies in obsessive-compulsive disorder. New York: Springer; 2005. p. 263–81.

[59] Van Oppen P, de Hann E, Van Balkom A, et al. Cognitive therapy and exposure in vivo in the treatment of obsessive compulsive disorder. Behav Res Ther 1995;33:379–90.

[60] Abramowitz J, Taylor S, McKay D. Potentials and limitations of cognitive treatments for obsessive-compulsive disorder. Cogn Behav Ther 2005;34:140–7.

[61] Steketee G, Frost R. Compulsive hoarding: current status of the research. Clin Psychol Rev 2003;23:905–27.

[62] Abramowitz J, Foa E, Franklin M. Exposure and ritual prevention for obsessive-compulsive disorder: effects of intensive versus twice-weekly sessions. J Consult Clin Psychol 2003;71(2): 394–8.

[63] Abramowitz J, Foa E. Does comorbid major depressive disorder influence outcome of exposure and response prevention for OCD? Behav Ther 2000;31:795–800.

[64] Benazon NR, Ager J, Rosenberg DR. Cognitive behavior therapy in treatment-naïve children and adolescents with obsessive compulsive disorder: an open trial. Behav Res Ther 2002;40:529–39.

[65] Cordioli A, Heldt E, Bochi D, et al. Cognitive-behavioral group therapy in obsessive-compulsive disorder: a randomized clinical trial. Psychother Psychosom 2003;72:211–6.

[66] Cottraux J, Note I, Yao S, et al. A randomized controlled trial of cognitive therapy versus intensive behavior therapy in obsessive compulsive disorder. Psychother Psychosom 2001; 70:288–97.

[67] Franklin ME, Kozak M, Cashman LA, et al. Cognitive behavioral treatment of pediatric obsessive compulsive disorder: an open clinical trial. J Am Acad Child Adolesc Psychiatry 1998;37(4):412–9.

[68] Freeston M, Ladouceur R, Gagnon F, et al. Cognitive-behavioral treatment of obsessive thoughts: a controlled study. J Consult Clin Psychol 1997;65(3):405–13.

[69] Fricke S, Moritz S, Andresen B, et al. Do personality disorders predict negative treatment outcome in obsessive compulsive disorders? A prospective 6 month follow-up study. European Psychiatry, in press.

[70] Gershuny B, Baer Lee, Jenike M, et al. Comorbid posttraumatic stress disorder: impact on treatment outcome for obsessive-compulsive disorder. Am J Psychiatry 2002;159(5):852–4.

[71] Jones M, Menzies R. Danger ideation reduction therapy (DIRT) for obsessive-compulsive washers. A controlled trial. Behav Res Ther 1998;36:959–70.

[72] McLean P, Whittal M, Thordarson D, et al. Cognitive versus behavior therapy in the group treatment of obsessive-compulsive disorder. J Consult Clin Psychol 2001;69(2):205–14.

[73] Piacentini R, Bergman R, Jacobs C, et al. Open trial of cognitive behavior therapy for childhood obsessive-compulsive disorder. J Anxiety Disord 2002;16:207–19.

[74] Rosqvist J, Egan D, Manzo P, et al. Home-based behavior therapy for obsessive-compulsive disorder: a case series with data. J Anxiety Disord 2001;15:395–400.

[75] Thienemann M, Martin J, Cregger B, et al. Manual-driven group cognitive-behavioral therapy for adolescents with obsessive-compulsive disorder: a pilot study. J Am Acad Child Adolesc Psychiatry 2001;40(11):1254–60.

[76] Vogel P, Stiles T, Gotestam G. Adding cognitive therapy elements to exposure therapy for obsessive compulsive disorder: a controlled study. Behav Cogn Psychother 2004;32:275–90.

[77] Wetzel C, Bents H, Florin I. High-density exposure therapy for obsessive-compulsive inpatients: a 1-year follow-up. Psychother Psychosom 1999;68:186–92.

[78] Wilhelm S, Steketee G, Reilly-Harrington N, et al. Effectiveness of cognitive therapy for obsessive-compulsive disorder: an open trial. Journal of Cognitive Psychotherapy: An International Quarterly 2005;19(2):173–9.

[79] McLean P, Whittal M, Thordarson D, et al. Cognitive versus behavior therapy in the group treatment of obsessive-compulsive disorder. J Consult Clin Psychol 2001;69(2):205–14.

[80] Steketee G, Eisen J, Dyck I, et al. Predictors of course in obsessive-compulsive disorder. Psychiatry Res 1999;89:229–38.

ELSEVIER
SAUNDERS

Psychiatr Clin N Am 29 (2006) 605–613

PSYCHIATRIC
CLINICS
OF NORTH AMERICA

Index

Note: Page numbers of article titles are in **boldface** type.

Changing Your Address?

Make sure your subscription changes too! When you notify us of your new address, you can help make our job easier by including an exact copy of your Clinics label number with your old address (see illustration below.) This number identifies you to our computer system and will speed the processing of your address change. Please be sure this label number accompanies your old address and your corrected address—you can send an old Clinics label with your number on it or just copy it exactly and send it to the address listed below.

We appreciate your help in our attempt to give you continuous coverage. Thank you.

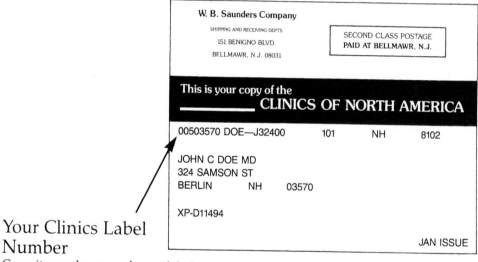

W. B. Saunders Company

SHIPPING AND RECEIVING DEPTS
151 BENIGNO BLVD.
BELLMAWR, N.J. 08031

SECOND CLASS POSTAGE
PAID AT BELLMAWR, N.J.

This is your copy of the
_____ CLINICS OF NORTH AMERICA

00503570 DOE—J32400   101   NH   8102

JOHN C DOE MD
324 SAMSON ST
BERLIN   NH   03570

XP-D11494

JAN ISSUE

Your Clinics Label
Number
Copy it exactly or send your label
along with your address to:
Elsevier Periodicals Customer Service
6277 Sea Harbor Drive
Orlando, FL 32887-4800
Call Toll Free 1-800-654-2452

Please allow four to six weeks for delivery of new subscriptions and for processing address changes.